Helping a Field See Itself

The perceived value of philosophy to medical education is increasing. But beyond the occasional application of philosophical concepts, what does it mean to be philosophical about medical education and to do philosophy—to create new concepts and ways of thinking about what medical education is? The complex and dynamic nature of academic medicine requires medical educators to reflect on their practices, to question assumptions, and to embrace the ambiguity of a world that cannot be captured by any one model or theory.

This volume explores philosophy as a practice in medical education. We use persistent problems that vex medical educators as a starting point to do philosophy, asking fundamental questions to probe them: How are teaching and learning related? How do we educate the value of personal experience relative to scientific evidence? We also challenge the assumptions underlying these problems with alternatives: What if teaching does not cause learning? What if we cannot divide our inner and outer world? We then explore ways forward: If we cannot cause learning, how do we reconceptualize the educational process? How do we help physician trainees critically reflect on medical epistemology throughout their professional development?

Each chapter explores one theme in medical education (e.g., education, science, inequality, technology, mortality) from a philosophical perspective, opening it up to fundamental re-examination and inviting readers to continue exploration beyond the printed words. This book is a step towards enabling medical educators to practice philosophy themselves at appropriate moments in their work. In this way, it aims to establish medical education as a mature field with its own philosophy. The chapters in this book were originally published in the journal *Teaching and Learning in Medicine*.

Mario Veen is Assistant Professor Educational Research at the Department of General Practice of Erasmus University Medical Center, interested in correspondences between philosophy and medical education. He has an interdisciplinary background in philosophy, social science, and the humanities. He hosts the podcasts *Let Me Ask You Something* and *Life From Plato's Cave*.

Anna T. Cianciolo is Associate Professor of Medical Education at Southern Illinois University School of Medicine, Editor-in-Chief of *Teaching and Learning in Medicine*, and a lover of questions. Her professional passion is to conduct and cultivate scholarship that empowers others to raise questions and explore answers together.

Helping a Field See Itself
Envisioning a Philosophy of Medical Education

Edited by
Mario Veen and Anna T. Cianciolo

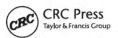

First edition published 2024
by CRC Press
4 Park Square, Milton Park, Abingdon, Oxon OX14 4RN

and by CRC Press
6000 Broken Sound Parkway NW, Suite 300, Boca Raton, FL 33487-2742

© 2024 selection and editorial matter, Mario Veen and Anna T. Cianciolo; individual chapters, the contributors

CRC Press is an imprint of Informa UK Limited

The right of Mario Veen and Anna T. Cianciolo to be identified as the authors of the editorial material, and of the authors for their individual chapters, has been asserted in accordance with sections 77 and 78 of the Copyright, Designs and Patents Act 1988.

Foreword © 2023 Megan E. L. Brown
Chapters 3–5, 8, 10–12 © 2023 Taylor & Francis
Chapter 14 © 2023 Anna T. Cianciolo and Mario Veen
Chapter 1 © 2020 Mario Veen and Anna T. Cianciolo. Originally published as Open Access.
Chapter 2 © 2020 Gert J. J. Biesta and Marije van Braak. Originally published as Open Access.
Chapter 6 © 2021 Chris B. T. Rietmeijer and Mario Veen. Originally published as Open Access.
Chapter 7 © 2022 Madeleine Noelle Olding, Freya Rhodes, John Humm, Phoebe Ross and Catherine McGarry. Originally published as Open Access.
Chapter 9 © 2022 Tim Fawns and Sven P. C. Schaepkens. Originally published as Open Access.
Chapter 13 © 2022 Sven P. C. Schaepkens and Thijs Lijster. Originally published as Open Access.

With the exception of Chapters 1, 2, 6, 7, 9 and 13, no part of this book may be reprinted or reproduced or utilised in any form or by any electronic, mechanical, or other means, now known or hereafter invented, including photocopying and recording, or in any information storage or retrieval system, without permission in writing from the publishers. For details on the rights for Chapters 1, 2, 6, 7, 9 and 13, please see the chapters' Open Access footnotes.

For permission to photocopy or use material electronically from this work, access www.copyright.com or contact the Copyright Clearance Center, Inc. (CCC), 222 Rosewood Drive, Danvers, MA 01923, 978-750-8400. For works that are not available on CCC please contact mpkbookspermissions@tandf.co.uk

Trademark notice: Product or corporate names may be trademarks or registered trademarks, and are used only for identification and explanation without intent to infringe.

British Library Cataloguing-in-Publication Data
A catalogue record for this book is available from the British Library

ISBN: 978-1-032-20414-7 (hbk)
ISBN: 978-1-032-20415-4 (pbk)
ISBN: 978-1-003-26346-3 (ebk)

DOI: 10.4324/9781003263463

Typeset in Minion Pro
by Newgen Publishing UK

Publisher's Note
The publisher accepts responsibility for any inconsistencies that may have arisen during the conversion of this book from journal articles to book chapters, namely the inclusion of journal terminology.

Disclaimer
Every effort has been made to contact copyright holders for their permission to reprint material in this book. The publishers would be grateful to hear from any copyright holder who is not here acknowledged and will undertake to rectify any errors or omissions in future editions of this book.

Contents

Citation Information	vii
Notes on Contributors	ix
Foreword	xi
Megan E. L. Brown	

1 Problems No One Looked For: Philosophical Expeditions into Medical Education   1
Mario Veen and Anna T. Cianciolo

2 Beyond the Medical Model: Thinking Differently about Medical Education and Medical Education Research   9
Gert J. J. Biesta and Marije van Braak

3 Teaching Medical Epistemology within an Evidence-Based Medicine Curriculum   17
Mark R. Tonelli and Robyn Bluhm

4 Language, Philosophy, and Medical Education   25
John R. Skelton

5 Contending with Our Racial Past in Medical Education: A Foucauldian Perspective   32
Zareen Zaidi, Ian M. Partman, Cynthia R. Whitehead, Ayelet Kuper and Tasha R. Wyatt

6 Phenomenological Research in Health Professions Education: Tunneling from Both Ends   42
Chris Rietmeijer and Mario Veen

7 Black, White and Gray: Student Perspectives on Medical Humanities and Medical Education   51
Madeleine Noelle Olding, Freya Rhodes, John Humm, Phoebe Ross and Catherine McGarry

8 Because We Care: A Philosophical Investigation into the Spirit of Medical Education   62
Camillo Coccia and Mario Veen

9 A Matter of Trust: Online Proctored Exams and the Integration of Technologies of Assessment
in Medical Education   71
Tim Fawns and Sven P. C. Schaepkens

10 Being-Opposite-Illness: Phenomenological Ontology in Medical Education and Clinical Practice   81
John Humm

11 The Lifecycle of a Clinical Cadaver: A Practice-Based Ethnography   90
*Anna MacLeod, Victoria Luong, Paula Cameron, George Kovacs, Molly Fredeen, Lucy Patrick,
Olga Kits and Jonathan Tummons*

12 Technical Difficulties: Teaching Critical Philosophical Orientations toward Technology 107
Benjamin Chin-Yee, Laura Nimmon and Mario Veen

13 Mind the Gap: A Philosophical Analysis of Reflection's Many Benefits 117
Sven P. C. Schaepkens and Thijs Lijster

14 Conclusions: Envisioning a Philosophy of Medical Education 127
Anna T. Cianciolo and Mario Veen

Index 137

Citation Information

The following chapters were originally published in various volumes and issues of the journal *Teaching and Learning in Medicine*. When citing this material, please use the original page numbering for each article, as follows:

Chapter 1
Problems No One Looked For: Philosophical Expeditions into Medical Education
Mario Veen and Anna T. Cianciolo
Teaching and Learning in Medicine, volume 32, issue 3 (2020), pp. 337–344

Chapter 2
Beyond the Medical Model: Thinking Differently about Medical Education and Medical Education Research
Gert J. J. Biesta and Marije van Braak
Teaching and Learning in Medicine, volume 32, issue 4 (2020), pp. 449–456

Chapter 3
Teaching Medical Epistemology within an Evidence-Based Medicine Curriculum
Mark R. Tonelli and Robyn Bluhm
Teaching and Learning in Medicine, volume 33, issue 1 (2021), pp. 98–105

Chapter 4
Language, Philosophy, and Medical Education
John R. Skelton
Teaching and Learning in Medicine, volume 33, issue 2 (2021), pp. 210–216

Chapter 5
Contending with Our Racial Past in Medical Education: A Foucauldian Perspective
Zareen Zaidi, Ian M. Partman, Cynthia R. Whitehead, Ayelet Kuper and Tasha R. Wyatt
Teaching and Learning in Medicine, volume 33, issue 4 (2021), pp. 453–462

Chapter 6
Phenomenological Research in Health Professions Education: Tunneling from Both Ends
Chris B. T. Rietmeijer and Mario Veen
Teaching and Learning in Medicine, volume 34, issue 1 (2022), pp. 113–121

Chapter 7
Black, White and Gray: Student Perspectives on Medical Humanities and Medical Education
Madeleine Noelle Olding, Freya Rhodes, John Humm, Phoebe Ross and Catherine McGarry
Teaching and Learning in Medicine, volume 34, issue 2 (2022), pp. 223–233

Chapter 8
Because We Care: A Philosophical Investigation into the Spirit of Medical Education
Camillo Coccia and Mario Veen
Teaching and Learning in Medicine, volume 34, issue 3 (2022), pp. 341–349

Chapter 9

A Matter of Trust: Online Proctored Exams and the Integration of Technologies of Assessment in Medical Education
Tim Fawns and Sven Schaepkens
Teaching and Learning in Medicine, volume 34, issue 4 (2022), pp. 444–453

Chapter 10

Being-Opposite-Illness: Phenomenological Ontology in Medical Education and Clinical Practice
John Humm
Teaching and Learning in Medicine, volume 35, issue 1 (2023), pp. 108–116

Chapter 11

The Lifecycle of a Clinical Cadaver: A Practice-Based Ethnography
Anna MacLeod, Victoria Luong, Paula Cameron, George Kovacs, Molly Fredeen, Lucy Patrick, Olga Kits and Jonathan Tummons
Teaching and Learning in Medicine, volume 34, issue 5 (2022), pp. 556–572

Chapter 12

Technical Difficulties: Teaching Critical Philosophical Orientations toward Technology
Benjamin Chin-Yee, Laura Nimmon and Mario Veen
Teaching and Learning in Medicine, DOI: 10.1080/10401334.2022.2130334

Chapter 13

Mind The Gap: A Philosophical Analysis of Reflection's Many Benefits
Sven Peter Charlotte Schaepkens and Thijs Lijster
Teaching and Learning in Medicine, DOI: 10.1080/10401334.2022.2142794

For any permission-related enquiries please visit:
www.tandfonline.com/page/help/permissions

Notes on Contributors

Gert J. J. Biesta, Centre for Public Education and Pedagogy, Maynooth University, County Kildare, Ireland; Moray House School of Education and Sport, University of Edinburgh, Edinburgh, UK.

Robyn Bluhm, Department of Philosophy, Lyman Briggs College and Michigan State University, East Lansing, Michigan, USA.

Megan E. L. Brown, Medical Education Innovation and Research Centre, The University of Buckingham, UK.

Paula Cameron, Department of Continuing Professional Development and Medical Education, Dalhousie University, Halifax, Nova Scotia, Canada.

Benjamin Chin-Yee, Schulich School of Medicine and Rotman Institute of Philosophy, Western University, London, Ontario, Canada.

Anna T. Cianciolo, Department of Medical Education, Southern Illinois University School of Medicine, Springfield, USA.

Camillo Coccia, Department of Medicine, University of Cape Town, Cape Town, South Africa.

Tim Fawns, Edinburgh Medical School, University of Edinburgh, Edinburgh, UK.

Molly Fredeen, Department of Continuing Professional Development and Medical Education, Dalhousie University, Halifax, Nova Scotia, Canada.

John Humm, Hull York Medical School, University of York, York, England, UK.

Olga Kits, Research Methods Unit, Nova Scotia Health, Halifax, Nova Scotia, Canada.

George Kovacs, Department of Emergency Medicine, Dalhousie University, Halifax, Nova Scotia, Canada.

Ayelet Kuper, Department of Medicine, University of Toronto, Toronto, Ontario, Canada.

Thijs Lijster, Faculty of Arts, University of Groningen, Groningen, The Netherlands.

Victoria Luong, Department of Continuing Professional Development and Medical Education, Dalhousie University, Halifax, Nova Scotia, Canada.

Anna MacLeod, Department of Continuing Professional Development and Medical Education, Dalhousie University, Halifax, Nova Scotia, Canada.

Catherine McGarry, Edinburgh Medical School, University of Edinburgh, Edinburgh, Scotland, UK.

Laura Nimmon, Centre for Health Education Scholarship Faculty of Medicine, University of British Columbia, Vancouver, British Columbia, Canada.

Madeleine Noelle Olding, Faculty of Life Sciences and Medicine, King's College London, London, England, UK.

Ian M. Partman, New York University, New York, USA.

Lucy Patrick, Department of Emergency Medicine, Dalhousie University, Halifax, Nova Scotia, Canada.

Freya Rhodes, Academic Unit of Medical Education, University of Sheffield, Sheffield, England.

Chris Rietmeijer, Department of General Practice/Family Medicine, Amsterdam University Medical Centers, Amsterdam, The Netherlands.

Phoebe Ross, Brighton & Sussex Medical School, University of Sussex, Brighton, England, UK.

Sven P. C. Schaepkens, Department of General Practice, Erasmus University Medical Center, Rotterdam, The Netherlands.

John R. Skelton, College of Medical and Dental Sciences, University of Birmingham, Birmingham, UK.

Mark R. Tonelli, Department of Medicine and Department of Bioethics and Humanities, University of Washington, Seattle, Washington, USA.

Jonathan Tummons, School of Education, Durham University, Durham, UK.

Marije van Braak, Department of General Practice, Erasmus Medical Centre, Rotterdam, The Netherlands.

Mario Veen, Department of General Practice, Erasmus University Medical Center, Rotterdam, The Netherlands.

Cynthia R. Whitehead, Department of Family and Community Medicine, University of Toronto, Toronto, Ontario, Canada.

Tasha R. Wyatt, Department of Medicine, Uniformed Services University, Bethesda, Maryland, USA.

Zareen Zaidi, Department of Medicine, University of Florida College of Medicine, Gainesville, Florida, USA.

Foreword

Best Things dwell out of Sight
The Pearl — the Just — Our Thought.

Most shun the Public Air
Legitimate, and Rare —

The Capsule of the Wind
The Capsule of the Mind

Exhibit here, as doth a Burr —
Germ's Germ be where?

Emily Dickinson, Best Things dwell
out of Sight (998)

When I first learned of the title of this book – 'Helping a Field See Itself: Envisioning a Philosophy of Medical Education' – I thought of this bewildering poem by Emily Dickinson. In passing (though I'm not convinced it's possible to read a Dickinson poem 'in passing'), you may surmise that, since the best things lie out of sight, including our thought, there is little point in trying to bring them into view. There is no one right way to interpret a poem, and there's joy in this multiplicity, but to me there's another meaning here.

The list of the best things that dwell out of sight speaks, to me, of Plato's work, which involves examining how forms (eternal truths) including concepts like beauty, justice, and goodness relate. The Pearl is beautiful – historically, Pearls were of great monetary value. The Just is what is right and fair. The good, for Plato, was perfection, the highest form that transcended all else. Plato illustrates the relationship between what exists in our physical world (which he calls 'particulars', imperfect physical objects), forms (perfect ideas which are universally true and exist in a different realm), and the good (the highest form), by drawing comparison with the light of the sun in the physical world. Like the sun, whose light allows our eyes to see and allows visible things to be seen, the form of the good allows the rational part of us – our soul – to understand the truths that are in the realm of the forms.

The best things – like beauty and justice – are unseen in that they are perfect ideals, not physically present in our world in their true forms. We do not know beauty in its true form, only a representation of beauty exists in our imperfect physical world. The same can be said of justice. But this does not mean that we should not try to see in other ways – to attempt to understand these truths in the realm of the forms by orientating our thinking towards eternal truths, rather than focusing solely on the empirical world. The inclusion of 'Our Thought' in the second line of the poem, rather than 'The Good' makes Dickinson's list *almost* Platonic, almost a summary of Plato's highest forms. This draws attention to 'Our Thought', it's the odd-one-out, not a perfect ideal like beauty or justice, yet it still makes the list of one of the 'best things'. Thought (when rational, when orientated towards truths) is most excellent, comparable to perfect ideals like beauty, and justice.

This book helps us to think about truths, to question established ideas, consider the implications for medical education of doing things differently, of seeing truth or ideals in different ways. In the second stanza of Dickinson's poem, there's a shift in language from 'Best Things dwell out of Sight', which implies *all* the best things are invisible in some way, to '*Most* shun the Public Air'. This suggests that some do not. The second line of the second stanza – Legitimate, and Rare – associates the Pearl (or beauty), which are (or were) rare, and the Just (justice), which ensures humankind conforms to law or rules, with the terms rare and legitimate, respectively. What is absent here, and so what Dickinson is suggesting is something that might not shun the Public Air, is Our Thought. Here, she aligns with Plato. Thought can be public, and it can help us to see when directed at truth. The thinking within this book, and the way in which it inspires its reader to think, makes public often unseen ideas or norms, and helps us to grasp what might, at first glance, seem out of sight.

To work within medical education is to walk a tightrope between theory and practice. Both are valuable, but too much of one, and not enough of another, causes struggle. Medical education, in my experience, tends to attract those with aspirations that their work will have practical application – we're less likely than some in other fields, perhaps, to sit lost in endless thought on the various interpretations of some theory or way of thinking. This speaks to the way in which our field is rooted in the natural sciences, in positivist ways of thinking that assert one truth, and do not guide their wielder to consider multiple interpretations. We're usually not aware, and our students often aren't aware, of the assumptions we make regarding the nature of knowledge (which Tonelli and Bluhm convincingly argue should form part of medical curricula).

If you've never had chance or cause to consider your position on knowledge, and how your background informs your assumptions, it would be worthwhile taking a moment to pause and consider this now. If you're from a natural sciences or medical background, rooted in positivism, and can still identify this position (or even traces of it) in the assumptions you make about knowledge and truth now, this book will challenge you to think differently. I have a medical background and, although I now don't practice and would like to consider myself an interpretivist who embraces the plurality and subjectivity of knowledge, this is a work-in-progress. Training runs deep, and it takes both time and a conscious desire to think in different ways about knowledge. As I read the chapters in this book, there were things that challenged my assumptions, questioned the truths I took as universal or self-evident. When I read the chapters a second time, I was able to add to the list of things I was beginning to think differently about.

Though we, in medical education, might consider ourselves practitioners, whose aim is to focus on affecting change for the field's stakeholders, we need to engage in conceptual work that challenges us to think differently about foundational questions within medical education – such as, what is knowledge (Chapter 3), what is language (Chapter 4), what is experience (Chapter 6), and what is care (Chapter 8). Though this book's chapters are theoretical, a masterclass in philosophical thinking, there are practical ramifications within each one – the authors walk the difficult tightrope between theory and practice deftly, with great skill. As you're guided to think about learning, technology, and power, for example, you'll find yourself moving from a focus on the physical, empirical world (which is very familiar to those of us who identify as scientists, or clinicians), to focusing on what Plato might frame as the realm of forms – on 'truths' or ideas that are more difficult to grasp, more challenging to comprehend, and then back to what these new ideas mean in practice.

I'm not sure I agree with Plato that any truths are universal and thinking within medical education is beginning to shift from this position also (as noted in Chapter 3) but looking at Dickinson's poem through the lens of Platonic forms can help us understand how and why considering such foundational questions is important (even if there isn't a universal answer), and why we often find this thinking so challenging. In the final two stanzas of the poem, Dickinson draws our attention to that both the Wind, and the Mind 'exhibit here'. It's unclear whether 'here' is the Public Air or the realm of the unseen, but to exhibit is to publicly display, again suggesting that what originally seems out of sight, or hidden, is there to view for those who seek it. The final line of the poem – Germ's Germ be where? – is playful, in that Germ can mean both a microorganism that causes disease, and the reproductive part of a plant which can grow into a new plant. 'Be where?' is a question of location – is the origin of disease (or perhaps, given the poem's focus on justice and thinking, bad thoughts, or inequality) in the realm of the unseen, or in Public Air? But it can also read as 'beware', a warning to the reader not to permit diseased thoughts or actions to reproduce. As readers of this book, you have taken a significant step towards examining the usually unseen, those thoughts and assumptions that could prove harmful if left unexamined. Germ's Germ is in the Capsule of the Wind, as harmful assumptions breeze unquestioned through our field, and in the Capsule of our Mind, as we bring our own backgrounds to our work as medical educators and researchers. As this book helps you to see the field, and to see yourself, you might begin to answer Dickinson's playful question: Germ's Germ be where?

Reference

Emily Dickinson's Poems: As She Preserved Them, edited by Cristanne Miller, Copyright © 2016 by the President and Fellows of Harvard College. Copyright © 1998 by the President and Fellows of Harvard College. Copyright © 1951, 1955 by the President and Fellows of Harvard College. Copyright © renewed 1979, 1983 by the President and Fellows of Harvard College. Copyright © 1914, 1918, 1919, 1924, 1929, 1930, 1932, 1935, 1937. 1942 by Martha Dickinson Bianchi. Copyright © 1952, 1957, 1958, 1963, 1965 by Mary L. Hampson. Used by permission. All rights reserved.

Megan E. L. Brown
Senior Lecturer in Medical Education
Programme Lead PGCert Medical Education
The University of Buckingham
Teaching Fellow in Medical Education Research
Imperial College London

⊗ OPEN ACCESS

Problems No One Looked For: Philosophical Expeditions into Medical Education

Mario Veen and Anna T. Cianciolo

ABSTRACT

Issue: Medical education has "muddy zones of practice," areas of complexity and uncertainty that frustrate the achievement of our intended educational outcomes. Slowing down to consider context and reflect on practice are now seen as essential to medical education as we are called upon to examine carefully what we are doing to care for learners and improve their performance, professionalism, and well-being. Philosophy can be seen as the fundamental approach to pausing at times of complexity and uncertainty to ask basic questions about seemingly obvious practices so that we can see (and do) things in new ways. *Evidence:* Philosophy and medical education have long been related; many of our basic concepts can be traced to philosophical ideas. Philosophy is a problem-creation approach, and its method is analysis; it is a constant process of shifting frames and turning into objects of analysis the lenses through which we see the world. However, philosophy is not about constant questioning for the sake of questioning. Progression in medical education practice involves recognizing when to switch from a philosophical to a practical perspective, and when to switch back. *Implications:* In medical education, a philosophical approach empowers us to "slow down when we should," thereby engaging us more directly with our subjects of study, revealing our assumptions, and helping us address vexing problems from a new angle. Doing philosophy involves thinking like a beginner, getting back to basics, and disrupting frames of reference. Being philosophical is about wonder and intense, childlike curiosity, human qualities we all share. Taking a philosophical approach to medical education need not be an unguided endeavor, but can be a dialog through which medical educators and philosophers learn together.

"When a clinical presentation is atypical, a postoperative patient goes off course, an unusual reaction occurs from medication, or an anatomical anomaly is confronted, will the clinician... take heed and recognize the intricacies and complexities of the case... or will that clinician plow through, oblivious to its uniqueness and unaware of its consequences?"[1(p.S110)]

Analysis of physicians' expert judgment suggests that optimal performance and patient outcomes depend on physicians' ability to recognize "muddy zones of practice,"[2(p.1019)] and "slow down" to attend to the situation, reframe the problem at hand, and take action accordingly.[1] Among surgeons, signs of slowing down include turning off background music in the operating room, silencing chatter, and pausing to regroup.[2]

Slowing down also may be proactively planned, prompted by the surgeon's anticipation of procedure- and patient-specific complexities and uncertainty.[2]

Medical education also has its muddy zones of practice, its own atypical presentations, unintended outcomes, and structural abnormalities for which to account. These areas of complexity and uncertainty likely feel familiar to many of us: they present as persistent challenges that frustrate the achievement of our intended educational outcomes, such as balancing learning and assessment or teaching and clinical service. Slowing down to consider context and reflect on practice are now seen as essential to medical education[3,4] as we are called upon to examine carefully

---

This is an Open Access article distributed under the terms of the Creative Commons Attribution-NonCommercial-NoDerivatives License (http://creativecommons.org/licenses/by-nc-nd/4.0/), which permits non-commercial re-use, distribution, and reproduction in any medium, provided the original work is properly cited, and is not altered, transformed, or built upon in any way.

what we are doing to care for learners and improve their performance, professionalism, and well-being. But what does "slowing down when we should"[1] look like in medical education?

Philosophy can be seen as the fundamental approach to pausing at times of complexity and uncertainty to ask basic questions about seemingly obvious practices so that we can see (and do) things in new ways. Whether we are aware of it or not, basic concepts we use in medical education can be traced to philosophy. For example, the idea that what we do – in medicine or in education – should be based on systematic empirical research whereby 'causes' and 'effects' are identified can be traced back to Hume and Locke.[5] Thinking about learners in terms of knowledge, skills, and attitudes can be traced back to Plato and Aristotle. Models of reflection, such as Kolb's,[6] can be traced back to John Dewey,[7] who in turn based his work on Hegel's philosophy. Slowing down with philosophy to reframe educational problems and take newly informed action may be seen as a kind of expedition – a journey of exploration with a particular purpose.

In this article, we illustrate a philosophical approach to slowing down in medical education, demonstrating how viewing a situation philosophically helps us pause to focus our attention, reframe the problem at hand, and take action accordingly. Next, we outline three philosophical practices that could be used to do philosophy in medical education. In this, we aim to support slowing down in the moment reactively to problems at hand. Finally, we describe what it means to be philosophical in our approach to teaching and learning and propose five themes as a starting point for dialog between philosophers and medical educators. These themes will be explored further in a series of articles published in *Teaching and Learning in Medicine* in the coming months. The aim of the series is to support proactive slowing down by identifying complexities and uncertainty in medical education that philosophers are wrestling with now.

A philosophical approach to the problem of resident teach back

Imagine an internal medicine residency program director faced with a problem: observation-based assessments reveal that before leaving the examination room, residents consistently fail to "teach back," or gauge their patients' understanding of their condition and what the next steps in their treatment plan will be.[8] Because teaching back has been shown to improve

patients' health-related behaviors[9] and is seen by the residency program as an important demonstration of the internal medicine sub-competency "communicates effectively with patients and caregivers,"[10(p20)] the program director decides to intervene.

The intervention the program director chooses depends on how they have formulated problem at hand. Let us say that the intervention comprises dedicating a resident conference to the teach back method and administering a simulated patient encounter to formally develop teach back skills. In this case, the problem has been diagnosed as a knowledge gap: 'Trainees do not know how.' But imagine that the intervention is not successful, residents still do not teach back, and the program director re-formulates the problem as a motivational deficit: 'Trainees know how, but they are not motivated to do it; they do not understand why it is important.' To convince residents of the value of teach back, the program director then selects a meta-analysis documenting the positive outcomes of teach back to be discussed at the next internal medicine journal club.

In our example so far, the program director has seen residents' failure to enact satisfactory doctor-patient communication as a lack of requisite knowledge, skills, and attitudes. This seems obvious. But being philosophical is about questioning the obvious, so let us do that together here and see what happens: How does the *resident* experience the task of teaching back? Do they see a problem, and if so, how do they define it? The resident may be seen as entering the exam room embodying multiple, potentially conflicting roles: learner and practitioner. Their relationship to the patient and whether this is conducive to teach back may depend on how they navigate these roles. For instance, in order to teach back, the resident may need to feel ownership of the patient's care,[11] yet residents know they must verify what they do with the attending, who is ultimately responsible. Moreover, the attending is the more experienced practitioner, who may disagree with the resident's plan. In this context, teaching back, especially if the plan later needs correcting, may constitute a breach of role boundaries: acting like a practitioner when one is in fact a trainee. If the problem of teach back is one of role conflict, it calls for an intervention aimed at clarifying and navigating role boundaries; intervention aimed at knowledge or motivation would not work.

This way of approaching the problem differs from the previous one in that it disrupts the program director's frame of reference, a classic philosophical move. The resident is no longer approached as an assemblage of knowledge, skills, and attitudes, but as a thinking, acting being, which has implications for what to do next. Instead of concluding 'We need an intervention,' the program director may step back and reimagine the problem, wondering 'Why don't residents teach back?' and, more generally, 'How can we help residents achieve high quality patient communication?' We already see numerous examples of this kind analysis in the medical education literature, which not only disrupt our assumptions about learners but also demonstrate that our community has a certain readiness to approach problems in medical education philosophically.

We now have three possible explanations for why a behavior expected of residents does not take place. Each of these explanations defines the problem in a certain way: as a communication knowledge/skill deficit, a motivational issue, and a role conflict. We may note that none of these definitions is necessarily truer than the other; after questioning the obvious and disentangling a problem from how it is viewed, philosophers are quick to disown the idea of finding the 'right' lens or framework, or to pretend that we can see the world 'as it is' without a lens or framework. The residents in our example may in fact need development of their teach back skills, but residents may not practice teach back because they are not motivated, and they may not be motivated because they seek to avoid role conflict.

(Some) new problems no one looked for

Let us imagine (perhaps readily) that despite identifying barriers to teach back and forming a response to address them, observational assessment of residents shows that their behavior still fails to meet expectations. Because medical education is interdisciplinary, the program director may recruit imported concepts and ways of thinking from medical science, cognitive psychology, educational science, and many other disciplines to solve this problem.[12–14] However, these different perspectives bring with them assumptions that might be incongruent with the aims of intervening or incompatible with each other. Raising philosophical questions about the interplay of power and knowledge, about the clash of learning and assessment priorities, even about the very nature of causality and progress may reveal buried and conflicting assumptions that underlie the recurrence of the teach back problem.

Through language, knowledge serves power

Perhaps our program director decides to examine resident-patient communication directly, approaching the project from the perspective of philosopher Michel Foucault (himself the son of a physician). A Foucauldian lens[15,16] would introduce two new perspectives on authority from which to view the problem at hand. The first perspective involves viewing authority in linguistic terms, as something that constrains who gets to say what and who can define key elements of the doctor-patient relationship, such as the diagnosis and the treatment plan. The second perspective involves viewing authority not as something one *has*, but something one *does*, and this depends on the kind of knowledge and information one can use. From this perspective we see the resident, patient, and attending as situated within a power-knowledge network;[15] knowledge is power enacted through what can be said and by whom.

Reconsidering our example now, the Shared Decision-Making framework,[17,18] of which teach back is one component, defines health care as a shared project of doctor and patient, but in the resident's situation the attending also participates. Examination of this group's communication may reveal that the attending physician is the one who leads the interaction when all three parties are in the room, defining how long the exchange lasts (e.g., by being the first person to say "goodbye") and what topics it covers (e.g., by being the one to ask questions). Viewing these interactions from the Foucauldian perspective may prompt the program director to shift the problem frame from 'How can we intervene to make residents teach back?' or 'Why does the resident not teach back?' to 'Why is it even a problem that residents, who lack power in this situation, do not teach back?'

Assessment or learning?

Taking a philosophical stance, the program director also may ask: 'Do we assess residents' teach back because it (1) ensures quality patient care; (2) facilitates the development of patient-communication competency; or (3) describes a resident behavior that we can evaluate readily with available instruments?' This question implies that it may not be enough for residents to *be* empathetic doctors,[19] or, in this case, effective communicators. They have to be *seen* as such, and this can only occur if they act in a way that is observable to the assessor. And even that is not enough; the assessor must translate their observations into the predefined structure of an assessment form.[20]

In this, we see the competition between two discourses, that of doctor-patient communication (what we want the resident to learn) and that of assessment (how we know the resident learned it).

The philosophical concept of 'instrumental thinking'[21,22] is relevant here. Philosophers have broadly distinguished two main ways of thinking: instrumental (or technical) rationality and value rationality. Instrumental rationality calls us to see the world in terms of ends that should be achieved as efficiently as possible. Value rationality, by contrast, calls us to relate to the world in a more holistic sense. These ways of thinking represent fundamentally different approaches of relating to the world, determining not just how we think but also how we feel and act. Our program director's question illustrates how instrumental thinking and value rationality may clash; teach back may reflect a more holistic notion of patient care, but its assessment may impose constraints on what constitutes teach back in order to evaluate trainees efficiently.

Recognizing this clash prompts the philosophical medical educator to slow down and analyze seemingly obvious practices and, buried beneath those, instrumental assumptions about skill and performance. We may discover that an assessment lens filters out resident practices that balance patient communication and skill development because they are not observable, measurable behaviors captured by assessment instruments.[23] Approaching teach back from a value rationality perspective may prompt the program director to ponder new questions: 'What is the ultimate purpose of teach back, and are there other practices that doctors in training can use to accomplish this goal?' 'Are our residents already doing these practices, but we fail to see it using our assessment instruments?'

Doing philosophy

There is a movement in medical education encouraging us to accept ambiguity as a part of becoming a doctor, rather than a sign that our training system is not working.[24,25] Modern philosophers like De Beauvoir have embraced ambiguity as a positive quality, potentially fundamental to human existence.[26] Perhaps tolerance for ambiguity is needed to become medical educators. Indeed, in medical education there is rarely a moment when we do not deal with ambiguity, and there is reason to suspect that one's ability to tolerate it is positively related to psychological well-being.[27] Hopefully, our illustration of viewing complexities and uncertainty in medical education philosophically has stimulated enthusiasm to slow down and wrestle with questions about why medical education is the way it is and, in so doing, see things anew and take productive action. Doing philosophy often involves engaging ambiguity by way of philosophical practices: points of entry for philosophizing helpfully about our educational efforts.

The first philosophical practice we suggest is to pay attention to what is happening and assume a beginner's mind, even if one is experienced. This is exemplified in the well-known saying (often misattributed to Socrates) "All I know is that I know nothing." Rather than achieving mastery, this first practice is aimed at the urge to "slow down" in the face of complexity or uncertainty, a hallmark of expertise.[1] In our example, when observational assessments continued to show, despite intervention, that residents were failing to teach back, the program director paused to question whether this was in fact attributable to knowledge, skill, or motivational deficits, and later, to question what made this 'problem' a problem in the first place. As another example, before asking the question 'How will we assess this new program?' this philosophical move—thinking like a beginner—gives us the space to ask 'Do we want to assess this program, and, if so – why?'[19]

A second philosophical practice is to lead a problem back to its most fundamental description, prompting assumptions to reveal themselves. If our program director kept seeing learners in terms of knowledge, skills, and attitudes, they would not have discovered the power dynamics in attending-resident relationships that might prevent residents from taking ownership of patient care. A guide in this practice is what Deleuze and Guattari call the first principle of philosophy: "Universals explain nothing, but must themselves be explained."[28 (p.6)] If a reason for intervening is because it is 'good,' because it is 'evidence-based,' or because that is how students 'learn,' doing philosophy involves asking: What do you mean by 'good,' by 'evidence,' or by 'learning?' In this way, the most obvious and basic concepts we have in medical education can become objects of analysis in themselves. This philosophical practice—getting back to the basics—could also be enacted by asking: '*What question* can be formulated that involves *me*, the questioner?' For instance, the question 'How can I get my trainees to learn?' if asked philosophically could become: 'How do I see myself as an educator and what are the implications of my perspective for what learning is?'

The third practice, served by the preceding two, is to disrupt frames of reference. Viewing something from a different perspective—whether by imagining what a problem looks like through someone else's eyes or by talking to someone with completely different sight—can reveal one's own assumptions or default lens. For example, in one of the Socratic Dialogs described by Plato, Socrates speaks with Euthypro, who is about to prosecute his father. Euthypro presents his case as obvious, but through a series of questions Socrates assumes an attitude of ignorance and invites Eurthypro, who claims "accurate knowledge of all such matters," to "teach" him.[29(p.6)] This disrupts Euthypro's frame of reference, forcing him to switch from a routine attitude in which values such as justice are taken as unproblematic to having to explain them. In our teach back example, it is the persistence of a problem that prompts the program director to take on different perspectives, to seek out residents' points of view, and finally to observe communication directly. Consequently, frames of reference were disrupted multiple times: from the resident as an object to a subject; from authority as something one has to something one does; and finally, from teach back as a problem the program director observes from a distance, to one that is shaped by their own views.

Being philosophical

> "The philosopher's treatment of a question is like the treatment of an illness."[30 (§255)]

Philosophy begins with the desire to understand something that is important to oneself, and with a dissatisfaction or even frustration with current ways of thinking. In this way, philosophy is an extension of those human qualities that are also at the root of scientific and technical advancement. However, philosophy remains close to questions, keeping them alive with intense, childlike curiosity and desire to understand. For example, in addressing a question such as 'What is good education?' a philosopher might invoke educational, psychological, neurological perspectives to consider instructional strategies, but then also go on to examine the terms 'good' and 'educational' from political, historical, linguistic, logical, and even spiritual perspectives. Philosophy can be seen as a form of inquiry that is not bound to any one lens or discipline. In this sense, it can act as a broker or negotiator between the different perspectives we have imported to medical education, leading us back to basic assumptions, providing common ground to think from rather than fueling debate between opposing views.

Plato's *Allegory of the Cave* illustrates how being liberated from the chains of our assumptions can be instrumental.[31] In this allegory, prisoners have been chained inside a cave for their entire lives, watching worldly forms dance on the cave wall. The prisoners do not realize that they are watching a projection, that they are seeing the shadows of objects being carried in front of a fire behind them. For them, the shadows are the objects. The prisoners learn that the world of shadows is an illusion only when they are released from their chains, turn around to discover the fire, and see the actual objects whose shadows they watched.[31] Being philosophical medical educators should prompt us to stand up, turn around, and see what objective we are trying to accomplish with education anew.

The aim of being philosophical is not to come up with 'a philosophy,' such as a theory or an ethical system to live by. If anything, philosophy is a problem-creation approach, and its method is analysis, a constant process of shifting frames and turning into objects of analysis the lenses through which we see the world. Being philosophical involves asking unanswerable questions and exploring ways in which one might go about answering them. The moment this process arrives at 'an answer,' the project becomes the charge of another discipline. For instance, the evidence-based medicine movement can be seen as a scientific answer to an epistemological question: What kind of knowledge can we rely on to guide our actions in patient care? Many thinkers have devoted their life to imagining how philosophy is a "pathway"[21(p.445)] for thinking, thinking that "does not come to a halt"[22(p.278)] in a theoretical or conceptual framework.

However, constant questioning also is a pitfall. We cannot constantly assume a philosophical attitude and be practical at the same time. As Nietzsche himself wrote: "I would die if I had to formulate the deepest reason for breathing before each breath I take."[32(p.21)] The challenge to a philosophical medical educator is to identify the point where progression necessitates applying incomplete, but compelling results of philosophical observation and analyses.

Moving forward

We offer here our undisguised hope that this article inspires more frequent philosophical analyses of the complexities and uncertainties that challenge medical education. Popular philosophy, such as the books by Alain de Botton[33] and *This is Water*,[34] and the podcasts Philosophize This![35] and the BBC's In Our

Time: Philosophy,[36] provide accessible, yet rigorous entry points for exploration. These are, however, general and likely require collaboration with philosophers to apply to medical education. For this reason, we aim to start a dialog between philosophers and medical educators via a series of articles that examine key areas in medical education using a philosophical approach. Five themes currently are planned for future discussion.

Perhaps the most fundamental theme connecting philosophy and medicine is mortality. The "questions intersecting life, death, and meaning, questions that all people face at some point, usually arise in a medical context."[37(p.70)] Moreover, mortality is the 'soil' in which medical education is grounded, for if we were not mortal, we would not need health care. Out of this ground rises the question: How can we support medical trainees in navigating professional/technical and empathetic/humane ways of thinking in medicine? Kalanithi eloquently expressed this dilemma with respect to cadaver dissection, writing that all of medicine "trespasses into sacred spheres. Doctors ... see people at their most vulnerable, their most scared, their most private... Seeing the body as matter and mechanism is the flip side to easing the most profound human suffering. By the same token, the most profound human suffering becomes a mere pedagogical tool."[37(p.49)] How could philosophy help us help trainees (and their educators) maintain humanity in the face of existential questions and taboos?[38]

The second theme concerns the 'hierarchy of evidence' and the concept of 'best' evidence—the foundations of evidence-based medicine[39] and medical education[40]—which link epistemology and philosophy of science to standards of medical care. The evidence-based movement rests upon these epistemological assertions, these claims regarding the appropriate kinds and relative value of knowledge. Students and physicians aiming to practice evidence-based medicine are instructed to integrate 'best' evidence, based on scientific research, with clinical expertise in order to reach clinical decisions. Yet, these people are given no clear guidance regarding how such integration should occur. How would analyzing medical epistemology help us reimagine evidence-based practice?[41]

Language is a third theme connecting philosophers and medical educators. As educators know, talk and interaction may be the most important pedagogical tools at their disposal. But language is pervasive: the words we use shape our world. From the standpoint of linguistic philosophy, the single most beneficial insight that still has to land in medical education is that language in the workplace is usually for *doing* things, for achieving goals.[30] Recognizing this involves a shift from seeing language as a neutral framework for representing the world and communicating cognitions to a view of language as performative: a way of accomplishing social action.[42,43] What are the implications of this for educational practice?

The fourth theme is control and causality. A core assumption underlying medical education is that we can control attention, motivation, learning, development, and patient care through pedagogy. What exactly is the relationship between teaching and learning in medicine? Does teaching cause learning 'in the student,' in the way that a clinical intervention causes a somatic effect in the patient? Because medical education exists at the intersection of medicine and education, this may be an area in which unhelpful assumptions have been imported from medical science.[44,45]

The fifth theme is the relationship between mind and world. The way we conceptualize the relationship between physicality, neurology, and psychology has implications for how we see physicians' (and patients') relationship to patients' bodies and related matters, such as patient autonomy and shared decision making.[46] Mind-body dualism, associated with Descartes' philosophy,[47] permeates the medical approach to health issues. But often, patients might experience this in a more holistic way; medical interventions such as prosthetics or brain surgery not only affect patients' bodies, but also the way they relate to their bodies and to themselves.[46] Similarly, our thinking about learning and the curriculum in medical education is shaped by seeing learners as minds enclosed bodies, making artificial distinctions between mind/body, emotions/thoughts, language/actions, and so on.[48] Reexamining medicine's philosophical heritage in Cartesian Dualism may allow us to expand our understanding of what it means to *be* a doctor rather than just doing what a doctor does.[49]

Conclusion

Medical education has long had a relationship with philosophy. A philosophical approach can advance medical education today by helping us slow down in the face of complexities and uncertainty, see old problems in new ways, and take productive action. Doing philosophy involves thinking like a beginner, getting back to the basics, and disrupting frames of reference. Philosophy is not about creating 'a philosophy,' i.e., settling on a useful conceptual frame with which to organize the world. Rather, it is a "pathway" for thinking that "does not come to rest." Yet, philosophy in medical education is not meant to question constantly simply for the sake of questioning. Instead, engaging with philosophy is meant to be helpful; it is about liberation from habitual ways of thinking and assumptions that underlie dissatisfying or even frustrating inability to progress. Ultimately, being philosophical is about wonder and intense, childlike curiosity, human qualities we all share. In identifying problems no one looked for, philosophy has empowered us for two and a half millennia to search ourselves.

Acknowledgements

We would like to thank Marije van Braak, Sven Schaepkens and Anne de la Croix for their helpful comments on an early draft of this manuscript, and the reviewers for their valuable feedback.

References

1. Moulton CA, Regehr G, Mylopoulos M, MacRae HM. Slowing down when you should: a new model of expert judgment. *Acad Med.* 2007;82(10 Suppl): S109–S116.
2. Moulton CA, Regehr G, Lingard L, Merritt C, Macrae H. Slowing down when you should': initiators and influences of the transition from the routine to the effortful. *J Gastrointest Surg.* 2010;14(6):1019–1026. Jundoi:10.1007/s11605-010-1178-y.
3. van der Vleuten C. When I say … context specificity. *Med Educ.* 2014;48(3):234–235. doi:10.1111/medu. 12263.
4. Koens F, Mann KV, Custers EJFM, Ten Cate OTJ. Ten Cate OT. Analysing the concept of context in medical education. *Med Educ.* 2005;39(12):1243–1249. Decdoi:10.1111/j.1365-2929.2005.02338.x.
5. Pearl J. Reasoning with cause and effect. *AI Magazine.* 2002;23(1):95–112.
6. Kolb DA. *Experiential Learning: Experience as a Source for Learning and Development.* Upper Saddle River, NJ: Prentice Hall; 1984.
7. Dewey J. *How We Think.* Boston, MA: DC Heath; 1910.
8. Tuckett DA, Boulton M, Olson C. A new approach to the measurement of patients' understanding of what they are told in medical consultations. *J Health Soc Behav.* 1985 ;26(1):27–38. Mardoi:10.2307/2136724.
9. Dantic DE. A critical review of the effectiveness of 'teach-back' technique in teaching COPD patients self-management using respiratory inhalers. *Health Educ J.* 2014;73(1):41–50. doi:10.1177/0017896912469575.
10. Abim A. The Internal Medicine Milestone Project. https://acgme.org/Portals/0/PDFs/Milestones/Internal MedicineMilestones.pdf?ver=2017-07-28-090326-787. Published July 2015. Accessed October 25, 2019.
11. Greenzang KA, Revette AC, Kesselheim JC. Patients of our own: defining "ownership" of clinical care in graduate medical education. *Teach Learn Med.* 2019; 31(4):393–401. doi:10.1080/10401334.2018.1556103.
12. Norman G. Fifty years of medical education research: waves of migration. *Med Educ.* 2011;45(8):785–791. Augdoi:10.1111/j.1365-2923.2010.03921.x.
13. Colliver JA. Constructivism: the view of knowledge that ended philosophy or a theory of learning and instruction? *Teaching and Learning in Medicine.* 2002; 14(1):49–51. doi:10.1207/S15328015TLM1401_11.
14. Hodges BD. Sea monsters & whirlpools: navigating between examination and reflection in medical education. *Med Teach.* 2015;37(3):261–266. Mardoi:10.3109/ 0142159X.2014.993601.
15. Hodges BD, Martimianakis MA, McNaughton N, Whitehead C. Medical education… meet Michel Foucault. *Med Educ.* 2014;48(6):563–571. Jundoi:10. 1111/medu.12411.
16. Ball SJ. *Foucault, power, and education.* New York, NY: Routledge; 2013.
17. Makoul G, Clayman ML. An integrative model of shared decision making in medical encounters. *Patient Educ Couns.* 2006;60(3):301–312. Mardoi:10. 1016/j.pec.2005.06.010.
18. Elwyn G, Frosch D, Thomson R, et al. Shared decision making: a model for clinical practice. *J Gen Intern Med.* 2012;27(10):1361–1367. doi:10.1007/ s11606-012-2077-6.
19. Veen M, Skelton J, de la Croix A. Knowledge, skills and beetles: respecting the privacy of private experiences in medical education. *Perspect Med Educ.* 2020; 9(2):111–116.
20. Tavares W, Ginsburg S, Eva KW. Selecting and simplifying: rater performance and behavior when considering multiple competencies. *Teach Learn Med.* 2016;28(1):41–51. doi:10.1080/10401334.2015.1107489.
21. Heidegger M. The end of philosophy and the task for thinking. In Krell DF, ed. *Basic Writings: Revised and Expanded Edition.* London: Routledge & K. Paul; 1993.
22. Adorno TW. *Negative Dialectics.* London: Routledge; 1973.
23. Koschmann T, Frankel R, Albers J. A tale of two inquiries (or, doing being competent in a clinical skills exam). *Teach Learn Med.* 2019;31(3):258–269. doi:10.1080/10401334.2018.1530597.
24. Tonelli MR, Upshur R. A philosophical approach to addressing uncertainty in medical education. *Acad Med.* 2019;94(4):507–511.
25. Teunissen PW, Westerman M. Opportunity or threat: the ambiguity of the consequences of transitions in medical education. *Med Educ.* 2011;45(1):51–59. Jandoi:10.1111/j.1365-2923.2010.03755.x.
26. de Beauvoir S. *The Ethics of Ambiguity.* New York, NY: Kensington Pub. Corp; 1976.
27. Hancock J, Mattick K. Tolerance of ambiguity and psychological well-being in medical training: A systematic review. *Med Educ.* 2020;54(2):125–137. Febdoi:10.1111/medu.14031.
28. Deleuze G, Guattari F. *What is Philosophy?* London: Verso; 1995.
29. Plato. *The Socratic Dialogues.* Kaplan M, Jowett B, eds. New York, NY: Kaplan Publishing; 2009.

30. Wittgenstein L. *Philosophical Investigations*. Oxford: Blackwell; 1953.
31. Plato. *Plato, Republic*. Emlyn-Jones CJ, Preddy W, eds. Harvard: Loeb Classical Library; 2013.
32. Nietzsche F. *Het Voordeel Van Een Slecht Geheugen: Een Kennismaking Met de Nagelaten Fragmenten. [The Advantage of a Bad Memory: Diary Fragments]*. Amsterdam: SUN; 2003.
33. Botton A. *The Consolations of Philosophy*. London: Penguin Books; 2014.
34. Wallace DF, Kenyon C. *This is water: some thoughts, delivered on a significant occasion, about living a compassionate life*. New York, NY: Hachette Audio; 2010. https://www.overdrive.com/search?q=B74517E5-B9F8-4521-BF66-7BDCD410E992.
35. West S. Philosophize This! http://www.philosophizethis.org/.
36. BBC In our Time: Philosophy. https://www.bbc.co.uk/programmes/p01f0vzr.
37. Kalanithi P. *When Breath Becomes Air*. New York, NY: Random House; 2016.
38. Callahan D. End-of-life care: a philosophical or management problem? *J Law Med Ethics*. 2011;39(2):114–120. Summerdoi:10.1111/j.1748-720X.2011.00581.x.
39. Howick J. *The Philosophy of Evidence-Based Medicine*. Chichester, West Sussex, UK: Wiley-Blackwell, BMJ Books; 2011.
40. Harden RM, Grant J, Buckley G, Hart IR. BEME guide no. 1: best evidence medical education. *Med Teach*. 1999;21(6):553–562.
41. Thornton T. Tacit knowledge as the unifying factor in evidence based medicine and clinical judgement. *Philos Ethics Humanit Med*. 2006;1(1):2.
42. Austin JL. *How to Do Things with Words*. Cambridge: Harvard University Press; 1975.
43. Searle JR. *Speech Acts: An Essay in the Philosophy of Language*. Cambridge: Cambridge University Press; 1969.
44. Cook DA, Beckman TJ. Reflections on experimental research in medical education. *Adv in Health Sci Educ*. 2010;15(3):455–464. Augdoi:10.1007/s10459-008-9117-3.
45. Biesta G. *The Rediscovery of Teaching*. New York, NY: Taylor & Francis; 2017.
46. Slatman J. *Our Strange Body Philosophical Reflections on Identity and Medical Interventions*. Amsterdam: Amsterdam University Press; 2014.
47. Descartes R. *Meditations on First Philosophy*. Lanham, MD: Dancing Unicorn Books; 2019.
48. Bleakley A. *Medical Humanities and Medical Education: how the Medical Humanities Can Shape Better Doctors*. New York, NY: Routledge; 2015.
49. Wald HS. Refining a definition of reflection for the being as well as doing the work of a physician. *Medical Teacher*. 2015;37(7):696–699.

🔓 OPEN ACCESS

Beyond the Medical Model: Thinking Differently about Medical Education and Medical Education Research

Gert J. J. Biesta 🆔 and Marije van Braak 🆔

ABSTRACT

Issue: In medical education, teaching is currently viewed as an intervention that causes learning. The task of medical education research is seen as establishing which educational interventions produce the desired learning outcomes. This 'medical model' of education does not do justice to the dynamics of education as an open, semiotic, recursive system rather than a closed, causal system. *Evidence:* Empirical 'evidence' of 'what works' – that is, what is supposed to affect 'learning' – has become the norm for medical educational improvements, where generalized summary outcomes of research are often presented as must-follow guidelines for myriad future educational situations. Such investigations of educational processes tend to lack an explicit engagement with the purposes of medical education, which we suggest to understand in terms of qualification (the acquisition of knowledge, skills, and understanding), socialization (becoming a member of the professional group) and subjectification (becoming a thoughtful, independent, responsible professional). In addition, investigations of educational processes tend to rely on causal assumptions that are inadequate for capturing the dynamics of educational communication and interaction. Although we see an increasing acknowledgement of the context-dependency of teaching practices toward educational aims, the currently prevailing view in medical education and educational research limits understanding of what is actually going on when educators teach and students participate in medical education – a situation which seriously hinders advancements in the field. *Implications:* In this paper, we hope to inform discussion about the practice of medical education by proposing to view medical education in terms of three domains of purpose (professional qualification, professional socialization, and professional subjectification) and with full acknowledgement of the dynamics of educational interaction and communication. Such a view implies that curriculum design, pedagogy, assessment, and evaluation should be reoriented to include and integrate all three purposes in educational practice. It also means that medical education research findings cannot be applied in just any teaching context without carefully considering the value of the suggested courses of actions toward the particular educational aims and teaching setting. In addition, medical educational research would need to investigate all three purposes and recognize the openness, semiotic nature, and recursivity of education in offering implications for teaching practice.

Introduction: medical education and the medical model of practice and research

In the wider field of educational research and practice it has become quite common to refer to a particular understanding of the dynamics of education as the 'medical model.'[1-5] This phrase is used to refer to the idea that teaching is an intervention to bring about learning in students. Some formulations even speak about teaching as the cause of such learning and see education as nothing but the production of measurable 'learning outcomes.'

This view of education, which actually relies on a rather simplistic understanding of the complexities of medical practice itself,[6] has generated a prominent line of educational research. In this research, the focus lies on finding the most effective ways in which

---

This is an Open Access article distributed under the terms of the Creative Commons Attribution-NonCommercial-NoDerivatives License (http://creativecommons.org/licenses/by-nc-nd/4.0/), which permits non-commercial re-use, distribution, and reproduction in any medium, provided the original work is properly cited, and is not altered, transformed, or built upon in any way.

teaching can bring about intended learning outcomes. The idea here is that research should find out 'what works' and that teachers should base their classroom practice on such evidence, either by simply following what the evidence tells them to do or by making sure that their actions are informed by the latest research evidence. Within the field of education there are ongoing discussions about the possibility and desirability of such an approach.[4–8] Policy makers nonetheless often seem quite keen to steer educational research and educational practice in the direction of such a medical model.

Medical education and its related research field have, over the past two decades, also adopted the medical model.[1,2,7,9] Medical educational *practice* relies heavily on the idea that teaching in some way causes learning. In this view, teaching is understood as an intervention that produces learning outcomes (see for example the definition of teaching as "the design and implementation of activities to promote learning" in Fincher and Work,[10(p293)] based on Smith[11]). The customary rationale here is that better teaching causes better learning, which provides for better patient care, which in turn improves patient outcomes (see for example, Chen, Lui, and Martinelli;[12] Harden et al.[9]).

In keeping with notions of teaching as an intervention and learning as the effect of that intervention medical educational *research*, following the logic of the medical model, looks for correlations between interventions and outcomes.[13] Current medical education research is predominantly designed to provide proof that particular teaching practices 'work'. It aims for "generalisable simplicity" to foster application in a wide range of contexts.[13(p31)] Despite being contested for their limited significance in educational contexts,[4–6,8,13,14] randomized controlled trials are still held in high regard in medical education research.[3,15] Building on analyses of teaching effects on learning, meta-analyses, and systematic reviews are frequently presented as guidelines for future educational situations[16,17] – see, for example, the field's renowned AMEE guides.

At one level the medical model of education looks quite plausible. After all, teachers do intervene with their teaching and they do so for good reasons as they want their students to learn. Moreover, if teachers can enhance the effectiveness of what they do, students definitely are to benefit. While at a superficial level this may make sense, a closer inspection begins to reveal several problems. In this paper we aim to identify two main problems of the medical model. The

first has to do with the rather bland reference to 'learning' as what education is supposed to bring about. The second concerns the rather simplistic assumption that there is some kind of causal connection between teaching and learning and that the main task of research is to make this connection more secure and more effective.

We are raising these two points within the context of medical education, first and foremost in order to inform discussion about the practice of medical education. We are also concerned, however, that because much *medical* research focuses on questions about effectiveness, there may be a strong pull for medical *education research* to emulate such an approach where it concerns matters of education. Our paper is therefore also meant to open up a discussion about adequate forms of research for informing the practice of medical education *beyond* the medical model.

What is education? And what is it for?

To suggest that the medical model amounts to a too simplistic representation of the dynamics of education, raises the question of what these dynamics actually are and, before that, what education actually *is*. The now ubiquitous language of 'teaching and learning' – used so easily that it often feels as if 'teachingandlearning' has become one word – seems to be a concise and meaningful summary of what education is about. After all, education involves teachers and thus some form of teaching and it seems plausible to assume that the activities of teachers are intended to bring about learning in their students.

However, one key problem with the suggestion that teaching is there to bring about student learning is that the language of learning is not sufficiently precise. After all, students can learn many things when they are in educational settings, just as they can learn many things outside of those settings. The whole point of education, however, is not to ensure that students learn, but that they learn *something*, learn it *for a reason*, and learn it *from someone*. Education thus always raises questions about content, purpose, and relationships – the three 'elements' that in a sense constitute education. These questions are often absent when we just describe education in terms of 'teaching and learning', or when, in research, we seek to find out which factors impact on 'student learning'.

With regard to content, purpose, and relationships it can be argued that the question of purpose is actually the first question that needs to be addressed. If one is not able to articulate what particular educational activities and arrangements are *for*, there is no way in which one can decide which content students should engage with and what kind of relationships will be most conducive for what one seeks to achieve. What makes education particularly interesting is that it is not oriented toward one purpose or domain of purpose, but that all education needs to engage with three 'domains of purpose'[1] (see, e.g., Biesta,[18] Bruner,[19] Egan,[20] and Lamm[21]). The first domain of purpose for education is that of *qualification*, which is about providing students with knowledge, skills, and understanding that will qualify them to do 'something.' This 'something' can be narrow, such as in the case of becoming qualified for a particular job or profession – which is, of course, key in the field of medical education – or it can be conceived more widely such as the role schools play in providing young people with the knowledge, skills, and understandings for living their life in complex modern societies.

The purpose of education is, however, not confined to qualification. Education also has an important role to play in the domain of *socialization*. Socialization is about providing students with an orientation in particular fields or domains including vocational and professional domains. It is about initiating students into the ways of being and doing, the norms and values of particular social, cultural, practical, or professional traditions. This is intended to give students a sense of direction in such traditions and practices and also contributes to developing a sense of identity by becoming part of particular traditions and practices. There are stronger forms of socialization where the ambition is to make sure that students follow the rules and regulations and adopt the particular norms and values of the practice or tradition. Here identities are prescriptive. Some medical specialist groups, for example, may be known for their specific ways of doing and being (e.g., Musselman, MacRae, Reznick, and Lingard[22] on surgical education). In those cases medical education plays a key role in students' becoming part of such ways of doing and being. There are, however, also more 'open' forms of socialization aimed at giving students a sense of direction, but giving them opportunities to find their own role and position within such traditions and practices. In addition to becoming competent – the acquisition of

knowledge and skills – such opportunities create room for questions about professional identity: how one wishes and should understand oneself as a competent practitioner.

It could be argued that qualification and socialization are, to a large degree, done 'to' students. We teach students knowledge, skills, and understanding and check through assessment whether they have acquired this successfully. Similarly, we teach them the ways of doing and being of particular practices and assess whether they have adopted these successfully. This, however, is not all there is to education. We do not want our students to end up as objects with knowledge, skills, values, and norms. We always aim for them to end up as subjects in their own right; as individuals who can make up their own mind, draw their own conclusions, and take responsibility for their actions. This is captured in the domain of *subjectification* where we encourage and support our students to become subjects of their own action. Subjectification thus has to do with key educational ideas such as agency, autonomy, and responsibility.[2]

The suggestion that all education needs to work in relation to three domains of purpose is not only relevant for general education, but also helps to get more precision vis-à-vis the purposes of professional education including medical education. It thus provides a much more helpful and precise discourse than the reference to 'learning.' Rather than asking whether students are learning, we need to ask whether their education addresses all three domains of purpose. The simple but nonetheless helpful insight here is that the purpose of such education is not confined to the presentation and acquisition of knowledge, skills, and understanding. In addition to *professional qualification* (becoming a competent doctor), there is also a need for *professional socialization*: providing and achieving orientation in a professional field. Professional socialization in medicine has to do with achieving a professional identity as a medical professional (which actually has been described by some as the main purpose of medical education).[23–26] Also, medical professionals do not just need to be qualified and socialized; they also need to become a subject of their own actions. That is, they need to be able to judge which knowledge, skills, and understandings need to be utilized in which situation and also when they should stick to the rules and when to question the rules or bend or sometimes even ignore them if a particular situation calls for this. There is, therefore, also always

---

[1]In this regard education differs from many other practices which are often oriented to only one purpose or domain of purpose. Think, for example, of the orientation of medical practice on (the promotion of) health (acknowledging that what counts as health and how one promotes this are complex questions) or the orientation of the legal domain on justice.

[2]For a more detailed discussion about the idea of subjectification as a core educational ambition, see Biesta.[33,34]

the need for medical education to focus on *professional subjectification*.

Instead of the bland and to a degree even meaningless suggestion that the task of medical education is to make students learn, we can now say that medical education needs to aim for *professional qualification*, *professional socialization*, and *professional subjectification*. It also needs to make sure that these do not remain separate compartments but actually become integrated in the knowing, doing, and being of professionals. This then suggests a framework for the development of curricula – the content and experiences that students should encounter and work with during their education. This includes a range of experiences students should 'meet' – one can think, for example, of the importance of encountering the limits of medical treatment, a first unexpected patient death, the ambiguity or uncertainty of a high stakes treatment decision, a first euthanasia, resistance (from patients or other medical professionals) to one's medical decision, a first consultation carried out independently and satisfactorily, etc. In addition to a framework for curricula, the proposed view on education also suggests a framework for the development of pedagogy – the ways in which medical teachers engage with their students in order to promote professional qualification, socialization, and subjectification.

How does education work? And how can we make it work?

To see that the point of medical education is not to make students 'learn' but to contribute to their professional qualification, socialization, and subjectification is helpful in overcoming the limitations of the language of learning but does not yet resolve the question of *teaching*. One could, after all, still argue that once we have a more refined understanding of what it is that we seek to achieve, we should focus our research efforts on finding out which teaching interventions work for each of the three domains. This conclusion is helpful to the extent that it shows that asking the general 'what works?'-question is actually not very meaningful. Rather, we need to begin by asking *for which particular purpose or domain of purpose* a particular teaching strategy may work.

With regard to this it is important to acknowledge that the three domains of purpose do not exist separately but are always all three at play in the concrete practice of education. Teaching a particular skill, for example, motivational interviewing in General Practice consultations, is not just about acquiring that skill (qualification). It also communicates something about the importance of the skill in the profession (socialization) and simultaneously has an impact on the agency of the student: by mastering a skill one is able to act differently, which raises the question when it is appropriate to utilize this skill and when not (subjectification).

Whereas there can be synergy between the three domains, there can also be tensions and even conflicts. Think for example how 'teaching to the test' does very little in supporting students becoming responsible practitioners (subjectification) and also sends out the message that what really matters is passing the test (socialization). So the question which of our teaching strategies or wider educational arrangements 'work' is actually much more complicated than that – not just because the question of 'working' is a threefold question, but also because what may work in relation to one domain of purpose may actually work differently, or may not work at all in another domain of purpose.

Much educational research that seeks to generate evidence about 'what works' couches its ambitions in terms of factors that impact on students. It is here that reference is often made to the medical model on the assumption that teaching is an intervention that produces particular effects. The important question for education, including medical education, is whether this understanding is adequate for capturing the dynamics of education. Can it be assumed that under ideal circumstances teaching is a cause and learning – or with the language we prefer: students' professional *formation*[27] – is the effect? And is the fact that we have *not yet* established certain and secure connections between educational 'input' (teaching) and educational 'outcome' (learning; formation), just a matter of time and money? That is, would investment in more research eventually lead us to the evidence that will tell us once and for all which interventions will produce which effects?

This, we think, is unlikely. The reason for that lies in the fact that the strong causality that is assumed in this way of thinking actually only occurs in very specific situations: in closed, deterministic systems that operate in unidirectional ways. The paradigm case for this is the clockwork where each cogwheel puts the next cogwheel into motion so that, if we know the initial situation of the clockwork and have perfect knowledge of all connections between the cogwheels, we can predict with one hundred percent certainty how the machine will operate, and will continue to operate until eternity. This, however, is not the reality of education.[28] So the first question to ask is what kind of system education actually is in order, then, to say something about how a system such as education works and can be made to work.[29]

The first thing to bear in mind here is that education is a relatively *open system*. What happens 'inside' education is significantly influenced by what happens 'outside' of it. Students have lives and experience outside of the classroom and are therefore influenced by much more than just the teaching they receive. What happens in the classroom is part of a wider social context with intended and unintended influences flowing in and out. Secondly, education is not a deterministic system of mechanistic 'push and pull,' but a *semiotic system*, that is, a system that works by means of communication and interpretation. Put simply, students need to make sense of what teachers tell them or present to them and this is a matter of interpretation, not of stimulus-and-predictable-response. Thirdly, unlike the unidirectionality of the clockwork, education systems are *recursive*, which means that the 'elements' in the system (teachers and students) can think for themselves, make up their own minds, and, based on this, can decide to act in a number of different ways. How the system evolves does, in other words, feed back into the system.

Acknowledging that education is an open, semiotic, and recursive system may make one wonder whether anything can work at all in education in that whether any connection between what teachers do and what students take from it can be established or secured. With so many uncontrollable factors, and so many complex, open dynamics, it seems as if education is almost impossible. Yet the point we wish to make is that understanding the dynamics of education in this way – that is, seeing education as an open, semiotic, and recursive system – is actually quite helpful because it allows to indicate with much precision what needs to be done to make such a system work in a more predictable way. Everything here comes to reducing the 'degrees of freedom' of the system: reducing the openness of the system (the influences from outside), reducing the semiotics of the system (the opportunities for interpretation), and reducing the recursivity of the system (that is, the way in which the system feeds back onto itself).

Interestingly, reducing openness, interpretation, and recursivity is exactly what educators do. We reduce openness, the interference from the outside, by putting students in classrooms or designated study spaces first and foremost in order to focus the attention of our students. The curriculum is a further step in reducing openness by specifying what students should focus on and what they should be doing. Similarly, while interpretation has, in a sense, no boundaries, the whole point of assessment is to limit the range of interpretations our students generate sometimes to make sure that they get it absolutely right, and sometimes to make sure that they remain within the boundaries of what is meaningful. Thirdly, as educators we also try to influence the recursivity that is happening in our classrooms, basically by helping our students to think in particular ways. In medical education, we encourage our students to think as medical professionals,[30] rather than 'just' as private persons so that, when they make up their minds about what to do with their education, for example, we try to 'frame' this within a particular context (medical practice) rather than let it go in any direction.

When we look at the dynamics of education in this way, we not just have an account of education that makes much more sense than the mistaken assumption that there is a causal connection between teaching and learning. Such connections simply do not exist in social systems such as education. We also have an account that shows how our educational endeavors – our school buildings, classroom settings, curricula, forms of assessment – all contribute to giving the whole process more direction and structure in light of what we seek to achieve with our students. Yet what this approach also brings into view is that if we go too far in all this by closing off the influences from the outside completely, telling our students that there is only one correct way to interpret the curriculum, and only one right way to think, act, and be, we have suddenly turned education into *indoctrination*. While this may be 'effective' from the perspective of qualification and strong socialization, indoctrination is the very opposite of what we should achieve vis-à-vis the domain of subjectification, that is, our ambition to make sure that our students can ultimately think and act for themselves and take responsibility for this. While it is of crucial importance that we generate structure and focus in our educational activities, it is also important that we never turn our students into objects of our control.

Lessons for medical education and medical education research

One important implication for medical education *practice* from the above discussion is that it provides a much more refined language for talking about what medical education is *for* than the rather empty but nonetheless prevalent language of learning. For *curriculum design* this approach raises helpful questions about what a medical education curriculum should look like. What kind of curricular content do we need to work toward the professional qualification, the professional socialization, and the professional subjectification of medical students? How can we design educational activities such that this content contributes to all three domains in an integrated fashion? The above discussion not just raises questions about particular content students should master in relation to the three domains, but also about what kind of experiences they should encounter during their medical education. Which encounters would create educational opportunities in terms of professional qualification, socialization, and subjectification? With curricular redesign would also come other forms of *assessment* to establish students' progress in light of each of the three domains. How can we design assessment in ways that address development in terms of qualification as well as socialization and subjectification? Can we address all three in an integrated assessment or do we need separate assessments for each? In addition, student *evaluations* of medical education would require a broader focus on all three domains of purpose. We would need to not just ask students about the knowledge, skills, and understanding they may have achieved, but also about ways in which the education has contributed to their professional identity formation[31] and their ability for thoughtful judgment and decision making. To look at medical education in this way rather than in terms of the language of 'student learning' thus gives more precision and more focus to the design and enactment of medical education. This is not to suggest, of course, that current medical education is devoid of these dimensions but the language of 'teaching and learning' is simply insufficient to have meaningful conversations about the aims, structure, and processes of medical education.

A second implication of this discussion is for teachers in medical education *practice* to carefully consider any research findings about the supposed effectiveness of particular teaching interventions or methods. What does existing research have to say in relation to each of the three domains of qualification, socialization, and subjectification? Also, any indication that a particular approach may work for one domain or aspect of a domain does not automatically mean that it will also work for the other domains or aspects of them and also not that it will be neutral with respect to (aspects of) the other domains. It may also be counterproductive, and this is crucially important in

considering any alleged evidence at all. For example, a disproportionate emphasis in the domain of qualification on, say, knowledge retention and reproduction, may do little for developing informed, self-confident professional identities just as checking long lists of acquired competencies may do little, and may actually hinder, the formation of robust professional judgment. While the point may be obvious, it is crucial also not to forget that what allegedly has worked in one setting – which also means: under the particular conditions of that setting – may not do anything at all in a different setting, under different conditions.[1,3,13,32] Dealing with the local contingencies of teaching, teachers cannot but approach research evidence as suggestions to be translated and applied flexibly according to circumstance and context, but as nothing more than that.[5]

For medical education *research*, the main lesson to draw from what we have presented above is the need to move beyond one-dimensional research designs that either focus on just one domain – qualification, socialization, or subjectification – and 'forget' to explore the interactions between the three or, even worse, that continue to investigate the 'impact' on 'learning' without specifying about and for what the learning is supposed to be. Moreover, the ideas outlined above suggest a different focus for medical education research – not a search for correlations in order to identify 'effective factors,' but rather a thorough and thoughtful exploration of the construction of educational 'ecologies,' that is, of how, through arranging the openness, semiosis, and recursivity of educational practices, meaningful education can be established. Such an approach cannot confine itself to just looking at education from the 'outside' or looking for collections between inputs and outcomes, but needs to engage with teachers and students and their own meaning making and interpretation. Such research would not only tell us whether a new (or, for that matter, an established) practice would influence students' grades or help them meet professional standards more quickly or efficiently (qualification). It would also give us insight into the ways that this practice helps students be, do, and feel like professionals of their sort (socialization) and is significant for their ability to act and judge in meaningful and responsible ways (subjectification).

Conclusion

In this paper we have argued that there is a need to move beyond the rather simplistic 'medical model' of education that sees teaching as an intervention and learning as its effect, and that suggests that the sole task of medical education research is to find out which interventions 'work' to produce the intended effects. We have raised questions about the narrowness of the language of 'learning' and have suggested that more precision can be reached if we begin to discuss the purposes of medical education in terms of professional qualification, professional socialization, and professional subjectification. We have also raised questions about the causal assumptions that seem to underlie the medical model and that suggest a particular approach for medical education research. Here we have suggested that it makes much more sense not to understand education as a closed, causal system but as an open system that works through communication and interpretation and the thoughtful actions of teachers and students. In such a view, teaching, curriculum, assessment, and evaluations no longer appear as 'factors' to produce 'outcomes' but become meaningful aspects of the practice of educators to steer the educational process toward particular purposes – always bearing in mind that too much steering runs the risk of reducing meaningful education to problematic forms of indoctrination. Along these lines we hope to have made a contribution to the discussion about the future of medical education and medical education research away from the simplicities of the 'medical model' toward approaches that are able to grasp what is really going on when medical educators teach and students take part in medical education.

Declaration of interest

The authors declare no competing interests.

Podcast

Let Me Ask You Something (iTunes, Spotify, Google Podcasts and letmeaskyousomething.podbean.com). https://letmeaskyousomething.podbean.com/

Previous installment

Mario Veen & Anna T. Cianciolo (2020) Problems No One Looked For: Philosophical Expeditions into Medical Education, Teaching and Learning in Medicine, DOI: 10.1080/10401334.2020.1748634

Twitter handle

@BraakMarije

ORCID

Gert J. J. Biesta http://orcid.org/0000-0001-8530-7105
Marije van Braak http://orcid.org/0000-0003-2938-1508

References

1. Davies P. What is evidence-based education? *Br J Educ Stud.* 1999;47(2):108–121. doi:10.1111/1467-8527.00106.
2. Slavin RE. Perspectives on evidence-based research in education—What works? Issues in synthesizing educational program evaluations. *Educ Res.* 2008;37(1): 5–14. doi:10.3102/0013189X08314117.
3. Pirrie A. Evidence-based practice in education: the best medicine? *Br J Educ Stud.* 2001;49(2):124–136. doi:10.1111/1467-8527.t01-1-00167.
4. Thomas G. After the gold rush: questioning the "gold standard" and reappraising the status of experiment and randomized controlled trials in education. *Harv Educ Rev.* 2016;86(3):390–411. doi:10.17763/1943-5045-86.3.390.
5. Davis A. It worked there. Will it work here? Researching teaching methods. *Ethics Educ.* 2017; 12(3):289–303. doi:10.1080/17449642.2017.1361267.
6. McKnight L, Morgan A. A broken paradigm? What education needs to learn from evidence-based medicine. *J Educ Pol.* 2019;34:1–17. doi:10.1080/02680939. 2019.1578902.
7. Simpson A. The evidential basis of "evidence-based education": an introduction to the special issue. *Educ Res Eval.* 2019;25(1-2):1–6. doi:10.1080/13803611. 2019.1617979.
8. Biesta GJJ. Why "what works" won't work: evidence-based practice and the democratic deficit in educational research. *Educ Theory.* 2007;57(1):1–22. doi:10. 1111/j.1741-5446.2006.00241.x.
9. Harden RM, Grant J, Buckley G, Hart IR. BEME guide no. 1: best evidence medical education. *Med Teach.* 1999;21(6):553–562. doi:10.1080/01421599978960.
10. Fincher RME, Work JA. Perspectives on the scholarship of teaching. *Med Educ.* 2006;40(4):293–295. doi: 10.1111/j.1365-2929.2006.02404.x.
11. Smith R. Expertise and the scholarship of teaching. In: Kreber C, ed. *Scholarship Revisited: Perspectives on the Scholarship of Teaching.* San Francisco, CA: Jossey-Bass; 2001:69–78.
12. Chen F, Lui AM, Martinelli SM. A systematic review of the effectiveness of flipped classrooms in medical education. *Med Educ.* 2017;51(6):585–597. doi:10. 1111/medu.13272.
13. Regehr G. It's NOT rocket science: rethinking our metaphors for research in health professions education. *Med Educ.* 2010;44(1):31–39. doi:10.1111/j.1365-2923.2009.03418.x.
14. Norman G. RCT = results confounded and trivial: the perils of grand educational experiments. *Med Educ.* 2003; 37(7):582–584. doi:10.1046/j.1365-2923.2003.01586.x.
15. Horsley T, Custers E, Tolsgaard MG. Fundamentals of randomized designs: AMEE Guide No. 128. *Med Teach.* 2020;52:486–492. doi:10.1080/0142159X.2019. 1681389.

16. Love JN, Messman AM, Merritt C. Improving the learning experience through evidence-based education. *West J Emerg Med.* 2019;20(1):1–5. doi:10.5811/westjem.2018.10.41320.

17. Hattie J, Nepper Larsen S. *The Purposes of Education: A Conversation between John Hattie and Steen Nepper Larsen.* New York, NY: Routledge; 2020.

18. Biesta GJJ. Good education in an age of measurement: on the need to reconnect with the question of purpose in education. *Educ Asse Eval Acc.* 2009;21(1):33–46. doi:10.1007/s11092-008-9064-9.

19. Bruner J. *The Culture of Education.* Cambridge, MA: Harvard University Press; 1996. doi:10.1007/s11092-008-9064-9.

20. Egan K. *The Future of Education: Reimagining Our Schools from the Ground up.* New Haven, CT: Yale University Press; 2008.

21. Lamm Z. *Conflicting Theories of Instruction: Conceptual Dimensions.* Berkeley, CA: McCutchan; 1976.

22. Musselman LJ, MacRae HM, Reznick RK, Lingard LA. 'You learn better under the gun': intimidation and harassment in surgical education. *Med Educ.* 2005;39(9):926–934. doi:10.1111/j.1365-2929.2005.02247.x.

23. Chandran L, Iuli RJ, Strano-Paul L, Post SG. Developing "a Way of Being": deliberate approaches to professional identity formation in medical Education. *Acad Psychiatry.* 2019;43(5):521–527. doi:10.1007/s40596-019-01048-4.

24. Cruess RL, Cruess SR, Boudreau JD, Snell L, Steinert Y. Reframing medical education to support professional identity formation. *Acad Med.* 2014;89(11):1446–1451. doi:10.1097/ACM.0000000000000427.

25. Irby DM, Cooke M, O'Brien BC. Calls for reform of medical education by the Carnegie Foundation for the Advancement of Teaching: 1910 and 2010. *Acad Med.* 2010;85(2):220–227. doi:10.1097/ACM.0b013e3181c88449.

26. Jarvis-Selinger S, Pratt DD, Regehr G. Competency is not enough: integrating identity formation into the medical education discourse. *Acad Med.* 2012;87(9):1185–1191. doi:10.1097/ACM.0b013e3182604968.

27. Biesta GJJ. How does a competent teacher become a good teacher? On judgement, wisdom and virtuosity in teaching and teacher education. In: Heilbronn R, Foreman-Peck L, eds. *Philosophical Perspectives on Teacher Education.* Oxford: Wiley Blackwell; 2015: 3–22.

28. Biesta GJJ. Why 'what works' still won't work: from evidence-based education to value-based education. *Stud Philos Educ.* 2010;29(5):491–503. doi:10.1007/s11217-010-9191-x.

29. Osberg DC, Biesta GJJ, (eds). *Complexity Theory and the Politics of Education.* Rotterdam, The Netherlands: Sense Publishers; 2010.

30. Fuks A, Boudreau JD, Cassell EJ. Teaching clinical thinking to first-year medical students. *Med Teach.* 2009;31(2):105–111. doi:10.1080/01421590802512979.

31. Goldie J. The formation of professional identity in medical students: considerations for educators. *Med Teach.* 2012;34(9):e641–e648. doi:10.3109/0142159X.2012.687476.

32. Cowen N. For whom does "what works" work? The political economy of evidence-based education. *Educ Res Eval.* 2019;25(1–2):81–98. doi:10.1080/13803611.2019.1617991.

33. Biesta GJJ. Risking ourselves in education: qualification, socialisation and subjectification revisited. *Educ Theory.* 2020;70(1):89–104. doi:10.1111/edth.12411.

34. Biesta GJJ. Can the prevailing description of educational reality be considered complete? On the Parks-Eichmann paradox, spooky action at a distance, and a missing dimension in the theory of education. *Pol Futures Educ.* 2020. doi:10.1177/1478210320910312.

Teaching Medical Epistemology within an Evidence-Based Medicine Curriculum

Mark R. Tonelli (iD) and Robyn Bluhm

ABSTRACT

Issue: Epistemology, the branch of philosophy that deals with the nature, value, and use of knowledge, receives little or no formal attention in medical education. Yet the understanding of medical epistemology - focused on what kinds of medical knowledge are relevant to clinical decisions, the strengths and limitations of those different kinds of knowledge, and how they relate to one another and to clinical expertise - represents a critical aspect of medical practice. *Evidence:* Understanding the meaning of the term "evidence" is one of the fundamental tasks of medical epistemology. Other foundations of the evidence-based medicine movement, such as the "hierarchy of evidence" and the concept of "best" evidence, rest upon epistemological assertions, claims regarding the appropriate kinds and relative value of knowledge in medicine. Here we rely upon the work of philosophers of medicine who have been engaged in debates regarding the epistemic tenets of the evidence-based medicine movement. We argue that medical students and physicians-in-training should learn basic terminology and methods of epistemology as they are being introduced to the concepts and techniques of evidence-based medicine. *Implications:* The skepticism and critical analysis encouraged by EBM can and should be applied to the underlying assumptions and primary tenets of EBM itself. It is not enough for philosophers to partake in this endeavor; students, trainees, and clinicians need to carefully and constantly examine the reasons and reasoning that coalesce into clinical acumen. Our role as medical educators is to give them the tools, including a basic understanding of epistemology, to do that over a lifetime.

Dr. Lee's first appointment of the afternoon, Mr. Jackson, was a frequent visitor to the general medicine outpatient clinic, primarily because he was not getting better. His problem list was extensive: Type II diabetes, hypertension, hyperlipidemia, coronary artery disease (CAD), congestive heart failure (CHF), chronic obstructive pulmonary disease (COPD), and a chronic pain syndrome. Mr. Jackson's chief complaint was usually some combination of fatigue, malaise, dyspnea, and pain. Mr. Jackson felt unable to do the things that he wanted to do; he was not living the life he wanted to live. Trying to deal appropriately with Mr. Jackson's medical issues always took time and today Dr. Lee had a medical student shadowing her, meaning she would also have to explain her clinical reasoning.

Dr. Lee was committed to practicing evidence-based medicine (EBM). This obligation required that she apply the best available evidence, generally meaning the results of rigorous clinical research, to decisions around the treatment of her patients. In Mr. Jackson, living up to this commitment was particularly challenging. The number of research studies and clinical practice guidelines that might reasonably apply to Mr. Jackson was staggering, and also often conflicting. Guidelines for COPD were developed using research subjects who did not have CAD, and vice versa. Treating his hypertension and hyperlipidemia might decrease his risk of cardiovascular complications in the long-term, but did nothing to make him feel better in the short-term. In fact, the medications for these diagnoses generally made him feel worse.

Dr. Lee knew that being an evidence-based practitioner did not mean that she should be slavishly devoted to following clinical practice guidelines, to practicing "cookbook" medicine. EBM allowed and even encouraged her to integrate her individual clinical expertise with the best available results of clinical research in order to make decisions for particular patients. But, practically, how was she supposed to do that? Her clinical expertise in large part derived from her experience taking care of patients, yet she had been taught early on that primary clinical experience was an unreliable guide. She had an excellent understanding of physiology and pathophysiology, but was unsure of the value of this kind of knowledge in making clinical decisions. While in medical school and residency training she had learned how to carefully and critically evaluate research methodologies and statistical analyses, but no one had ever really taught her anything about integrating her clinical expertise into her practice. And if she could not articulate how she was reasoning, what knowledge she was relying upon and why, her medical student would be no wiser either.

Introduction

Like all physicians, Dr. Lee has spent many years acquiring a tremendous body of medical knowledge from a wide variety of sources, knowledge that provides not only the basis of her professional qualifications but is meant to serve as a foundation for all of her clinical decisions. Yet a strong knowledge base alone is insufficient for clinical practice, as clinicians must be able to "judge which knowledge, skills, and understandings need to be utilized in which situation, when they should stick to the rules and when to question the rules or bend or sometimes ignore them if a particular situation call for this."[1] This component of medical education, referred to as "professional subjectification" by Biesta and van Braak in an earlier contribution to this series,[1] requires a deep understanding of knowledge itself, of how it is developed, how it is categorized, when it is useful, and when it is unreliable or inappropriate. Without the ability to negotiate between variable, incomplete, and often conflicting sources and kinds of knowledge, a clinician cannot benefit her patients.

Epistemology is the branch of philosophy that deals with the nature, value, and use of knowledge. Currently, however, epistemology receives little or no formal attention in medical education. As part of this series on the value of philosophy in medical

education, we argue that a basic understanding of medical epistemology, focused on what kinds of medical knowledge are relevant to clinical decisions, the strengths and limitations of those different kinds of medical knowledge, and how they relate to one another, represents a critical aspect of medical education and practice. Students and clinicians should develop the ability to perform an epistemic analysis of clinical decisions, making explicit the specific kinds of knowledge they are relying upon for individual clinical decisions and how they are weighting the value of that knowledge. In order to develop this basic understanding in students and physicians, we believe the best approach involves the longitudinal introduction and incorporation of epistemology throughout undergraduate and graduate medical education. We suggest that one nearly universal aspect of modern medical education, the teaching of the fundamentals of evidence-based medicine (EBM), offers a convenient opportunity for epistemology to be integrated into the medical curriculum.

Evidence-based medicine has for some time now been the dominant medical epistemology, or theory of medical knowledge. Virtually all North American medical schools have dedicated time within their curriculum to teach the foundations of EBM.[2] EBM entails much more than the simple claim that medicine should be based on evidence; the enterprise of EBM makes strong claims about the kind of evidence required and the process of clinical decision making. The foundations of EBM, such as the "hierarchy of evidence" and the concept of "best" evidence, rest upon epistemological assertions, claims regarding the appropriate kinds and relative value of knowledge in medicine. Examining these claims is important for medical educators and medical students, not just to ensure that clinical practice is based on sound knowledge, but to clarify what EBM does well and what challenges it still faces. Leaving the epistemic assumptions of EBM unexamined and unchallenged invites the practice of "rubbish" EBM, the misguided and mindless misuse of misinterpreted clinical research.[3]

As EBM represents a school of medical epistemology, salient epistemic questions arise and become relevant at specific points in medical training. Integrating medical epistemology into the EBM curriculum will allow students to evaluate the various kinds of knowledge that rightly influence clinical decisions and examine various approaches to integrating knowledge at the bedside. Here we will outline three underlying assumptions of EBM, noting when in the medical curriculum examining them is most appropriate, and offer concrete suggestions for helping trainees examine each.

Pre-clinical studies: knowledge, evidence, and hierarchies

The concept of evidence-based medicine is generally introduced to medical students very early, often as part of an introduction to epidemiology and research methodology. Students coming from a variety of backgrounds in the physical sciences, social sciences, or humanities will bring with them different understandings of the term "evidence," making it necessary to examine what constitutes "evidence" for medicine in particular.

EBM rests upon claims regarding evidence in medicine that have not always been well elucidated or defended.[4,5] Specifically, while acknowledging that evidence comes from a variety of sources, EBM consistently endorses the notion that some evidence is "best" when it comes to medical decision making. This claim regarding the relative value of evidence is made manifest in an evidence hierarchy central to any understanding of EBM.[6,7] While there are multiple hierarchies of evidence promulgated by EBM, including different hierarchies for different tasks (e.g., treatment studies, studies of prognosis, studies that assess how well clinical decision rules work in practice),[8] the hierarchy for treatment studies is the most widely discussed and the one we will focus on here. In general, hierarchies of evidence related to a particular kind of study tend to be similar. For example, for studies of treatments, they are structured as below.[7]

- Systematic reviews of randomized trials
- Single randomized trial
- Systematic review of observational studies addressing patient-important outcomes
- Single observational study addressing patient-important outcomes
- Physiologic studies
- Case reports/Unsystematic clinical observations

The hierarchy of evidence is intended to provide initial guidance as to the strength of a study of the efficacy of a treatment by ranking study methods; studies higher on the hierarchy will (generally) provide stronger evidence. As the hierarchy above shows, studies that compare treatment outcomes in an experimental and a control group are held to provide better evidence than an individual physician's own clinical experiences with a treatment or studies that focus on physiological mechanisms rather than clinical outcomes. But the assignment of tiers represents an epistemic assertion rather than a necessary ordering.

The hierarchies of EBM also contain subsidiary epistemic assumptions. One is that random allocation is considered to be the best way to maximize the probability that the treatment and the control groups are similar with regard to patient characteristics that may affect treatment outcomes (e.g., age, sex, presence of comorbid conditions). Another is that concealing (blinding) whether an individual has been assigned to the treatment or to the control group, both from the participant themselves and from the study personnel who assess clinical outcomes is crucial because knowing which treatment (including, in many studies, placebo) an individual is receiving may influence perceptions of their response to therapy. Proponents of the hierarchy of evidence say that randomized and blinded studies are less likely to be biased, in the statistical sense of giving results that systematically deviate from the truth, than non-randomized, non-blinded studies.[7]

When learners are first exposed to the hierarchy of evidence during their pre-clinical training, a program in medical epistemology will encourage them to examine these underlying assumptions rather than simply accept the hierarchy as a pyramid of truth. Students examining the assumptions contained within the hierarchy will find that much of this work has already been done by philosophers of science. One major criticism of EBM, for instance, is that it overstates the value of some research methodologies, particularly the value of randomization.[9,10] While random allocation may be a useful tool and can achieve important epistemological goals, critics of EBM have worried that its importance has been overemphasized, to the detriment of other important sources of evidence. In a classic paper, Worrall argues that, while it is true that randomization is a good way to ensure allocation concealment and to balance potential confounding variables between the experimental and control groups, there are other ways to achieve these ends in designing a study.[9] Others have emphasized that not all clinical questions (for example, the risk of cigarette smoking) are best answered by randomized trials.[10] (In making these philosophical points accessible to medical students, the use of a fictional and satirical RCT may be helpful.)[11]

Moving from randomization to other aspects of study design opens up the question of whether (and when) a poorly-designed randomized trial might be of overall lower quality than a well-designed non-randomized study, which some versions of the hierarchy of evidence do allow. Students might also be asked to think about situations in which a case report might be more useful than a randomized trial. For example, a report on a patient similar to Mr. Jackson, in the case that opens this paper, may give Dr. Lee better guidance than a randomized trial involving patients with only a single illness, without co-morbidity.

Pre-clinical students will likely need little prompting to wonder why they are studying principles of physiology and pharmacology if these represent only the lowest form of evidence for clinical decision making. Challenging them to *answer* this question will lead them to consider how these principles are related to the results of clinical research, and how both kinds of knowledge might work together in clinical decision making. The relationship between pathophysiologic understanding and studies that compare clinical outcomes in treatment and control groups is of great epistemic significance in medicine. Within the philosophy of science, Russo and Williamson have argued that mechanistic evidence is generally required along with difference-making evidence (e.g. clinical trials) in order to establish causality in medicine.[12] Howick, a philosopher who is very sympathetic toward EBM, has argued that it is sometimes possible to establish the efficacy of a therapy without doing a controlled trial, because the mechanism of action is so well understood. Although rare, these cases show we should not rule out using evidence of a mechanisms linking a treatment and an outcome.[13] More recently, Tonelli and Williamson have shown that knowledge of mechanisms is essential for several aspects of clinical decision making, including using the results of population-level studies to make decisions about the care of individual patients (an issue we will return to below) and assessing the results of population-level reports.[14] As with the relationship between randomized and non-randomized trials, always putting mechanistic evidence at the bottom of the hierarchy means that clinicians may not be willing to make use of good evidence when it would be helpful. Rather than a hierarchy, the relationship between knowledge derived from epidemiological and laboratory research may best be viewed as a network.[15]

Similarly, the methodologies occupying the pinnacle of the evidence hierarchy have their own epistemic limitations. Systematic reviews and meta-analyses use well-defined and explicit methods to identify, select, synthesize, and appraise all high quality research evidence relevant to a particular question; a meta-analysis also statistically combines the results of these studies to provide an overall estimate of the effect of a treatment. These systematic studies have largely replaced an older style of "narrative" review, in which an expert clinician surveyed the literature and offered their own, often idiosyncratic, judgment of the evidence. Yet the apparent objectivity of systematic reviews and meta-analyses should be questioned. Stegenga, among others, has pointed out that many methodological decisions need to be made when conducting a meta-analysis.[16] These include decisions about which studies to include in the review, which effects (both intended effects and side effects) of a treatment to include, how to determine the quality of these studies, and how to statistically combine them. In fact, these choices can have such a strong effect on the results of the review that two meta-analyses may come to opposite recommendations about the use of a therapy; Stegenga gives several such examples. While some philosophers have responded to criticisms like Stegenga's by defending meta-analyses,[17] others have argued that the problems with these quantitative studies mean that we should reconsider the value of narrative reviews, which have the distinct strength of providing interpretation and critique of the evidence.[18]

Upon this philosophical examination of the notion of evidence in medicine, some students may come to the (very defensible) conclusion that we should abandon the idea that evidence can be ranked on a hierarchy at all. This conclusion does not necessarily mean, however, that evidentiary support for clinical decisions is not necessary or that thinking in terms of hierarchies has no value at all. Even authors who have been critical of EBM and the hierarchy of evidence have acknowledged that it has made positive epistemic contributions, including raising awareness of the varying quality of research studies.[19,20] Moreover, as we noted above, examining the assumptions underlying the hierarchy will give students a deeper understanding of its strengths and weaknesses and enable them to be more thoughtful users of evidence from clinical research.

Introduction to clinical medicine: appraising, or accepting, evidence

The first introduction of EBM to the broader medical community was made in the context of medical education. A 1992 article published in JAMA by the EBM Working Group contrasts EBM's "Way of the Future" with the unsatisfactory "Way of the Past".[21] It describes a medical resident, pre-EBM, treating a previously-healthy patient who has just experienced a first grand mal seizure and who asks her about his risk of seizure recurrence. She brings this question to her senior resident and the attending physician, who tell her to inform her patient that his risk of a seizure recurrence is high. Once given this information, her patient "leaves in a state of vague trepidation" about his prognosis. By contrast, the way of the future has the resident go to the library and conduct a literature search, sifting through a couple dozen search results to find a study that is directly relevant to her patient's situation. According to this study,

> the patient risk of recurrence at one year is between 43% and 51% and at three years the risk is between 51% and 60%. After a seizure-free period of 18 months, his risk of recurrence would likely be less than 20%.

When she tells her patient about these results, he "leaves with a clear idea of his likely prognosis."

Leaving aside the question of whether the patient is really likely to find the latter description of his prognosis more helpful than the former, there is much to like about this scenario. We are told that the resident has already learned how to judge the quality of a study of prognosis, and she is also able to conduct a literature search and retrieve the results. (Note that, in 1992, this required her to actually go to the library, search the stacks for the relevant journal, and photocopy the results, though we are told that this entire process took only half an hour.)

Similarly, Upshur talks about his medical training at McMaster University, at the same time that EBM (then called clinical epidemiology and critical appraisal) was being developed.[22] People proposing a specific course of clinical action during rounds were frequently challenged to provide their evidence for and reasoning behind a recommendation, to explicitly justify what they proposed to do. At its best, EBM has drawn attention to the importance of clinical research for practice, fostered skills of critical appraisal, and (as part of a broader group of movements including the Cochrane Collaboration and the CONSORT Group), improved the conduct, or at least the reporting, of clinical trials. Yet in practice, and increasingly over time, EBM has shifted from encouraging individual engagement with the medial literature (as depicted in the original JAMA article) to espousing reliance on aggregated and curated summaries, representing the kind of unquestioned, and frequently disappointing, authority that it aimed to replace.

The amount of time available and the amount of clinical research published ensure that situations like the one depicted in the JAMA article's "Way of the Future" will be, at best, rare. As early as 1996, the proponents of EBM recognized this problem. Sackett et al. calculated that British medical consultants had about an hour a week to keep up with reading, and

that the volume of articles published in general medicine meant that, to actually keep up, a clinician would have to read approximately 19 articles per day.[23] Four years later, Guyatt et al. acknowledged that clinician interest in engaging directly with the literature would also be a limiting factor.[24] They recognized that becoming adept at the skills of EBM "requires intensive study, and frequent, time consuming, application." They therefore distinguished between "evidence-based practitioners", who are able to independently find and appraise evidence "from scratch", and "evidence users", who have some training in the skills of EBM, but who generally rely on published guidelines and pre-appraised evidence published as secondary sources. Since then, the developers of EBM have increasingly promoted the use of these kinds of resources. Such a reliance on processed knowledge, however, raises additional epistemic challenges.

Students and clinicians seeking definitive guidance from curated sources, such as Up to Date and the Cochrane Collaboration, should understand that the process of curating, even when based upon explicit criteria, is subjective and value-laden. Students should be encouraged to examine the sources of bias, including funding source and academic advancement, that enter into the what is often promoted as an objective collation and synthesis of published research.[25] For instance, the Cochrane Collaboration has been embroiled in a very public controversy that centers on competing claims of what represents a fair and objective assessment of evidence. While attention has been paid to these issues in philosophical publications,[26] students may find discussions more accessible by reading reports in the lay and scientific press.[27]

The ability to properly assess individual reports of clinical research is a fundamental skill of any health care provider. But given that it is impossible for an individual physician to perform the kinds of patient-specific searches depicted in the original article describing EBM, or to be familiar with all of the research relevant to their practice, some form of evidence summary is not merely useful, but necessary. Students being introduced to clinical medicine should develop a similar level of skepticism for curated research guidance as they have been encouraged to develop for individual research reports or the proclamations of attending physicians.

Graduate medical education: integrating evidence into clinical practice

After graduation, physicians-in-training must increasingly make independent clinical decisions, creating a period of trepidation that offers the opportunity to build on the foundation of medical epistemology developed during medical school. As seen in Dr. Lee's encounter with Mr. Jackson, the primary epistemic challenge of clinical practice relates to what knowledge can and should be brought to bear in arriving at a particular diagnostic or therapeutic decision. EBM provides an idealized version of clinical decision making, but little in the way of real-world guidance, leaving this intractable epistemic challenge to clinicians.

In the most widely cited definition of EBM, Sackett and colleagues state that:

> "Evidence based medicine is the conscientious, explicit, and judicious use of current best evidence in making decisions about the care of individual patients. The practice of evidence based medicine means integrating individual clinical expertise with the best available external clinical evidence from systematic research. By individual clinical expertise we mean the proficiency and judgment that individual clinicians acquire through clinical experience and clinical practice."[23]

This attempt at a simple definition belies the complexity of negotiating between research evidence and the myriad other things that doctors know, the knowledge that serves as the foundation of clinical expertise. EBM has an integration problem, a problem created by the ethical imperative of clinicians to individualize care along with the acknowledgment that the results of clinical research alone can never be prescriptive. The integration problem is made manifest to trainees in a number of ways, from realizing that extrapolating from a population to a particular individual is not straightforward (in epistemology, this is known as the reference-class problem) to wondering how much weight and deference to give the judgments of senior clinicians explicitly based upon their experiential knowledge, sometimes in seeming opposition to published research results. The acknowledgment of the value of clinical expertise raises the crucial question of what constitutes that expertise. Sackett and colleagues make clear that it derives, in large part, from knowledge gained by experience in direct patient care, yet EBM provides no guidance as to how to balance this experiential evidence with evidence from research. In fact, experiential knowledge is routinely denigrated as anecdotal within EBM.

The focus of the epistemology curriculum at this stage should be on understanding the strengths and weaknesses of various kinds of medical knowledge.[28] Reflecting back upon the epistemology learned in the pre-clinical years, house staff will recall that the hierarchy of evidence fails to provide a model for integration. By following the recommendations of Sackett and colleagues to make clinical decision making explicit, trainees should be able to categorize the kinds of knowledge being invoked in support of a clinical assessment or decision. For instance, the results of clinical research may be alternatively augmented or challenged by pathophysiologic rationale or by the personal experience of the clinician. Knowledge regarding the particular patient, including understanding their goals and values, will also be crucial to any decision. In addition, knowledge of the context (e.g. legal, cultural, financial) in which healthcare is being provided also facilitates or constrains certain decisions. One of us has argued that all relevant medical knowledge falls into one of these five categories: clinical research, mechanistic reasoning, experiential, individual patient characteristics, and contextual features.[29] (While we are focused solely on medical epistemology here, this framework acknowledges the ethical, emotional, and cultural complexity of clinical decisions.) Having trainees reason out loud, performing an epistemic analysis regarding the knowledge they are utilizing in support of their choices, allows for discussion about the relative weight given to different kinds of knowledge in specific cases.

Elucidating and mitigating the integration problem, we would suggest, is best taught through case-based formats. Cases can be either actual, analyzed in real-time, or standardized. Published literature offers a wide-variety of cases that can be used for such purposes, including some specifically chosen to illustrate epistemic challenges.[30] Case-based reasoning encourages trainees to bring to the table multiple kinds of knowledge relevant to a particular decision. When clinicians disagree about the differential diagnosis or the preferred treatment recommendation in a case, an epistemic analysis can determine whether the disagreement comes from a lack of knowledge, a difference in interpretation of information, or a different weighting of the relevant knowledge in the case. This approach helps to both repudiate the notion that clinical expertise is a "black box" and reinforce the value of multiple sources of knowledge in arriving at sound clinical conclusions. Each kind of medical knowledge has its own strengths and weaknesses in terms of making decisions for patients. In approaching any specific case, a clinician should utilize and incorporate all of the relevant knowledge available to her. While EBM explicitly claims that there is some "best" evidence that should be relied upon in clinical medicine, in clinical practice physicians need to evaluate the totality of evidence used to justify a clinical decision, which means negotiating an "untidy epistemic pluralism."[31] A formal approach to examining clinical decision making based upon an understanding of epistemology can help make this pluralism a bit more tidy for trainees.

Conclusion

A basic understanding of medical epistemology serves as an operator's manual for students, trainees, and clinicians, guiding the use clinical research results, pathophysiologic understanding, and experiential knowledge in medical practice. To provide this philosophical foundation, medical educators, with the aid of philosophers of medicine, can incorporate the teaching of the language, principles, and understanding of medical epistemology into parts of the medical curriculum where they fit naturally. In particular, the curriculum focused on evidence-based medicine represents an ideal opportunity to explore the philosophical questions related to medical knowledge, as EBM represents a school of medical epistemology. Philosophers of science have been examining the epistemic assertions and assumptions of EBM since its inception. The insights provided are not abstract musings, but are highly relevant to medical education and practice. The skepticism and critical analysis encouraged by EBM can and should be applied to the underlying assumptions and primary tenets of EBM itself. It is not enough for philosophers to partake in this endeavor; students, trainees, and clinicians need to carefully and constantly examine the reasons and reasoning that coalesce into clinical acumen. Our role as medical educators is to give them the tools, including a basic understanding of epistemology, to do that over a lifetime.

Disclosure statement

No potential conflict of interest was reported by the authors.

ORCID

Mark R. Tonelli ⓘ http://orcid.org/0000-0001-8402-922X

References

1. Biesta GJJ, van Braak M. Beyond the medical model: thinking differently about medical education and medical education research. *Teach Learn Med.* 2020; 32(4):449–456. doi:10.1080/10401334.2020.1798240.
2. Maggio LA, Tannery NH, Chen HC, ten Cate O, O'Brien B. Evidence-based medicine training in undergraduate medical education: a review and critique of the literature published 2006–2011. *Acad Med.* 2013;88(7):1022–1028. doi:10.1097/ACM.0b013e3182951959.
3. Greenhalgh T, Howick J, Maskrey N, Evidence Based Medicine Renaissance Group. Evidence based medicine: a movement in crisis? *BMJ.* 2014;348:g3725 doi:10.1136/bmj.g3725.
4. Feinstein AR, Horwitz RI. Problems in the "evidence" of "evidence-based medicine. *Am J Med.* 1997;103(6):529–535. doi:10.1016/s0002-9343(97)00244-1.
5. Goldenberg MJ. On evidence and evidence-based medicine: lessons from the philosophy of science. *Soc Sci Med.* 2006;62(11):2621–2632. doi:10.1016/j.socscimed.2005.11.031.
6. Montori V, Guyatt G. What is evidence-based medicine and why should it be practiced? *Respiratory Care.* 2001;46(11):1201–1214.
7. Guyatt G, Rennie D, eds. *Users' Guides to the Medical Literature.* 2nd ed. Chicago: AMA Press; 2008.
8. Blunt C. Hierarchies of evidence in evidence-based medicine [PhD]. London: Philosophy, London School of Economics; 2015. http://etheses.lse.ac.uk/3284/.
9. Worrall J. What evidence in evidence-based medicine? *Philosophy of Science.* 2002;69(S3):S316–S330. doi:10.1086/341855.
10. Grossman J, Mackenzie FJ. The randomized controlled trial: gold standard, or merely standard? *Perspect Biol Med.* 2005;48(4):516–534. doi:10.1353/pbm.2005.0092.
11. Study of Maternal and Child Kissing (SMACK) Working Group. Maternal kisses are not effective in alleviating minor childhood injuries (boo-boos): a randomized, controlled and blinded study. *J Eval Clin Pract.* 2015;21(6):1244–1246.
12. Russo F, Williamson J. Interpreting causality in the health sciences. *Int J Phil Sci.* 2007;21(2):157–170. doi:10.1080/02698590701498084.
13. Howick J. *The Philosophy of Evidence-Based Medicine.* Oxford: Wiley-Blackwell; 2011.
14. Tonelli MR, Williamson J. Mechanisms in clinical practice: use and justification. *Med Health Care Philos.* 2020;23(1):115–124. doi:10.1007/s11019-019-09915-5.
15. Bluhm R. From hierarchy to network: a richer view of evidence for evidence-based medicine. *Perspect Biol Med.* 2005;48(4):535–547. doi:10.1353/pbm.2005.0082.
16. Stegenga J. Is meta-analysis the platinum standard of evidence? *Stud Hist Philos Biol Biomed Sci.* 2011; 42(4):497–507. doi:10.1016/j.shpsc.2011.07.003.
17. Holman B. In defense of meta-analysis. *Synthese.* 2019;196(8):3189–3211. doi:10.1007/s11229-018-1690-2.
18. Greenhalgh T, Thorne S, Malterud K. Time to challenge the spurious hierarchy of systematic over narrative reviews? *Eur J Clin Invest.* 2018;48(6):e12931 doi:10.1111/eci.12931.
19. Glasziou P, Vandenbroucke J, Chalmers I. Assessing the quality of research. *BMJ.* 2004;328(7430):39–41. doi:10.1136/bmj.328.7430.39.

20. Goldenberg MJ. Iconoclast or creed? Objectivism, pragmatism, and the hierarchy of evidence. *Perspect Biol Med.* 2009;52(2):168–187. doi:10.1353/pbm.0.0080.

21. The Evidence-Based Medicine Working Group. Evidence-based medicine: A new approach to teaching the practice of medicine. *JAMA.* 1992;268(17): 2420–2425.

22. Upshur RE. Looking for rules in a world of exceptions: reflections on evidence-based practice. *Perspect Biol Med.* 2005;48(4):477–489. doi:10.1353/pbm.2005.0098.

23. Sackett D, Rosenberg W, Gray J, Hynes R, Richardson W. Evidence based medicine: what it is and what it isn't. *BMJ.* 1996;312(7023):71–72. doi:10.1136/bmj.312.7023.71.

24. Guyatt GH, Meade MO, Jaeschke RZ, Cook DJ, Haynes RB. Practitioners of evidence based care. Not all clinicians need to appraise evidence from scratch but all need some skills. *BMJ.* 2000;320(7240): 954–955. doi:10.1136/bmj.320.7240.954.

25. Fuller J. Meta-research evidence for evaluating therapies. *Philosophy of Science.* 2018;85(5):767–780. doi:10.1086/699689.

26. Greenhalgh T, Ozbilgin MF, Prainsack B, Shaw S. Moral entrepreneurship, the power-knowledge nexus, and the Cochrane "crisis". *J Eval Clin Pract.* 2019; 25(5):717–725. doi:10.1111/jep.13124.

27. Kolitz D. 'Evidence-based medicine' and the expulsion of Peter Gotzsche. *Undark.* 2020. https://undark.org/2019/12/30/peter-gotzsche-cochrane/.

28. Tonelli MR. The challenge of evidence in clinical medicine. *J Eval Clin Pract.* 2010;16(2):384–389. doi:10.1111/j.1365-2753.2010.01405.x.

29. Tonelli MR. Integrating evidence into clinical practice: an alternative to evidence-based approaches. *J Eval Clin Pract.* 2006;12(3):248–256. doi:10.1111/j.1365-2753.2004.00551.x.

30. Tinetti ME, Fried T. The end of the disease era. *Am J Med.* 2004;116(3):179–185. doi:10.1016/j.amjmed.2003.09.031.

31. Solomon M. *Making Medical Knowledge.* Oxford: Oxford University Press; 2015.

Language, Philosophy, and Medical Education

John R. Skelton

ABSTRACT

Issue: When medical schools began to recognize, a generation ago, that clinical "communication skills" could not be taken for granted among students, a process began of researching them, and introducing the results into curricula. This allowed for a discussion, for the first time, about how doctors should talk to patients, and manage interviews with them. However, there was a focus on a set of behavioral processes which were often unsophisticated with respect to the role of language in communication, or of language as a means of sustaining and describing ambiguity, or language as the primary impetus for educational reflection. *Evidence:* This paper looks at literature from language studies, the philosophy of language and the philosophy of education to establish the point that, where natural languages are concerned, it is possible and useful to talk of the purposes for which language is used. It is also important to recognize that the meaning of a particular language use is to a substantial extent defined by context: and that languages are excellent vehicles for maintaining and describing ambiguity, where it is impossible to reduce a state of affairs to the well-defined conclusion of empirical research. *Implications:* In the light of this understanding, there is a need for "communication," and particularly the methodologies through which it is taught, to reflect these points. Simulation exercises, designed to develop clinical communication, should be clear that there is no single correct way of "talking to patients," no set of behavioral processes which is always effective. It is, in the end, the awareness and wisdom of the doctor, selecting from among a range of available approaches, which is at stake. In addition, methodologies should account for the recognition that awareness comes only from reflection, and that helping medical students and doctors alike to reflect is central to good practice.

Introduction

In this paper I offer some thoughts about the relationship between philosophy, language, and my own job, as a teacher and researcher in clinical communication.

I began professional life as a teacher of English to second and foreign language learners, and then spent some years as a teacher trainer/educator, and academic applied linguist. I came to Medical Education in 1992 with a remit to teach and research what was known as "communication skills."

At that time, Erwin Mishler's book,[1] still perhaps the best qualitative study of language and medicine, had been around for some years, as had a number of others studies, from a variety of traditions.[2-5] Yet the lion at the gate for communication skills in medicine was the Toronto Consensus statement, as it was called.[6] It declared that "[communication] skills can be defined with behavioral criteria and can be reliably taught and assessed" (The "behavioral criteria" in this tradition were things like "open questions"). This seemed to me a misunderstanding of how language works (I have discussed the details elsewhere).[7] So, for example, when Ong et al.[8] published an early state of the art paper on the field, subsequently much cited, not a single qualitative study was mentioned.

What I came to understand more clearly was the need for medical students and doctors to have a more sophisticated understanding of a number of things. For example, there was a need to emphasize professional language as *doing things with words*, to borrow a phrase from Speech Act Theory,[9] and therefore as being task-focused. There was a need to emphasize that meaning is defined by the context in which language is used, a fundamental point covered in part by the concepts of *communicative competence* and *community meaning*. And finally there was a need to emphasize the ability of language to help us manage and discuss the *ambiguity* of professional and personal life, and to discuss also the relationship between language, *self-awareness* and the *power* these things bring.

It is these areas which I look at below.

Language is about doing things with words: The importance of *aims*

A useful starting place is to consider when purposes are unfulfilled. To take an example from a very well-researched field, [10] imagine Mr Jack Smith, aged 44, a heavy smoker. His doctor thinks: "Right, next time, I'm going to get him to stop." A month later, Mr Smith walks in. "Now listen, Jack," says the doctor, "You've just got to stop this smoking nonsense. It's madness. For God's sake stop!"

The result? Mr Smith thinks, as so often before, "My grandad smoked like a chimney and lived past 90. I'm not going to see that doctor again. All he does is nag me." Then one day Mr Smith begins to cough more, to lose weight, to feel weak….and when he does go to his doctor again, it's too late. "Well," says the doctor virtuously to his wife, "some people just won't listen…."

So, did the doctor achieve his aim? Clearly not. It matters not at all that he was right, nor that he truly wished to help his patient. He failed. He did not get things done. A central point for all teaching in clinical communication is: what is your purpose? What do you want to *do*?

The concept of "doing things with words," and Austin's original study (Austin 1962), blossomed into a field of research of considerable depth – and even greater complexity. I want to touch, very briefly, on just two aspects of it: the focus on how words come to "do things," and the division (details have been the subject of more than 50 years of discussion) between what we appear to mean on the surface, what we actually intend to mean, and what others take us to mean.

Austin, in the original study, looked at something very specific: a type of verb he called "performative" because, if uttered by a person in authority, they actually do ("perform") the action they mention. Thus, a judge may say "I sentence you to five years," and so it is: the vicar may "pronounce you man and wife," and so you are.

In itself this is a linguistic curiosity of marginal interest, at least for our purposes. But it led to a detailed discussion about the other things we can do with language, and how we do them. Thus we can request, promise, describe the world, express our feelings, and so on. Sometimes the authority of the speaker is very considerable, and is made to sound so. Indeed, it seems in some circumstances, by virtue of our office, that we can change the world by *fiat*. Note the similarity between the Biblical "Let there be light," and the utterance "Make it so," as Jean-Luc Picard so often says in *Star Trek*. In this respect, see Searle's remark on what he calls "extra-linguistic declarations": "we do more than represent: we create."[11(p114)] (See also Hansson Wahlberg[12] for a detailed discussion of this quotation, and other aspects of the issue.)

However, there are more quotidian ways in which we use language to create new states of affairs. For our purposes, the question is: how do we do so effectively? And for that matter, why is it that we fail?

There are many ways of looking at this. Within Speech Act theory, it is worth picking up the simple yet profound distinctions between the apparent, or purely propositional, meaning of an utterance, what one intends to achieve through it, and whether the person one is speaking to understand the intention. Consider Mary, say, who looks ruefully at her friend and says, "It's cold in here." Clearly, a statement about temperature is intended to be a request, perhaps to close the window (Searle[13] would call this an "indirect speech act"). If the friend says, "Oh sorry – let me…." and jumps up and closes the window, she has understood the intention. To nod judiciously and respond, "Yes Mary, you're quite correct" is not.

On a bigger scale, with more at stake, the question of purpose is central. The first clinic I ever observed was an ENT doctor who was dealing with a succession of patients with tonsillitis. In perhaps 10 out of fifteen cases, he concluded by saying, "I think you'd be better off without those [ie, the tonsils], don't you?" All of the patients agreed, some willingly but one or two with a degree of surprise. What was the doctor's purpose? He might say it was to see if the patient consented to a tonsillectomy. But the question, posed in just this way, made a refusal very difficult. It seemed the real purpose was to move the clinic along briskly by getting consent without discussion. (For an exploration of the sociolinguistics of what we now know as "Shared Decision-making" see Robertson et al.)[14]

Language is meaning in context: Different things work for different people

Underpinning the previous section is one fundamental principle about how we convey meanings when we speak or write: it is context which defines meaning.

The ENT doctor above took advantage of a kind of creative ambiguity. As a linguist would say, he used a grammatical *interrogative*, but he did not functionally ask a *question*. Rather, he – let's say – sought to maneuver the patient into swift acquiescence (about what was the best thing anyway).

All languages have endless opportunities for ambiguity, though usually context removes it. This incidentally is a major function of such phrases as "he said sarcastically" in novels: to disambiguate text by providing a context (the context of intonation, here) lost in the written language.

Conveying the meaning you want, and having it correctly understood, is recognized in language studies, particularly language in education, as "communicative competence." The central ideas are set out in Hymes: he summed them up by saying that "There are rules of use without which the rules of grammar would be useless."[15(p278)] A "rule of grammar" is, for example, that one says "You aren't" but "He isn't." A rule of use is that "He ain't" is commonplace particularly in the USA and therefore, through Hollywood and popular song, known around the English-speaking world. So, if I want to sound American, particularly perhaps blue-collar American, I might use "ain't": if I want to sound British, professional, etc, I will use "isn't."

Many of these issues have to do with politeness, particularly across cultures (as above, this might include working-class versus middle-class culture, as well as cultures in different areas of the world). If you are British and travel abroad, for example, you might find east Europeans worryingly direct, the Japanese worryingly oblique – and of course, the converse is true: a British person risks being thought of as too indirect ("no offence, but you're all a bit two-faced, you know?" an east European doctor once said to me), or too direct, as a Japanese person would probably *not* tell you for fear of causing offense. Everyone needs an understanding of communicative competence: including, most relevantly, International Medical Graduates (IMGs). It is an excellent thing to introduce them to the idea, to rules of use, and help them to repackage what may almost seem character flaws – rudeness, concealment – as just matters of language.

There are other ways too of considering the relationship between what one says and what one means.

Consider pain, for example – it is, by definition, something which cannot be shared with someone else (you can't say: "Here, sample some of my pain"). This is where Wittgenstein's famous "beetle" paradox comes in.[16] Let us suppose that we all have something we call a "beetle" in a box. How do we know, just by using language, that we are describing the same thing – that the beetle in my box is identical to the beetle in yours? We cannot, suggests Wittgenstein – or, given the gnomic nature of his writing, so people have argued. Certainly, if our view of language is that it merely communicates concepts ("my pain"), then it seems we have a problem. But if we see in language the potential for using language itself to negotiate and agree a meaning, it is not. (This, like all aspects of Wittgenstein's work, is hugely contested. For a detailed but technical discussion see Kripke,[17] in a very much discussed paper. For a discussion of the beetle analogy as it applies to medical education, see Veen et al.)[18]

So it is too, we might argue, with all kinds of abstract concepts. Is the idea of "duty" or "love" which I have in my mind the same as the idea you have in yours? If you and I talk about "a doctor's duty," are we talking about the same thing?

One purpose of discussion is to refine the meaning of the term in one's own mind as one hears how others use it, and so reach a consensus. In effect it is through use that words come to have moderately clear meanings, and also how it is that meanings come to change. No-one now can use the word "gay" to mean happy, the word "square" to mean "old-fashioned": the consensus, simply, is otherwise. One must aim, in other words, for the community view. And understanding the community view is – though this, like all abstractions, is up for discussion – an aspect of communicative competence.

A final point here. The very existence of such words as *irony, nuance, ambiguity* make it clear that what we say or write cannot always be taken at face-value. Foreign language textbooks, for many years, worked on the presumption that their role was to describe and teach prototypical, unambiguous language, with sections linked by grammatical similarity. The result was famously odd. Indeed, a point which should be a great deal more widely known, Eugene Ionesco was inspired partly by the *Assimil* English language textbooks of the 1930s, and the bizarre nature of their language, to create the Theater of the Absurd.[19]

Reductionism and ambiguity: Language helps to capture the world's complexity

Science asks us to clear away the fog, to identify what can be proven (a hypothesis), to test it and see what "the facts" are. Do more people get better more quickly on this new drug, than on that old drug? Test it and see. Has this patient got a bacterial infection or not? Find out. As Hobbes said, science is "the knowledge of consequences and the dependence of one fact upon another."[20(p25)]

We are all as patients – of course – much safer because of the increasingly sophisticated way that cause and effect links are understood, isolated, and explored, most recently through the work of the EBM (Evidence-based Medicine) movement. (Tonelli and Bluhm[21] have an excellent discussion of epistemology in an EBM world). There are, however, two well-established caveats. One dates perhaps from the skeptical arguments put forward by Hume. He asked how we know – how we really know – that just because cause and effect relationships have held true in the past, they will do so in future. How can we be sure that tomorrow we will perceive the sun as rising in the east? We cannot. It is only "custom" which "makes us expect for the future, a similar train of events with those which have appeared in the past."[22(p44)]

Well, we must muddle through somehow. Either one is completely skeptical about knowledge in general (in which case, why bother with research), or one may take the view that repeated co-occurrences of the same set of phenomena amount to something one may *assume* to be "a fact." Formally, observations reach a conventionally applied standard of statistical significance.

The other caveat is, quite simply, that experience tells us we cannot understand all aspects of the human condition empirically. How does Jane know her husband loves her? "Well," she may say, "he buys me nice things, he always rings if he's away from home, he remembers my birthday……" But we all accept that reducing love to a set of empirical behaviors in this way does not answer to our own experience. How does Jane know? She just does. She is a mature woman, with a good understanding of human nature, and can therefore recognize that her husband's behavioral attentions to her are proxies – if we stick with the parlance of the scientist – for something deeper and less tangible. Love as we know it to be: not a disposition merely to behave in such and such a way. After all, as Hamlet knew, "One may smile and smile and be a villain."[23(p690)]

A central theme of the Sherlock Holmes stories is the tension between Holmes' brilliant deductive mind, and his oddity as a human being. Talking of his craft, he asks Dr Watson: "How often have I said to you that when you have eliminated the impossible whatever remains, *however improbable*, must be the truth?" (Italics in original). Actually, Holmes gives a version of this thought more than once – this is one of two such aphorisms in *The Sign of the Four*.[24(p111)] Holmes was created, of course, by Arthur Conan Doyle, a qualified doctor, and his "methods" were based on a real doctor who was one of Conan Doyle's teachers as a medical student. (For an interesting modern defence of Holmes's abilities as a scientist, see O'Brien 2013.)[25]

So, in every one of the stories, Holmes ends with what he and everyone else is happy to claim is new knowledge. We did not know who killed the victim: now we do. This is satisfactory, however, only because Holmes asks a clear question (how do we account for the empirical phenomena?) to which it turns out there is a single, unambiguous answer.

This brings us to the role of language. "Science" offers facts: language however offers us a way of thinking about and discussing life as we live it, in all its complexity. If we want to determine whether a doctor has good professional values, it is not enough to look at overt behavior, but at whether the doctor's character and values shine through, in ways which we cannot easily measure. Performance in the workplace and when on display in the simulated surgery are not identical.[26] Aristotle (in Roberts' translation)[27(p7)] suggested:

> It is not true, as some writers assume in their treatises on rhetoric, that the personal goodness revealed by the speaker contributes nothing to his power of persuasion; on the contrary, his character may almost be called the most effective means of persuasion he possesses.

How doctors professionalize virtue – to borrow an excellent phrase from Garver[28] – is not open to statistical analysis. If we want to decide what we mean by an abstract term like "professionalism" then, as with Wittgenstein's beetle, we must discuss it together and arrive at a community view. In other words, we must use language, and we must understand that language has meaning as it used – that the context of use determines the meaning.

This is at the heart of communicative competence, but more broadly it is at the heart of a view of the world, and of research, which is not reductionist, and which we think of, loosely, as "qualitative."

One of the seminal texts in medical sociology is Glaser and Strauss's *Awareness of dying*.[29] It studies how awareness of the fact of impending demise affected the interactions between those concerned: and it is beautifully written. This seems relevant to me: excellent use of language is the way in which ambiguities can be understood but not dissolved. Good use of language – a sense of style, one might colloquially say – gives life to one's meanings. (The great American anthropologist, Clifford Geertz, once remarked, "I'm probably a closet rhetorician, although I'm coming out of the closet a bit.")[30(p245)] Or, as Scott Fitzgerald famously put it, "the test of a first-rate intelligence is the ability to hold two opposed ideas in the mind at the same time, and still retain the ability to function."[31(p1)]

This perspective lends itself well to the contemporary focus on holistic, or humanistic, medicine. In one sense, this is a discussion which has been couched in terms of a contrast between a mechanistic approach to medicine (the body is a machine which sometimes breaks down), and the holistic approach (illness affects a person, not a machine). The debate has been pushed back as far as Ancient Greece, with early physicians from Cnidos said to be in favor of the former and those from Cos the latter – the distinction gained some currency in the 1990s when it was discussed by Ian McWhinney,[32] one of the founding fathers of family medicine, and a strong advocate of holistic care.

In addition, perhaps particularly in North America, a "humanistic" approach to may involve an understanding of the arts, where a degree of ambiguity is at the heart of the endeavor. A successful work of art means multiple things at the same time, but all the meanings, all the contradictions, nevertheless hang together. A work of art on this basis may be treated as a single statement irreducible in its ambiguities. So: what is *Hamlet* about? Everything. Nothing. It just is. Is Vermeer's *View of Delft*[33] a view of Delft? Of course it is. And of course it isn't: it's a meditation on silence, and peace and the human condition. When we explore such things, we do so on the clear understanding that we don't get to the bottom of them. We understand: but we don't know.

Language and power: Develop the ability to understand ourselves

The relationship between language and power has been extensively discussed (as regards medicine, Foucault [2003] is an obvious influence). A standard general account is Fairclough,[34(p2)] who demonstrates how a "common sense" view creates power relationships without us being aware of them. He illustrates this with medicine:

....the conventions for a traditional type of consultation between doctors and patients embody 'common sense' assumptions which treat authority and hierarchy as natural – the doctor knows about medicine and the patient doesn't; the doctor is in a position to determine how a health problem should be dealt with and the patient isn't; it is right (and 'natural') that the doctor should make the decisions and control the course of the consultation and of the treatment, and that the patient should comply and cooperate, and so on....assumptions of this sort are embedded in the forms of language which are used.

Presumptions about hierarchical position might flow from something as simple as a prestigious accent, or the ability to speak an international language in addition to a local language. This is true of English today in many parts of the world. (For a detailed discussion of the issues here, see Salager-Meyer).[35] However, I would like to put a slightly unusual twist on this.

The distinguished Brazilian educationist, Paulo Freire, looked at language and the underprivileged – children from the *favelas*, illiterate adults. His ideas have been influential from the 70s. A central metaphor is that of banking[36(p72)]:

Education....becomes an act of depositing, in which the students are the depositories and the teacher is the depositor....This is the "banking" concept of education, in which the scope of action allowed to the students extends only as far as receiving, filing and storing the deposits.

In more familiar terms, this is an image of education as information transfer. The expert, as it were, hands down the oracle – and the oracle says what the privileged believe. The teacher describes the world.

In contrast to the banking metaphor, Freire[36(p40)] offers "problem-posing education." The echoes of "problem-based learning" (PBL), as the term is used in Medical Education, are obvious, but the resemblance is not complete. PBL is used to encourage students to find solutions, but often there is a single right answer to the problem posed, so that once more the task is to disambiguate. For Freire, his methodology is designed to encourage learners to become more empowered, through raising their awareness (*conscientização*, in Portuguese). As he expresses it in *The pedagogy of indignation*[37(p15)]: "education makes sense because women and men learn that through learning they can make and remake themselves."

Freire's starting point is then empowerment through having a voice in society. But, privileged or not, most of us been exposed to education as banking, and we all struggle to articulate new ideas and ways of thinking. Medical students, and qualified doctors, are not necessarily more articulate than anyone else at specifying why someone "communicates well" or badly, for instance, nor at setting out and developing a position on medical ethics

– justifying a position for or against abortion, say. Language as a means of exploration, of probing and discussing ideas, of looking at things (perhaps a doctor-patient consultation) and talking about them in a manner which helps us build and reflect on ideas, is a key aspect of education. The process enables us to understand and shape more fully the community view, as well as our own.

Long before Freire, John Locke wrote at length both of knowledge and how we come by it, and by extension about education.[38] (Locke, famously, introduced the term *tabula rasa*, the blank slate, to the educational debate). On this basis, how do we come by knowledge? By sensation (we see and hear, and so on), and by reflection – we make sense of what we see and hear. And part of what is at stake is the liberty that stems from the ability to reflect:

The idea of liberty, so crucial to all of Locke's writings on politics and education, is traced in the *Essay [Concerning Human Understanding]* to reflection on the power of the mind over one's own actions, especially the power to suspend actions in the pursuit of the satisfaction of one's own desires until after a full consideration of their objects (II.21.47, N: 51–52)[39(p16)]

Liberty is, I would suggest, particularly pertinent to medical education. Education is about liberation, for the poor and desperate, but also for those who seek to be the best they can be at their chosen profession – the liberty to think and talk, and thereby to understand effectively oneself and one's patients and the world around one.

Language then is task-focused, defined by context, an ideal vehicle for expressing the world's complexity, and for offering the awareness that empowers the user.

But this is not quite the conclusion. Here is a conundrum.

Consider the concept of "patient-centeredness" through this exchange (invented, but it seems commonplace):

Doctor: So – what do you want to do?

Patient: Oh, I don't know – I'll leave all that up to you doc.

In this case, is it patient-centred to do what the patient asks? Patient-centred, therefore, to be doctor-centred? (In a not dissimilar vein, I once – slightly joking – asked a first year nursing student at a Medical School in Pakistan why she and her very capable classmates were so eager to think for themselves. "Because we were told to," she responded, perfectly seriously).

We might think of the patient-centred conundrum in terms of one of the key philosophical studies of liberty, Mill's *On Liberty*.[40] We are, Mill says, free to do what we want (with the usual caveat that my liberty must not infringe yours): but we are not free to sell ourselves into slavery – not at liberty, in other words, to yield up liberty. On this basis, it would seem the patient cannot choose to abrogate the right to choose. But I would argue that trust may trump liberty at the patient's discretion. If the doctor is trusted to be competent, and of good character, then "loss of liberty" is less relevant. Perhaps in moments of frailty it is the possibility of willing surrender which makes power within medicine different. Surrender, that is, even about something which matters utterly to us. Our life, our health and the lives and health of those we love.

In the workplace, then, it is (see comments on Aristotle above) the use of language to represent our character which matters.

Conclusion

I have tried to suggest a number of ways in which an understanding of language, and of the history of ideas, can enrich teachers of healthcare and, appropriately managed for level, of students as well. I would suggest the following by way of examples:

1. Healthcare students are taught a reductionist model of "knowledge" (this is a good thing). They are not, however, taught to value the discussion and exploration of ideas nor, despite the focus on holistic medicine, are they really taught to value ambiguity and the creation of community meaning. A central role of language and communication is to give students a context (a role-play with a patient refusing a cervical smear, eg) where they must reflect on their values. And when they say "the right thing" – when they act as if they were repositories of knowledge, in Freire's terms, one must challenge them, and invite students to challenge themselves.

2. "Uncertainty" in medical education, if it is taught at all, tends to be taught in the context of managing and explaining risk. This too is a good thing. However, there are wider issues, to do with the uses and abuses of ambiguity in our personal and professional lives. If at all possible, help students to study the arts, and to discuss. In communication classes, create scenarios which are ambiguous, perhaps because of the ramifications for more general patient welfare, the doctor's relationship with the patient, and so on. Present and discuss unusual case histories, unusual narratives either through simulation exercises (the ideal), or at least as paper cases. Think, just think. Where simulation exercises are concerned, spend as little time as possible on behavioral criteria. There is a hierarchy of questions for feedback, [41] from "What did you do?" at one end of the scale to a question

perhaps never explicitly asked, but always there: "What is it to be a doctor?"

3. Language is power. Help students to recognize this is a truth of relevance to them, that they have the right to be supported to become more articulate. Reflection happens through language. Patient care improves through reflection, or at the very least, this is the current educational presumption. It is not unreasonable to discuss just these issues with medical students, and qualified doctors, and to introduce them to such ideas as communicative competence, or the "community view."

4. Drawing the attention of students and doctors to the light touch version of Speech Act Theory I offer above can be very powerful. The distinction between propositional meaning, what one intends and how one is understood is easy to grasp, and offers a way of reflecting on, eg about why a colleague or patient might have been offended. And most people can see that doctors, too, may be seen as talking ex cathedra, not only when they say "you have diabetes," but when they use the same language for more uncertain propositions: "You're just a bit fed up…"

Language is, then, a powerful element of medicine and medical education. As teachers and course designers, we should transcend the idea of seeing language as merely the communication of ideas. Through reflection on our own language use, we can become aware of the way that language is doing things with words, that the meaning of those words depend on the context in which they are used, that through careful and precise language use we can do justice to complexity, and that the choices we make in all of these have implications for whether our language use empowers or disempowers.

References

1. Mishler EG. *The Discourse of Medicine: Dialectics of Medical Interviews*. Norwood, NJ: Ablex Publishing Corp; 1984.
2. Fisher S, Todd AD, eds. *The Social Organization of Doctor-Patient Communication*. Washinton DC: Center for Applied Linguistics; 1983.
3. Coulthard M, Ashby M. Talking with the doctor, 1. *J Commun*. 1975;25(3):140–147. doi:10.1111/j.1460-2466. 1975.tb00616.x.
4. Candlin C, Bruton CJ, Leather JH. *Doctor-Patient Communication Skills. Working Papers 1-4*. Lancaster: University of Lancaster Institute of Education; 1974.
5. Foucault M. *The Birth of the Clinic* (Tr: Sheridan AM). Abingdon: Routledge Classics. 2003. (Originally published in French as Naissance de la Clinique 1963).

6. Simpson M, Buckman R, Stewart M, et al. Doctor-patient communication: the Toronto consensus statement. *BMJ.* 1991;303(6814):1385–1387. doi:10.1136/bmj.303.6814.1385.

7. Skelton JR. *Language and Clinical Communication: This Bright Babylon.* Abingdon: Radcliffe; 2008.

8. Ong LML, de Haes JCJM, Hoos AM, Lammes FB. Doctor-patient communication: a review of the literature. *Soc Sci Med.* 1995;40(7):903–918. doi:10.1016/0277-9536(94)00155-M.

9. Austin JL. *How to Do Things with Words: The William James Lectures Delivered at Harvard University 1955.* Oxford: Clarendon Press; 1962.

10. Lindson N, Klemperer E, Hong B, Ordóñez-Mena J, Aveyard P. Smoking reduction interventions for smoking cessation. *Cochrane Database Syst Rev.* 2019;7. doi:10.1002/14651858.CD006936.pub4.

11. Searle JR. *Making the Social World: The Structure of Human Civilization.* Oxford: Oxford University Press; 2010.

12. Hansson Wahlberg T. The creation of institutional reality, special theory of relativity, and mere Cambridge change. *Synthese.* 2019. doi:10.1007/s11229-019-02435-y.

13. Searle JR. Indirect speech acts. In: SearleJR, ed. *Expression and Meaning: Studies in the Theory of Speech Acts.* Cambridge: Cambridge University Press; 1979:30–57.

14. Robertson M, Moir J, Skelton JR, Dowell J, Cowan S. When the business of sharing treatment decisions is not the same as shared decision making: a discourse analysis of decision sharing in general practice. *Health.* 2011; 15(1):78–95. doi:10.1177/1363459309360788.

15. Hymes DH. On communicative competence. In: Pride JB, Holmes J, eds. *Sociolinguistics. Selected Readings.* Harmondsworth: Penguin, 1972:269–293.

16. Wittgenstein L. *Philosophical Investigations.* Oxford: Blackwell, 1972:293. (First published 1953).

17. Kripke S. *Wittgenstein on Rules and Private Language.* Harvard: Harvard University Press; 1982.

18. Veen M, Skelton JR, de la Croix A. Knowledge, skills and beetles: respecting the privacy of private experiences in medical education. *Perspect Med Educ.* 2020;9(2):111–116. doi:10.1007/s40037-020-00565-5.

19. Elsky J. Rethinking Ionesco's absurd: *The Bald Soprano* in the interlingual context of Vichy and postwar France. *Publ Mod Lang Assoc Am.* 2018;133(2):347–363. Retrieved from Loyola eCommons, Modern Languages and Literatures: Faculty Publications and Other Works, doi:10.1632/pmla.2018.133.2.347.

20. Hobbes T. *Leviathan.* 1651. See Curley E, ed. *Leviathan.* Indianapolis: Hackett; 1994.

21. Tonelli MR, Bluhm R. Teaching medical epistemology within an evidence-based medicine curriculum. (In press).

22. Hume D. *An Enquiry Concerning Human Understanding.* 1748. See *Enquiries Concerning Human Understanding and Concerning the Principles of Morals.* Selby-BiggeLA,

ed, 3rd ed. revised by P. H. Nidditch. Oxford: Clarendon Press; 1975: 5.1.6/44.

23. Shakespeare W. *Hamlet.* 1600-1601. In WellsS, ed, *William Shakespeare: The Complete Works.* Oxford: OUP; 2005:681–718. Act I Sc V:109.

24. Conan Doyle A. *The Sign of the Four* 1890. In *The Complete Sherlock Holmes.* Harmondsworth: Penguin; 1981:111.

25. O'Brien J. *The Scientific Sherlock Holmes: Cracking the Case with Science and Forensics.* Oxford: OUP; 2013.

26. Atkins S, Roberts C, Hawthorne K, Greenhalgh T. Simulated consultations: a sociolinguistic perspective. *BMC Med Educ.* 2016;16:16. doi:10.1186/s12909-016-0535-2.

27. Aristotle. *Rhetoric.* (Tr Roberts WR). 1:1356a. Available eg in Aristotle, *Poetics and Rhetoric.* Houston, TX: Barnes and Noble Classics. Originally published c350BCE. http://classics.mit.edu/Aristotle/rhetoric.1.i.html. Accessed October 22, 2020.

28. Garver E. *Aristotle's Rhetoric: An Art of Character.* Chicago: University of Chicago Press; 1994.

29. Glaser BG, StraussAL. *Awareness of Dying.* Chicago: Aldine Publishing Co; 1965.

30. Olson GA. The social scientist as author: Clifford Geertz on ethnography and social construction. *J Adv Compos.* 1991;11(2):245–268.

31. Fitzgerald S. The crack up. Esquire Feb;1. https://www.esquire.com/lifestyle/a4310/the-crack-up/. Published 1936. Accessed July 13, 2020.

32. McWhinney IR. *An Introduction to Family Medicine.* Oxford: OUP; 1981.

33. Vermeer J. *Gezicht op Delft (View of Delft).* Mauritshuis: The Hague;c1660-1661.

34. Fairclough N. *Language and Power.* 2nd ed. London: Longman; 1989 (2001):2.

35. Salager-Meyer F. Scientific publishing in developing countries: challenges for the future. *J English Acad Purposes.* 2008;7(2):121–132. doi:10.1016/j.jeap.2008.03.009.

36. Freire P. *Pedagogy of the Oppressed* (Tr RamosM). New York: Continuum: 2005:72. (First published 1970).

37. Freire P. *Pedagogy of Indignation.* Abingdon: Routledge2016. (First published 2004):15.

38. Locke J. In: NidditchPH, ed. *Essay Concerning Human Understanding.* 1689. Oxford: Clarendon; 1975. doi:10.1093/actrade/9780198243861.

39. Grant R, TarcovN, eds. *Some Thoughts Concerning Education and the Conduct of the Understanding.* Indianapolis: Hackett Publishing Co., 1996:xvi.

40. Mill JS. On liberty. In: Mill JS, ed. *On Liberty and Other Writings* Collini (ed). 1859. Cambridge: Cambridge University Press; 1989:102–103.

41. Skelton JR. Clinical communication. In: DentJA, Harden RM, Hunt D, eds. *A Practical Guide for Medical Teachers.* 5th ed. London: Elsevier. 2017:188–194.

Contending with Our Racial Past in Medical Education: A Foucauldian Perspective

Zareen Zaidi, Ian M. Partman, Cynthia R. Whitehead, Ayelet Kuper, and Tasha R. Wyatt

ABSTRACT

Issue: Practices of systemic and structural racism that advantage some groups over others are embedded in American society. Institutions of higher learning are increasingly being pressured to develop strategies that effectively address these inequities. This article examines medical education's diversity reforms and inclusion practices, arguing that many reify preexisting social hierarchies that privilege white individuals over those who are minoritized because of their race/ethnicity. *Evidence:* Drawing on the work of French theorist Michel Foucault, we argue that medical education's curricular and institutional practices reinforce asymmetrical power differences and authority in ways that disadvantage minoritized individuals. Practices, such as medical education's reliance on biomedical approaches, cultural competency, and standardized testing reinforce a racist system in ways congruent with the Foucauldian concept of "normalization." Through medical education's creation of *subjects* and its ability to normalize dominant forms of knowledge, trainees are shaped and socialized into ways of thinking, being, and acting that continue to support racial violence against minoritized groups. The systems, structures, and practices of medical education need to change to combat the pervasive forces that continue to shape racist institutional patterns. Individual medical educators will also need to employ critical approaches to their work and develop strategies that counteract institutional systems of racial violence. *Implications:* A Foucauldian approach that exposes the structural racism inherent in medical education enables both thoughtful criticism of status-quo diversity practices and practical, theory-driven solutions to address racial inequities. Using Foucault's work to interrogate questions of power, knowledge, and subjectivity can expand the horizon of racial justice reforms in medicine by attending to the specific, pervasive ways racial violence is performed, both intra- and extra-institutionally. Such an intervention promises to take seriously the importance of anti-racist methodology in medicine.

"How can the free gaze that medicine, and, through it, the government, must turn upon the citizens be equipped and competent without being embroiled in the esotericism of knowledge and the rigidity of social privilege?" – Michel Foucault, *The Birth Of The Clinic*

Amidst ongoing national conversations about the systemic and structural racism deeply embedded in the fabric of American society and institutions, there is growing pressure for educational institutions – in particular, colleges and universities – to reckon with their own racist histories, practices, and biases and develop strategies for mitigation. With this pressure comes increasing recognition that preexisting methods employed to discuss or decrease racial inequality within institutions, including medicine and medical education, are insufficient or, in some instances, problematic.[1] How and why do these institutions only superficially address systemic racism within their institutional architectures? What is preventing medical education and their institutions from mitigating and ultimately rectifying these failures?

In this invited article, we argue that these failures are neither neutral nor accidental, but the direct result of a deeply entrenched systematic hierarchy that privileges specific individuals over others. We take up the dual questions of: (a) how we can understand this hierarchy and (b) how we can identify steps to dismantle systemic racism in medical education drawing upon the theoretical work of French theorist Michel Foucault. This Foucauldian approach to the analysis of the racial politics of medical education enables us to propose theory-driven answers to our questions that lead to practical, actionable solutions.

Why Foucault?

Michel Foucault is no stranger to medicine and medical education, yet his work has perhaps greater visibility in other disciplines, such as medical sociology and anthropology.[2] As a theorist, Foucault is interested in understanding how power is constituted through accepted forms of knowledge, scientific understanding, and what is considered *truth*. Of particular concern is how "helping" professions, such as education and medicine exercise power in an attempt to serve their clients' needs. Specifically, Foucault examines how, when professionals create new knowledge and use it in practice, they affect how individuals view themselves, their relationship to others, and the reality in which they live. Foucault's ideas are particularly relevant now as our field grapples with how to address the deep-seated systemic racism in our profession; racism that affects both patients and trainees.

The making of a subject

Foucault's exploration of the relationship between power and knowledge was central to his academic work. He was clear, however, that his goal was not the study of power itself, but of the ways that humans are made into *subjects* that interested him most.[2] *Subjects* are created through a process of *objectification*. In his work, Foucault describes three different *modes* or techniques, of *objectification* in which individuals are acted upon and influenced by an "effect of power."[3(p.375)] This objectification process recasts individuals and groups as objects where they are named, sorted, and reclassified to serve the organizational and functional needs of others.

The first technique deals with "**modes of inquiry**" or ways of creating and codifying knowledge.[4(p.777)] Medicine's *mode of inquiry* has primarily been biomedical, in which physicians focus on biological factors and explanations for disease to the exclusion of psychological, environmental, and social influences. As such, medical education is concerned with issues related to aligning their training curriculum with biomedical sciences, and then training physicians in practices that reinforce this approach to patient care.

This biomedical approach has had far reaching consequences for how physicians see patients and their diseases and has pushed other forms of knowing to the periphery. Elsewhere in the world, physicians use different ways of knowing, thinking about health, supporting healing within human bodies, and treating disease beyond just the biomedical approach that dominates North America.[5] Such *modes of inquiry* within disciplines and professions are rarely scrutinized as a means of objectification, yet they are the process by which knowledge is created and shapes the way we see *subjects*. In medicine, this has had consequences for how we see patients and the way we train physicians.

The second technique occurs through "**dividing practices**," which is the process by which people are labeled, grouped, and then separated from others in accordance with that labeling and grouping. From a Foucauldian perspective, the very term, underrepresented minorities (URM) is steeped in a project of racist objectification. In medical education, the category of URM is now ubiquitously used to represent protected racial groups within the profession (e.g., Black, Latinx, Indigenous) even though there are important differences between these groups. The phrase appears mostly in American institutional, academic language to describe nonwhite students, however, many of these communities do not self-identify in this way. This is because the experience of a Black medical student is vastly different from that of a Hispanic student, differences that are washed away by this grouping. Even though both students experience forms of subjugation by nature of their underrepresented and nonwhite status, their experience of such subjugation is contingent on the different historical and social contexts of their oppression. The problem with "dividing practices," then, is not so much that they are used, but *how* and *why*. We see – in the very iteration of the term URM – that even when the aspiration to frame diversity and inclusion efforts through historical underrepresentation of certain identities and individuals is well-intended, the consequences of these aspirations can be negative precisely for those whom they are supposed to benefit. Rather than allow for more robust accounts of representation within medical institutions, the framework of URM codifies dividing practices by generalizing the term to minorities without attention to overlapping systems of discrimination associated with intersectionality and, subsequently, erasing the very historically specific nature of their collective subjugations. *Dividing practices* is one of the ways that individuals are objectified and then become *subjects* for others to think about and act upon, a technique that is deeply embedded in our institutional policies, practices, and discourses. In turn, using these terms maintains power relations and legitimizes preexisting social hierarchies. Dividing practices help to illuminate how norms are codified through the virtue of selective inclusion and exclusion.

The third technique is the process by which specific groups of human beings become subjects through "subjectification" with certain categories of being, such as race, class, sexuality, or gender. Here, a person takes up their label as part of their identity. For example, those labeled by others as URMs begin to identify themselves as part of the URM group. This mode of objectification, by which subjects form and associate themselves with identities that were handed to them is paramount to the success of maintaining power relationships within institutions. For example, embedded in the phrase URM is an assumption about the person's identity and how that identity is placed within the matrices of power in an institution. It raises questions around: Who counts as represented and who counts as underrepresented? What are the thresholds for representation and underrepresentation? The phrase URM also conjures questions of who makes the decision about representation, and under what terms. Identification affects how subjects learn to think of themselves from an outside perspective, which in turn affects their internalization of these labels.

Foucault's understanding of these techniques of *objectification* raise deeper questions such as who counts as a *subject* and how do they navigate institutional landscapes. Applied to medical education, Foucault's work raises other questions, such as: Who gets to be a *subject* within medical education? Which *subjects* have authority over knowledge? How is that authority linked to power, and what is the effect of this power on those who cannot become *subjects*? And finally, how do *subjects* continue to be objectified within our institutions? And perhaps, most importantly, how might these processes of objectification be contested and challenged within the institutions that befit and codify them.

Normalization in medical education

Normalization is the process whereby something that is socially constructed comes to be considered normal.

This could be a standard created by science against which people are measured (e.g., the sane man or the law-abiding citizen are "normal" people). But the idea of "normal" also implies the existence of the abnormal (i.e., the madman or the criminal).[6] In other words, an idea of deviance is possible only where norms exist. For Foucault, norms are techniques of objectification that are constantly used to evaluate and control us because they exclude those who cannot conform to "normal" categories. As such, the process of normalization is unavoidable, but an insidiously harmful feature of modern society.

Normalization is employed by reinforcing behaviors, beliefs, and practices, which legitimatize certain forms of knowledge, and the creation of certain kinds of subjects. The process of normalization is inextricably linked to Foucault's other ideas of power. By establishing what is normal and abnormal, it makes it possible to qualify, classify, and punish those who behave in ways outside the norm in a system of surveillance.[6] In turn, this system shapes subjects and coerces them into engaging in standardized ways of being and thinking.

The process of normalization exists in the introduction of standardized education, the organization of the medical profession, and systems that continue to perpetuate general norms of health, such as teaching hospitals. For example, in medical education, the professional identity formation (PIF) literature is replete with studies that have framed research in ways that help to reinforce the image of a certain kind of physician, one that has a professional identity that is in line with those espoused by white men.[7] In contrast there is only one study that explores experiences of PIF in URM physicians and there was an almost complete absence of critical stances used to study PIF.[8] This narrow construction of what it means to be a physician influences norming practices, and conflicts with the ways in which Black/African American physicians see themselves.[8]

Within any institution, dominant perspectives and ideas exist as the basis for authorizing and normalizing certain subject positions. These perspectives become the basis for granting entry to some and denying entry to others based on their relationship to the "norm." Normalization is thus used to reinforce preexisting sites of domination and oppression.[7] To this end, normalization can be seen as playing a central role in upholding, creating, and shaping the white supremacist norms that organize contemporary American society.[9] Other examples include the ways of speaking and accessing the multiple meanings embedded in medicine that white students bring to the profession.[10] Understanding subtle meaning shifts in language use within a medical context puts white learners at an advantage because it helps them join the medical community in ways that are not available for minoritized learners who have not had access to the language of medicine.

In medical education, the process of normativity also benefits some medical students by equipping them with the skills that result in better Medical Student Performance Evaluation letters (MSPE)[11] from mentors, and other skills that increase their likelihood of selection for the Alpha Omega Alpha Honor Medical Society (AOA).[12,13] These resources increase learners' likelihood of securing prestigious training positions,[14] but may also have influence further along in learners' careers. For example, because white learners have access to the language and framing of medicine, white individuals are more likely than minoritized individuals to secure their first R01 research grants.[15] This is because achieving insider-status is much easier when learners have prior access to high-quality preparatory education, previous work experience, and other modalities of privilege.[16] What often goes unrecognized is that when an individual grows up in a society that is calibrated around their values, beliefs, and practices, they are placed at an advantage almost anywhere in that society.

Ultimately, what is underlying the process of normalization is the unspoken notion that white people are the norm whereby all other populations are compared. American institutions harbor discrete forms of domination, such as these which are designed to govern and manage minoritized populations.[17] Therefore, institutions are complicit in this process because they work by sanctioning discriminatory acts against certain individuals in order to maintain the authority of others. For example, by normalizing a clear distinction between underrepresented and overrepresented groups, medical education continues to sidestep the issues and systems that have led to the so-called underrepresentation.[18] This sidestep reinforces the very dynamic of overrepresentation-as-power. Other examples include pre-medical education assessments like the MCAT and medical admission practices,[19] which are used to screen physicians, many of whom are not a part of the norming group. Other practices include medical curricula, which treats race as a biological variable in medical education,[20] essentially erasing larger issues of sociohistorical context on the health and lived experiences of minoritized patients and learners. Even well-intentioned initiatives to combat racism in medical institutions, such as cultural competency curricula and diversity programs fail to meaningfully challenge deeply entrenched practices in medical education, and as such deploy processes of normalization.[21-23]

While the process of normalization is harmful to all students, it is particularly difficult for minoritized physicians who are most noticeably asked to conform to the norms set by white individuals. In other words, by norming what is expected from physicians using norms endemic to white society, medical education uses its power and knowledge of what is expected to shape minoritized physicians into subjects of their choosing. Combating normalization requires that institutions confront their policies and procedures, which can be challenging because their origins are eventually subsumed into the "just the way things are." For example, in 2020, the Trump administration created an executive order that functionally prohibits federally funded institutions from engaging in, sponsoring, and/or funding implicit bias training within those institutions.[24] The White House labeled implicit bias training as fundamentally an anti-American exercise, which could have consequences for race relations for some time to come. In time, institutions would run the risk of not addressing issues of race, and this avoidance would feel "normal." Deployed at the societal and institutional and educational level, policies and practices like these perpetuate racist structures in our society.

Contextualizing Foucault into medical education

Clearly, medical education, like all educational institutions is deeply enmeshed in the process of normalization as a means to uphold power. As Foucault writes, "the disposal of its space, the meticulous regulations which govern its internal life, the different activities which are organized there, the diverse persons who live there or meet one another, each with his own function, his well-defined character – all these things constitute a block of capacity-communication-power." [4(p.787)] Normalization of systemic and systematic racism in medicine is not just a contemporary issue. It has deep roots in American society and is often most easily seen in the historical exclusion of Black and other minoritized physicians. In 1910, when Abraham Flexner was commissioned by the Carnegie Foundation to survey medical schools across North America, his report closed all but two historically Black medical schools essentially leaving Black would-be physicians without an opportunity to train.[25] He is often credited for being the grandfather of standardizing modern medicine, yet in justifying his recommendations for closing these schools, his comments toward the training Black physicians were overtly racist, insisting that the function of medical education for Black doctors was not only to train future physicians to be a service to "[their] own race" but also to protect white populations from diseases contracted from African American communities:

> The negro must be educated not only for his sake, but for ours. He is, as far as human eye can see, a permanent factor in the nation. He has his rights and due and value as an individual; but he has, besides, the tremendous importance that belongs to a potential source of infection and contagion. [25](p.180)

Flexner's belief that Black populations posed an inherent health risk to the safety of white communities, and his suggestion to close the majority of historically Black medical schools, demonstrates the pervasiveness of how normalization works to maintain asymmetrical power relations in society and within our institutions. In the name of improving medical education, Flexner's report committed forms of racial violence against Black physicians for nearly a century and since then, Black physicians remain unrepresented in the workforce at levels incommensurate with white physicians.

Even though there have been multiple attempts to enfold Black individuals into the profession, these legislative reforms have had only slightly countered these inequalities. For example, some of these rebalancing initiatives included forcing medical schools and hospitals to desegregate if they were to receive federal funding. Others proposed programs through US anti-discrimination legislation improved academic support systems for under-represented minorities in health. The 1977 U.S. Supreme Court case *University Of California Regents vs. Bakke* authorized affirmative action practices designed to increase diversity in admissions.[26] At the professional level, the Association of American Medical Colleges (AAMC) oversaw affirmative action policies, which resulted in an increase in minority enrollment in medical schools from 3 to 10%.[27] Then later, the AAMC implemented the "3000 by 2000" Health Professional Partnership Initiative, which created pipeline programs nationally to double the number of URMs in medical schools by the year 2000.[28] While falling short of its goal, the initiative led to a further increase in minority enrollment to 12% by 1995.[24] However, since 1996, affirmative action programs have been under attack in the U.S., which has resulted in a decline in URM medical student admissions.[29]

These initiatives to rebalance power within medical education are important. However, viewed from the Foucauldian lens, even if medical schools' race-conscious admissions policies increase the enrollment and admissions rates of minority students, this will not change the racist norms, biases, and policies that exist within the profession. Racism does not go away simply by admitting more minoritized medical students into training. Racism is itself a form of power that persists precisely because of its normalization within institutions, and thus, cannot be rectified without accounting for – in the case of admissions – the practices that shape underrepresentation in the first place. What is needed is for the profession to interrogate the *norms* used by institutions that work to shape individuals into the right kind of *subject* at the expense of nonwhite *subjects*. It is the norming practice that must be addressed, so that minoritized physicians can be the kind of physician that upholds their own values, beliefs, and racial norms.[8]

However, this is challenging because as noted earlier, white individuals are the norm against which all other groups are compared, and it is the white norming group that works as an organizing force in our educational systems. The existence of a white norm at work in higher education was recently revealed in the *Regents of California vs. Bakke* case where the Supreme Court ruled that a university's use of racial quotas in its admissions process was unconstitutional, but a school's use of affirmative action to accept minoritized applicants was constitutional. In the Supreme Court, "Bakke argued that the minority admissions plan abridged Fourteenth Amendment guarantees for whites, who although not historically oppressed, were nevertheless 'persons' within the meaning of the Equal Protection Clause."[30](p.1772) This ruling upholds white normativity by setting a precedent for the abandonment of special-admissions programs which would otherwise have aided the nonwhite beneficiaries of race-conscious admissions.[31] Cases like these demonstrate that white normativity is powerful in the creation and treatment of *subjects*. It does not exist solely outside of or on the edges of institutions; it is deeply embedded within them.

The racial contract as hidden curriculum

Lurking under the surface of medicine's curriculum are hidden practices, which mask the structural conditions of medicine, the cultural history of medical education, and the ways in which medical knowledge is stratified along lines of power. These hidden practices might be viewed as part of the hidden curriculum[32] that socializes medical students in ways of being, thinking, and feeling that are unwritten and unofficial, exerting influence over all aspects of medicine and call into question: Who decides what is to be included and prioritized in the curriculum? Who is charged with curricular development and assessment, and how do they make decisions about what is included?

The hidden curriculum is tacit and powerful as it transforms and organizes institutions in ways that reinforce and legitimatize asymmetrical power relationships. It is implicated in normalization processes and in the creation of *subjects*. For example, the hidden curriculum is a powerful force in shaping medicine's social contract with society. These are more implicit than explicit agreements between institutions and society that serve to regulate what kinds of physicians are suitable. On one side, physicians are expected to uphold the values of professionalism, care for the sick, and fulfill their role as a professional. In return, society grants them and their profession respect, autonomy in practice, self-regulation, and financial rewards.[33] However, social contracts serve the hidden curriculum by shaping of *subjects* into an idealized version of a physician. In this way, they always harbor *racism* at its core because they were created to protect white people and their genetic descendants.[34] Essentially, medicine's social contract attempts to shape trainees into the *right* kind of physician,[35] thereby oppressing minoritized individuals in ways that are rarely made explicit, yet fall along the lines of Foucault's notions of power, knowledge, and processes of normativity.

For example, when nonwhite students enter institutions of learning they are taught within "the limits of the identities and aspirations that school and society make available to them."[36(p.470)] This limiting environment is one that trains minoritized students to accept educational inequities and stratifications by denying them access to possibilities available to white students. Other examples are found in medical schools' pedagogy in which students are taught primarily through lectures, seminars, and clinical research,[37] which impart particular values and beliefs, such as biomedicine's underpinning constructs of positivism and objectivity. Use of these pedagogical practices reinforces the very form of objectification that creates *subjects*. This is further reified as students employ objective modes of inquiry and divisive practices in their interactions with patients. As Foucault writes, "the exercise of power is not a naked fact, an institutional right, nor is it a structure which holds out or is smashed: it is elaborated, transformed, organized; it endows itself with processes which are more or less adjusted to the situation."[38(p.792)]

Seen in this perspective, curricular projects are organized in service of elite groups with a primary function to preserve the elite's social hegemony.[39] Although not often spoken of in this way, the hidden curriculum is a means to assimilate learners into a normative space, which unevenly prepares learners for entrance into an already oppressive and deeply racist society.[40]

Resisting existing power structures in medical education

Given the pervasive effects of hidden curricula in contemporary medical education, developing counter-methodologies and pedagogies to reveal and undermine systemic racism is imperative for reducing the scale and scope of racial violence.[41] What is needed is what Foucault refers to in "The Subject and Power" as a "new economy of power relations"; [4(p.779)] that is, methodologies and agendas that encompass a broad understanding of the distribution and interaction of power relations within medical institutions. In developing counter-methodologies, it is important to understand that the aim is not to reform medical education, rather to resist existing power structures and upend it altogether.

In the process of upending medical education, the profession needs to focus on the recruitment of racially diverse faculty because the lack of diversity within medicine "hampers learning and professional development". [42(p.251)] Great efforts have been made to increase the diversity of medical students, however faculty members remain majority white.[43] Following a Foucauldian analysis, a lack of faculty diversity may also limit and hamper pedagogical diversity. Because white faculty experience a society that regards them and their experiences, practices, and values as the dominant norm by which all other experiences, practices, and values are circumscribed, the kinds of knowledge they have about their curriculum is limited in regards to the complex shape of systemic racism in American society – and particularly, how systemic racism actively constitutes their knowledge.[24] Certainly, a more diverse medical faculty doesn't directly translate into an anti-racist medical curriculum. However, the lack thereof is problematic that preserves existing power relations and undermines an institutions ability to develop well-intentioned reformation efforts.

Additionally, medical education privileges quantitative research and experiential, clinical-based education over qualitative, critical-frame approaches to education.[44–46] Didactic instruction, like lectures and small groups, grant little space for exploring and engaging in these approaches, and multiple-choice question banks have been shown to reinforce a naturalized understanding of race-as-biological and perpetuate harmful stereotypes.[47] These practices produce a ceiling on the content of the curriculum and limit the possibility for interdisciplinary approaches to biomedicine. Medical education programs are increasingly shaped by the Competency Based Medical Education (CBME) framework. While CBME helps deliver curriculum content efficiently questions have been raised about whether the approach is appropriate for all aspects of medical education.[5] There have been calls to decolonize medical education and focus on practical wisdom (phronesis) which, when embodied in the physician, links the knowledge and skills of the biomedical and clinical sciences with a moral orientation and call.[48] What is needed is a curriculum that emphasizes "recognition of the web of interpersonal networks, environmental factors and political/socioeconomic forces that surround clinical encounters," and further, the way that these variables produce the conditions for poor health.[49(p.684)]

Reimagining medical education through Foucault

Foucault's work draws attention to the ways power and the creation of knowledge uphold a system that is unbalanced in favor of those in positions of authority. Through power, knowledge, objectivation, and normativity, physicians are enfolded into the profession in ways that turn them into *subjects* that enable them to be controlled *by* institutions. If we are to address systemic racism and its structures that uphold the mistreatment of minoritized individuals, continuing to make minor adjustments to the medical education enterprise are insufficient to reach this goal.[50] What are needed are proposed solutions capable of disrupting the structures that keep the system in place. A Foucauldian approach would not just focus on individuals, but insist on a coordinated effort in which everyone in medicine (i.e. physicians, scientists, administrators, educators, staff, and trainees), including those in leadership positions at the American Association of Medical Colleges (AAMC) be involved in addressing systemic racism.[51]

To this end, we propose three strategies that we believe Foucault would support. First, medical education must begin by recognizing and positioning medical education as historically constructed and socially negotiated, and then work to understand how these constructions are maintained.[50] To achieve this, educators must reconceptualize their role in academic

medicine and shift their pedagogical methods to incorporate elements of *critical consciousness*.[52] Critical consciousness raises individuals' understanding of their social current conditions and the forces that have created them in an effort to critique and therefore change these conditions.[53] There have been multiple calls to incorporate critical consciousness into health professions education,[21] and in all of these efforts, educators are attempting to place medical schools in a "social, cultural, and historical context... [coupling it] with an active recognition of societal problems and a search for appropriate solutions".[53(p.782)] Incorporating critical consciousness would create a platform for trainees to identify the underlying structures that maintain systemic racism and learn how to resist them as physicians in training. Further, its integration would help trainees grapple with medicine's "culture of no culture," so that they can develop sensitivities to how the system unfairly advantages some groups over others.[54]

There are many tools available to promote critical consciousness in medical education, but successfully doing so will necessitate different kinds of professional development than what is currently recommended.[21, 55] For example, educators should incorporate activities that elicit trainees' personal histories and lived experience, to assist trainees' understanding how an individuals' context impacts the creation of new knowledge.[21, 56] Additionally, by incorporating curricula from marginalized groups' experiences, students will be exposed to patients and their needs that are often taken for granted.[57]

Second, medical education has long supported the idea that physicians must be resilient in a system that overburdens them with long working hours, grueling amounts of content, and patient care expectations that are unreasonable.[58] However, attempts to boost physician resilience without correcting broken system borders on the disingenuous.[59] A Foucauldian perspective would suggest that medical education needs to refocus its efforts to better help students understand when individuals should resist current structures, rather than conform to current expectations that keep the current system in place.

For this reason, medical education needs to recast advocacy efforts as productive and integral to their training as physicians. Currently, advocacy training in medical education is controversial. On one side, physicians believe that it is outside the professional responsibility of physicians to engage in political issues,[60] whereas on the other, physicians are thought to be uniquely qualified to observe and delineate links between social factors and health.[61] A

Foucauldian analysis would support trainees' direct instruction on how to engage in advocacy to improve societal conditions. There are several small studies and examples on various websites that show the efficacy of advocacy training other medical schools might use as inspiration.[41, 62-64] Additionally, there are other structural actions that institutions can take to address systemic racism throughout medical education's clinical and learning environments that would help create a healthier system for trainees.[51]

Third, in medical education, curricula writing and delivery is one way that individuals are objectified. Therefore, educators should co-construct curricula with minoritized students so that content is reimagined and reflective of the lived experiences of minoritized individuals. To only teach dominant perspectives is to reify the processes that continue to objectify minoritized trainees and patients. Therefore, educators should develop strategies that invite students and educators into a shared space to reimagine the educational process, methods of assessment, and targeted outcomes of medical education.[65]

Conclusion

The historical and theoretical work of Michel Foucault provides a generative lens from which to analyze the matrices of power and systemic racism within medical education and its institutions. Our goal has been to demonstrate the importance of re-imagining medical education, resisting the tending-toward power and race-neutral projects of contemporary medical curricula broadly defined. An explicitly radical, anti-racist medical pedagogy should inform institutional and educational practices within medical education and avoid the material shortcomings of status-quo diversity initiatives.

The stakes of such a practice are large, but the consequences of its foregoing are much larger. By placing hidden curricula, race-conscious diversity initiatives, and assessment bias squarely in the schema of white normativity, as intentional and consequential forms of power and knowledge, we can better understand how and why medical education fails minoritized students. Further, we can develop the methodologies necessary to mitigate these failures in meaningful and impactful ways. As institutions across the country face great reckoning for the damage caused by systemic anti-Black racism, we would be remiss not to consider how specific technologies of power are enacted within medical institutions that reinforce, legitimate, and normalize such racist violence. As Foucault reminds us, "where this is power,

there is resistance."[66(p.95)] We all need to be part of that resistance, and it starts by examining our institutions for the ways in which it continues to harbor larger historical, cultural, and political acts meant to maintain systems of oppression.

Acknowledgements

Tasha R Wyatt was affiliated with the Medical College of Georgia at the time this paper was written.

Disclaimer

The views expressed herein are those of the authors and do not necessarily reflect those of the U.S. Department of Defense or other federal agencies.

ORCID

Zareen Zaidi (iD) http://orcid.org/0000-0003-4328-5766
Tasha R. Wyatt (iD) http://orcid.org/0000-0002-0071-5298

References

1. Dobbin F, Kalev A. Why diversity programs fail. *Harv Bus Rev.* 2016;94(7):14.
2. Foucault M, Faubion JD, Hurley R. *Power.* London: Penguin Classics; 2020.
3. Foucault M. *The Hermeneutics of the Subject: Lectures at the Collège de France 1981–1982.* New York: Macmillan; 2005:375.
4. Foucault M. The subject and power. *Critical Inquiry.* 1982;8(4):777–795. doi:10.1086/448181.
5. Naidu T. Southern exposure: levelling the Northern tilt in global medical and medical humanities education. *Adv in Health Sci Educ.* 2020;26(2):739–752. doi:10.1007/s10459-020-09976-9.
6. Foucault M, Sheridan A. *Discipline and Punish: The Birth of the Prison.* London: Penguin modern classics; 2020.
7. Wyatt TR, Balmer D, Rockich-Winston N, et al . 'Whispers and shadows': A critical review of the professional identity literature with respect to minority physicians. *Med Educ.* 2021;55(2):148–158. doi:10.1111/medu.14295.
8. Wyatt TR, Rockich-Winston N, Taylor TR, White D. What does context have to do with anything? A study of professional identity formation in physician-trainees considered underrepresented in medicine. *Acad Med.* 2020;95(10):1587–1593. doi:10.1097/ACM.0000000000003192.
9. Borger J. Insurrection Day: when white supremacist terror came to the US Capitol. 2021. https://www.theguardian.com/us-news/2021/jan/09/us-capitol-insurrection-white-supremacist-terror. Accessed January 16, 2021.
10. Wong BO, Blythe JA, Batten JN, et al. Recognizing the role of language in the hidden curriculum of under-

graduate medical education: Implications for equity in medical training. *Acad Med.* 2020;96(6):842–847. doi:10.1097/ACM.0000000000003657.

11. Ross DA, Boatright D, Nunez-Smith M, Jordan A, Chekroud A, Moore EZ. Differences in words used to describe racial and gender groups in Medical Student Performance Evaluations. *PLoS One.* 2017;12(8):e0181659. doi:10.1371/journal.pone.0181659.

12. Boatright D, Ross D, O'Connor P, Moore E, Nunez-Smith M. Racial disparities in medical student membership in the Alpha Omega Alpha Honor Society. *JAMA Intern Med.* 2017;177(5):659–665. doi:10.1001/jamainternmed.2016.9623.

13. Wijesekera TP, Kim M, Moore EZ, Sorenson O, Ross DA. All other things being equal: exploring racial and gender disparities in medical school honor society induction. *Acad Med.* 2019;94(4):562–569. doi:10.1097/ACM.0000000000002463.

14. Davis G, Allison R. White coats, black specialists? Racial divides in the medical profession. *Sociol Spectr.* 2013;33(6):510–533. doi:10.1080/02732173.2013.836143.

15. Ginther DK, Kahn S, Schaffer WT. Gender, race/ethnicity, and National Institutes of Health R01 research awards: is there evidence of a double bind for women of color?*Acad Med.* 2016;91(8):1098–1107. doi:10.1097/ACM.0000000000001278.

16. Lawrence C, Mhlaba T, Stewart KA, Moletsane R, Gaede B, Moshabela M. The hidden curricula of medical education: a scoping review. *Acad Med.* 2018;93(4):648–656. doi:10.1097/ACM.0000000000002004.

17. Foucault M. *Society Must Be Defended.* trans. D. Macey. *New York:Picador.* 2003.

18. Page KR, Castillo-Page L, Poll-Hunter N, Garrison G, Wright SM. Assessing the evolving definition of underrepresented minority and its application in academic medicine. *Acad Med.* 2013;88(1):67–72. doi:10.1097/ACM.0b013e318276466c.

19. Lucey CR, Saguil A. The consequences of structural racism on MCAT scores and medical school admissions: The past is prologue. *Acad Med.* 2020;95(3):351–356. doi:10.1097/ACM.0000000000002939.

20. Hoffman KM, Trawalter S, Axt JR, Oliver MN. Racial bias in pain assessment and treatment recommendations, and false beliefs about biological differences between blacks and whites. *Proc Natl Acad Sci USA.* 2016;113(16):4296–4301. doi:10.1073/pnas.1516047113.

21. Halman M, Baker L, Ng S . Using critical consciousness to inform health professions education: A literature review. *Perspect Med Educ.* 2017;6(1):12–20. doi:10.1007/s40037-016-0324-y.

22. Frambach JM, Martimianakis MAT . The discomfort of an educator's critical conscience: the case of problem-based learning and other global industries in medical education . *Perspect Med Educ.* 2017;6(1):1–4. doi:10.1007/s40037-016-0325-x.

23. Zaidi Z, Verstegen D, Naqvi R, Morahan P, Dornan T. Gender, religion, and sociopolitical issues in cross-cultural online education. *Adv Health Sci Educ Theory Pract.* 2016;21(2):287–301. doi:10.1007/s10459-015-9631-z.

24. Nivet MA. Minorities in academic medicine: review of the literature. *J Vasc Surg.* 2010;51(4):S53–S58. doi:10.1016/j.jvs.2009.09.064.

25. Flexner A, Updike DB. Carnegie Foundation for the Advancement of T, Merrymount P. Medical education in the United States and Canada: a report to the Carnegie foundation for the advancement of teaching. 576 Fifth Avenue, New York City: [publisher not identified]; 1910.

26. Epstein L, Knight J. Brennan's Account of Regents of the University of California v. Bakke. *Yale L. & Pol'y Rev.* 2000;19(341).

27. Cohen JJ, Gabriel BA, Terrell C. The case for diversity in the health care workforce. *Health Aff (Millwood)).* 2002;21(5):90–102. doi:10.1377/hlthaff.21.5.90.

28. Nickens HW, Ready TP, Petersdorf RG. Project 3000 by 2000–Racial and ethnic diversity in US medical schools. *Mass Medical Soc.* 1994;472–476.

29. Cohen JJ. The consequences of premature abandonment of affirmative action in medical school admissions. *JAMA.* 2003;289(9):1143–1149. doi:10.1001/jama.289.9.1143.

30. Harris CI. Whiteness as property. *Harvard Law Review.* 1993;106(8):1707–1791. 1772. doi:10.2307/1341787.

31. Bhandaru D. Is white normativity racist? Michel Foucault and post-civil rights racism. *Polity.* 2013;45(2):223–244. doi:10.1057/pol.2013.6.

32. Hafferty FW. Beyond curriculum reform: confronting medicine's hidden curriculum. *Acad Med.* 1998;73(4):403–407. doi:10.1097/00001888-199804000-00013.

33. Cruess SR, Cruess RL, Steinert Y. Linking the teaching of professionalism to the social contract: a call for cultural humility. *Med Teach.* 2010;32(5):357–359. doi:10.3109/01421591003692722.

34. Mills CW. *The Racial Contract.* Ithaca: Cornell University Press; 1997.

35. Frost HD, Regehr G . "I am a doctor": negotiating the discourses of standardization and diversity in professional identity construction. *Acad Med.* 2013;88(10):1570–1577. doi:10.1097/ACM.0b013e3182a34b05.

36. De Lissovoy N. Education and violation: Conceptualizing power, domination, and agency in the hidden curriculum. *Race Ethnicity and Education.* 2012;15(4):463–484. 470 doi:10.1080/13613324.2011.618831.

37. Jackson P. *Life in Classrooms.* New York. *Holt Rinehart Winston.* 1968.

38. Foucault M. *An aesthetics of Existence.* London: Routledge; 1988:792.

39. McLaren P. *Life in Schools: An Introduction to Critical Pedagogy in the Foundations of Education.* London: Routledge; 2015.

40. Apple M, Apple MW. *Ideology and Curriculum.* London: Routledge; 2018.

41. Paton M, Naidu T, Wyatt TR, et al . Dismantling the master's house: new ways of knowing for equity and social justice in health professions education. *Adv Health Sci Educ Theory Pract.* 2020;25(5):1107–1126. doi:10.1007/s10459-020-10006-x.

42. Braun L. Theorizing race and racism: preliminary reflections on the medical curriculum. *Am J Law Med.* 2017;43(2–3):239–256. doi:10.1177/00988588 17723662.

43. Nunez-Smith M, Ciarleglio MM, Sandoval-Schaefer T, et al. Institutional variation in the promotion of racial/ethnic minority faculty at US medical schools. *Am J*

Public Health. 2012;102(5):852–858. doi:10.2105/AJPH.2011.300552.

44. Tilley S. The role of critical qualitative research in educational contexts: A Canadian perspective. *Educ Rev.* 2019;35(75):155–180. doi:10.1590/0104-4060.66806.

45. Farghaly A. Comparing and contrasting quantitative and qualitative research approaches in education: the peculiar situation of medical education. *EIMJ.* 2018;10(1):3–11. doi:10.21315/eimj2018.10.1.2.

46. Morse JM, Dimitroff LJ, Harper R, et al. Considering the qualitative-quantitative language divide. *Qual Health Res.* 2011;21(9):1302–1303. doi:10.1177/1049732310392386.

47. Ripp K, Braun L. Race/ethnicity in medical education: an analysis of a question bank for step 1 of the United States Medical Licensing Examination. *Teach Learn Med.* 2017;29(2):115–122. doi:10.1080/10401334.2016.1268056.

48. Kumagai AK. From competencies to human interests: ways of knowing and understanding in medical education. *Acad Med.* 2014;89(7):978–983. doi:10.1097/ACM.0000000000000234.

49. Metzl JM, Roberts DE. Structural competency meets structural racism: race, politics, and the structure of medical knowledge. *AMA J Ethics.* 2014;16(9):674–690.

50. Whitehead CR, Hodges BD, Austin Z . Captive on a carousel: discourses of 'new' in medical education 1910-2010. *Adv Health Sci Educ Theory Pract.* 2013;18(4):755–768. doi:10.1007/s10459-012-9414-8.

51. Ross PT, Lypson ML, Byington CL, Sánchez JP, Wong BM, Kumagai AK. Learning from the past and working in the present to create an antiracist future for academic medicine. *Acad Med.* 2020;95(12):1781–1786. doi:10.1097/ACM.0000000000003756.

52. Freire P. *Pedagogy of the oppressed (Rev. ed.).* New York: Continuum; 1993:1970.

53. Kumagai AK, Lypson ML. Beyond cultural competence: critical consciousness, social justice, and multicultural education. *Acad Med.* 2009;84(6):782–787. doi:10.1097/ACM.0b013e3181a42398.

54. Taylor JS. Confronting "culture" in medicine's "culture of no culture". *Acad Med.* 2003;78(6):555–559.

55. Triemstra JD, Iyer MS, Hurtubise L, et al. Influences on and characteristics of the professional identity formation of clinician educators: A qualitative analysis. *Acad Med.* 2020;96(4):585–591. doi:10.1097/ACM.0000000000003843.

56. Zaidi Z, Verstegen D, Naqvi R, Dornan T, Morahan P. Identity text: an educational intervention to foster cultural interaction. *Med Educ Online.* 2016;21(1):33135. doi:10.3402/meo.v21.33135.

57. Dogra N, Bhatti F, Ertubey C, et al. Teaching diversity to medical undergraduates: curriculum development, delivery and assessment. AMEE GUIDE No. 103. *Med Teach.* 2016;38(4):323–337. doi:10.3109/0142159X.2015.1105944.

58. West CP, Dyrbye LN, Sinsky C, et al. Resilience and burnout among physicians and the general US working population. *JAMA Netw Open.* 2020;3(7):e209385. doi:10.1001/jamanetworkopen.2020.9385.

59. Goroll AH . Addressing burnout-focus on systems, not resilience. *JAMA Netw Open.* 2020;3(7):e209514. doi:10.1001/jamanetworkopen.2020.9514.

60. Huddle TS. Perspective: Medical professionalism and medical education should not involve commitments to political advocacy. *Acad Med.* 2011;86(3):378–383.

61. Earnest MA, Wong SF, Federico SG, Federico SG. Perspective: Physician advocacy: what is it and how do we do it? *Acad Medicine.* 2010;85(1):63–67.

62. Huntoon KM, McCluney CJ, Wiley EA, Scannell CA, Bruno R, Stull MJ. Self-reported evaluation of competencies and attitudes by physicians-in-training before and after a single day legislative advocacy experience. *BMC Med Educ.* 2012;12(1):47. doi:10.1186/1472-6920-12-47.

63. Cole McGrew M, Wayne S, Solan B, Snyder T, Ferguson C, Kalishman S. Health policy and advocacy for new mexico medical students in the family medicine clerkship. *Fam Med.* 2015;47(10).

64. Metzl JM, Hansen H. Structural competency: Theorizing a new medical engagement with stigma and inequality. *Soc Sci Med.* 2014;103:126–133. doi:10.1016/j.socscimed.2013.06.032.

65. Ferenchak KS, Wyatt TR. From the Hawaiian classroom to the wards: A model of effective pedagogy for clinicians, trainees, and patients. *The Clinical Teacher.* 2020;

66. Foucault M. *The history of sexuality. Vol 1: An Introduction.* New york: Random house; 1978.

8 OPEN ACCESS

Phenomenological Research in Health Professions Education: Tunneling from Both Ends

Chris Rietmeijer and Mario Veen (ID)

ABSTRACT

Issue: The term "phenomenology" is increasingly being used in Health Professions Education research. Phenomenology refers to a philosophical tradition or discipline. For researchers in Health Professions Education without a philosophical or humanities background, there are two practical problems. The first is that it is not always clear how studies that call themselves "phenomenological" are distinct from studies that use other methods; phenomenology as a label seems to be used for any study that is interested in the experiences of participants. The second problem is that a more in-depth study of phenomenology in the literature yields either abstract definitions such as "examining the underlying structures of consciousness," or contrasting translations of phenomenology to concrete research tools. What would phenomenology in medical education research look like that is both true to its philosophical roots and yields research findings that contribute to the quality of medical education? *Evidence*: Two medical education researchers, one with a medical background and the other with a philosophy background, engaged in a dialogue with the purpose of formulating an approach for phenomenology in medical education research. The first departed from the practical demands of his research project in which phenomenology was suggested as a methodology, but guidance was lacking. The other departed from the philosophical tradition of phenomenology with the purpose of exploring how phenomenological insights can be valuable for medical education research. The paper presents these journeys and the results of this dialogue where they formulate starting points for an approach to conducting HPE research that has scientific phenomenological integrity and yields practical results. *Implications*: Phenomenology has been one of the defining developments in philosophy and the humanities in the 20th century. A basic grasp of its insights is useful for medical education researchers since any research today takes place in the light of these insights. Within medical education, there are certain types of phenomena, research questions, and research goals that call for an explicitly phenomenological approach. Rather than prescribing specific methods or methodologies, phenomenology offers signposts for how to think about the relationship between our research object, methods, and data, and our own role as researchers. We suggest that researchers in HPE, when reporting a phenomenological study, instead of claiming to have followed a certain phenomenological method, explain how their research question, methods, and results fit the purposes and standards of phenomenology. We illustrate this with an example of how to use phenomenology in an interview study.

Introduction

What follows is the substrate of an e-mail dialogue between CBTR (Chris) and MV (Mario). We started this dialogue at the 2019 Association for Medical Education in Europe conference in Vienna, and it has been ongoing since then. The purpose was to connect our two perspectives to a common ground: phenomenology in health professions education (HPE) research. We share an interest in conducting

meaningful research from a phenomenological perspective, as well as a frustration with the current "pointers" that are available for educational researchers. Chris is a general practitioner (GP) and GP training program director, who is conducting PhD research on direct observation of GP trainees by their supervisors. Mario is an interdisciplinary philosopher and educational researcher, with no medical background. Tunneling from both ends is how we experienced this

This is an Open Access article distributed under the terms of the Creative Commons Attribution-NonCommercial-NoDerivatives License (http://creativecommons.org/licenses/by-nc-nd/4.0/), which permits non-commercial re-use, distribution, and reproduction in any medium, provided the original work is properly cited, and is not altered, transformed, or built upon in any way.

attempt to meet on common ground. During this process Mario joined Chris's research project on patients' experiences in direct observation situations, which helped us concretize the phenomenological principles we were discussing. True to the phenomenological approach, our dialogue is still continuing. In this paper, we present our current understanding. While this text is – partly – written as a dialogue, we discussed and wrote subsequent drafts of all sections and the final paper together.

Introduction Chris

A few years ago, my PhD supervisor suggested a phenomenological approach for a patient interview study.[1] We had finished two constructivist grounded theory focus group studies on the residents' and the supervisors' perspectives on direct observation (DO) in general practice training.[2,3] My supervisor argued that since we were interested in the patients' experiences with DO situations, a phenomenological approach seemed appropriate. This confused me and I asked him what the difference would be from the constructivist grounded theory approach we had used to study the experiences of residents and supervisors. Was that not already phenomenological?

This was the beginning of my quest to understand the value of phenomenology for my research, and to learn how a phenomenological approach differs from what I had been doing so far. I embarked on a search of the literature on phenomenology in and outside HPE. In HPE literature, I found overviews of distinct phenomenological schools.[4–6] This literature often explains the differences between Husserl's Descriptive or Transcendental phenomenology and Heidegger's Interpretive or Hermeneutic phenomenology. It provides descriptions of phenomenology and trademark terms such as "bracketing," "phenomenological reduction," and "pre-reflective experience." Unfortunately, I found these descriptions complex and at times contradictory. They did not provide concrete guidance for my project.

I therefore decided to read works by some contemporary phenomenologists.[7,8] This helped me start to grasp some phenomenological principles, but also added to my confusion. I encountered many disagreements among seasoned scientists in this field: Van Manen attacks Smith's Interpretive Phenomenological Analysis.[9] Zahavi accuses van Manen of "getting it quite wrong."[10] Apparently, phenomenologists themselves disagree on what phenomenology is. Moreover, I hardly found any practical guidelines on how to apply phenomenology in research, such as in the

context of an interview study. Indeed, this literature made clear to me that one of the core elements of phenomenology is the absence of fixed rules, let alone a research method.

As a third strategy, I studied examples of research papers in the HPE domain that claim a phenomenological approach. Ajjawi and Higgs[11] conducted research on how physical therapists learn clinical reasoning and how to communicate about this. Bynum and colleagues investigated shame experiences of residents.[12] McLachlan and colleagues studied patients' experiences of medical student teaching encounters.[13] There are more examples.[14,15] The authors of these interview studies describe their phenomenological methods in detail, and I saw evidence of meticulous analyses through immersion in data and thorough reflexivity. Alas, although I was impressed by the quality of many of these papers, to me, the type of results they provided seemed quite similar to the results of other qualitative inquiry methods. I found descriptions of the phenomenological stance and methods somewhat confusing, and was unable to discern any kind of "phenomenological magic," or at least a workable ingredient that would distinguish phenomenological from "non-phenomenological" interview studies.

I concluded that, in HPE literature, phenomenology is often presented as synonymous with investigating subjective experiences that people have with some phenomenon. But other types of qualitative research, such as constructivist grounded theory, can also investigate this. The thought occurred to me that perhaps, 120 years after Husserl, all qualitative researchers have integrated insights from phenomenology so that the term has become superfluous.

So, here I found myself after these three searches, fascinated, overwhelmed, empty handed, and annoyed. Fascinated and overwhelmed by phenomenology as a promising world in itself, but incomprehensible to outsiders. It was clear to me by now that in my lifetime, as a GP, I was never going to really understand classical phenomenology in depth, in the same way that most philosophers, in their lifetime, are never going to master clinical reasoning. I felt empty handed because I had not found a clear practical research methodology, and a bit annoyed with confusing descriptions of phenomenology in research papers that, as far as I could see, did not deliver results that fundamentally differed from some other qualitative approaches.

Nevertheless, phenomenology intrigued me and I saw beauty in its promise to reveal what people basically experience when exposed to a phenomenon. So, instead of throwing in the towel, I became determined to find out how a phenomenological approach differs from other qualitative approaches, such as constructivist grounded theory, and how that can be captured in understandable language and methods. Somewhere in this process I met you, Mario, at the AMEE conference in Vienna. It was a relief that you, as a philosopher, understood my confusion. It was also a consolation, though inconvenient for the short term, that you yourself were struggling with the application of phenomenology in HPE research; you had no brief answers. That is when we started this tunneling project through an extensive exchange of letters.

Introduction Mario

When you approached me with questions about phenomenology, this was confronting in the sense that I recognized your questions as relevant but could not answer them easily. My background is in the Humanities and I started working in medical education about ten years ago. This was an interesting experience and culture shock. I found out that the approach to research I was used to in the Humanities was referred to as "phenomenology" in medical education research. Often, this was contrasted with "empirical" research. But, to my confusion, I also found out that phenomenology was presented as a "method" for conducting empirical research.

In the Humanities, when someone makes a claim about phenomenology, the first question is "whose phenomenology?" Phenomenology can be seen as an intellectual tradition in which different thinkers respond to each other and differ with regard to what phenomenology is and how to put it into practice. Husserl is generally seen as the founder of philosophical phenomenology. But he responded to earlier thinkers such as Kant and Hegel, who also used the term. His student, Heidegger, in turn responded to Husserl, but also criticized some fundamental assumptions that Husserl had made about phenomenology. In the historical tradition of phenomenology, each thinker both develops notions of their predecessor and criticizes others. For instance, Butler[16] develops de Beauvoir's notion of gender[17] in a way that was hugely influential in gender studies and cultural theory. All of these thinkers have in common that they first define either what they see as phenomenology, or *whose* phenomenology they are using, rather than treating it as an out-of-the-box method.

When you approached me with questions, I had, as you say, no easy answers. This is an ongoing struggle with philosophy and medical education research.

But phenomenology faces an additional challenge; as a science of studying everyday phenomena, it uses words that are familiar to us in a technical way for instance: experience, meaning, and intention. In our everyday language and HPE research, we often use words such as "experience" as if we know exactly what they mean. Phenomenology calls these into question (what is experience?). Since HPE research is practically oriented, we simply do not have the bandwidth to elaborate on each of these terms in depth.

Let us start with a technical definition of phenomenology nonetheless, although what this definition means in practice will have to become clear as we go along. Doing phenomenology means describing that which arises in consciousness (phenomena). Phenomenology treats phenomena as objects worthy of description in their own right, rather than only as manifestations of an underlying objective or subjective reality. Whether there is such a reality and whether we can ever get to it, is a question that phenomenology "brackets" (sets aside) rather than trying to answer it, in order to focus on describing phenomena exactly how and when they occur to us, and looking for recurrent patterns or structures in their occurrence. Whether these structures can be called *essences*[18] of phenomena or are contingent manifestations of our *being-in-the-world*[19] is one of those fundamental questions phenomenologists debate.

Here is my version of the problem that you stated: while we both see benefits of phenomenology in HPE research, phenomenology is not an out-of-the-box "method" or even "methodology" that we can simply apply. It is an *approach* to research that requires a certain attitude of the researcher. This attitude permeates all levels of the research: research question, data collection, fine-grained analysis, how you report your results, and reflexivity on your own position as a researcher. Without this attitude, one can use methods that are labeled as phenomenological in a way that is inconsistent with phenomenology as a philosophical approach – which does not mean it is not good research; it is just not phenomenology. And conversely, one can use methods that are not labeled as phenomenology in a phenomenological way. Adding to this complexity, one can take a phenomenological approach to only one aspect of the research – e.g. phenomenological interviewing[20] – but not to others.

To avoid getting bogged down in a debate between different phenomenological approaches, let us confine ourselves to understanding some basics of phenomenology that are directly relevant to HPE research.

What is phenomenology?

Let me share - with a minimum of jargon - how I see phenomenology. Phenomenology has a radically different *starting point* from approaches to research that investigate the world as an objective reality that we can have biased or unbiased knowledge of. Its key feature is that it focuses on the world as it *occurs* to human beings, and asserts that it is impossible to describe the world as it objectively "is" independent of how it occurs.

Phenomenology is the analysis of phenomena as we encounter them. The way the world presents itself to us human beings in ordinary life is its starting point. A phenomenon can be anything from a thing to a situation to a thought or experience that we become aware of as we go about our day. *Phenomenon* means that which shows itself, or that which occurs. Phenomen*ology* therefore means to study that which shows itself to us *as* it shows itself to us.[19] In this way, phenomenology is contrasted with approaches to science and research that do not take everyday life as a starting point, and with those that examine everyday life occurrences not on their own terms, but within preset analytical frameworks.

As an example, think of waking up and remembering a dream you had that night. The dream is the phenomenon. Perhaps, in the dream, you were flying. You could think about the dream and analyze it, writing your thoughts down and examining how it makes you feel, whether this is a recurring dream and if the dream means anything to you. You could even perform a phenomenological analysis of your dreams by writing them down each morning, comparing them, looking for patterns, and examining (e.g. by keeping a diary) whether there are other events in your day that seem to co-occur with certain elements in dreams. Notice that in this phenomenological analysis, you have not concerned yourself with whether dreams are real or not, whether they have predictive value, or what causes them. You are simply aiming to describe what occurs to you.

The moment we start to look at neurological or psychological theories about dreams, for instance by seeing dreams as the processing of unfinished cognitive activities during the day, we have left phenomenology. This does not mean that, in phenomenology, we deny the possibility of neurological or other explanations; we simply suspend this option in order not to be distracted from how the phenomenon shows itself to us as a meaningful event. This suspending of explanations or theory in phenomenology is called "bracketing": we are not concerned with whether the phenomenon - in this case the dream - is "real" or with what "caused" it. Instead, we remain focused on describing the "things themselves".[18(p168)] This is both the core and the major challenge of phenomenology, to capture how a phenomenon occurs before we analyze it through interpretive frameworks. This is the ideal of capturing pre-reflective awareness: the raw way in which the world presents itself to us, rather than a "processed" version of it. This is so challenging because we (especially researchers) are used to instantly analyzing phenomena by categorizing them within analytical frameworks.

Some basic principles of phenomenology

Immediate access to phenomena

With this example in mind, we come to a basic description of phenomenology as being concerned with that to which we have *immediate access*. Only the dreamer has direct access to the dream. Others (including researchers) only have access to the dream through what dreamers report. Non-phenomenological approaches usually attempt to go beyond that which we have immediate access to, and instead analyze phenomena from a pre-defined theoretical position, such as psychology or neurology. Realist evaluation, as another example of a non-phenomenological approach, attempts to identify "underlying, generative mechanisms that give rise to causal regularities".[21(p1)] Phenomenology does not make any claim about whether these kinds of mechanisms exist or what they consist of, but only that they are not immediately available when we simply observe what occurs to us. Applying this principle of phenomenology to our interview study on how patients experience direct observation (DO) situations,[1] our goal was to study participants' immediate access to the phenomenon in an everyday life context, looking for recurring patterns in the relationship between the DO situation and the patient.

However, in the practice of HPE research, the question is not just what the *participants* have direct access to, but through which data and methods *we* as researchers can gain access to the situation. There is no obvious answer to that question. Our DO study could have been done using methods of autoethnography, in which the researcher *is* the participant and describes and reflects on their own experience. Or alternatively, through recording actual DO situations and analyzing the video recordings. In that case, we would have had immediate access to what is visible and audible during DO: what happens in terms of verbal interaction, but also in terms of eye contact, who sits where, etc. We opted for conducting interviews with participants. But whatever data collection method one adopts, it should be focused on the phenomenon, or part of the phenomenon, being able to show itself on its own terms, rather than through a filter of interpretation, memory, or any other categorization we impose on it from the start.

Although in the practice of empirical research "pre-reflective" is an idealization, we tried as much as possible to capture the "raw" experience of what it was like for the participant to have been part of that DO situation. We performed the interviews immediately after the DO situation, so that the experience was still "fresh" and the participants did not have much time to reflect on it. In the interviews, we gently steered participants to the "how" of the experience, rather than focusing on their opinions about DO or their own interpretations of it – as might be done in an interview study that explicitly asks participants about perceived barriers and enablers with regard to a certain phenomenon. Instead of introducing interpretive frameworks through elaborate questions, we stimulated participants with non-directive prompts, like nodding and repeating the last words of a sentence.

Meaningfulness and bracketing the natural attitude

As a second basic principle, phenomenology considers meaning to be an integral *part* of phenomena and not something that we have to do away with in order to have an "objective" research object. Phenomena occur to *someone* and point to *something*. For instance, there is no such thing as "knowledge" that is not knowledge *by* someone and *about* something. The research objects that HPE research concerns itself with are almost always meaningful. Unlike medical science, for instance, we do not study chemical processes but human processes. We study relationships between objects and subjects. In our research project, the patient was the subject and we studied their relationship to the DO situation that they were in. Phenomenology treats subjects, objects, and the relationships between them as essential parts of phenomena without which we cannot understand them. These relationships are part of a phenomenological investigation instead of taking them for granted.

Husserl called this taking for granted of relationships the natural attitude: the attitude of everyday life in which we do not question the existence of an objective reality or our relationship to it.[22] It is also the attitude we have in non-phenomenological HPE research, in which we conduct research from the perspective that there is an empirical reality outside of us that we can investigate without being part of it. From the perspective of the natural attitude, the resident has a consultation with a patient, and the supervisor is "just there" to observe. Of course we know this is an ideal, but the more the supervisor can conform to this role and be a "fly on the wall," the more successful the observation will be.[2] From the natural attitude, we could, for instance, hold interviews with the participants and code them.

But from a phenomenological attitude (bracketing the natural attitude), we called the idea of "direct observation" into question. We did not assume that we knew beforehand what the relationship was between the supervisor and the other people present. In fact, this was precisely what we wanted to investigate. As part of this investigation, we wanted to interview patients about how they experienced the situation. In the analysis of these interviews, we then focused on how patients constructed their relationship to the situation as a whole and their relationship to the two other people that were present.

Importantly, one can only bracket what one is aware of. Becoming aware of the dispositions we already have toward the phenomenon is just as important as placing them to one side. In phenomenology, we recognize that the objects we are aware of are imbued with our perspective, our judgements, and our values.[3] Anything we see is already colored by our fundamental attitude to the world. However, becoming aware of one's own fundamental assumptions is one of the most challenging philosophical practices.[23] It is an ongoing practice throughout phenomenological research, rather than a one-time reflection before or after the research. In our study, prior to conducting interviews the two main researchers each wrote an essay on their own assumptions about being the patient in a DO situation. They then interviewed each other about these essays. This session was recorded, transcribed, and analyzed, and this process served as the start of a reflexive diary that both researchers kept throughout the study.

While researcher reflexivity is a part of all qualitative approaches, it usually comes down to reflecting on one's own positionality to look for ways in which one's own background as a researcher might have biased their perspective. However, bracketing is not so much about the *opinions* (or other "biases") one might have, but on assumptions about the *relationships*, such as, in this case, for example, the relationship between the patient and the resident and supervisor in the DO situation, and about what underlying mechanisms one assumes are at work in DO.

Describing phenomena on their own terms

As a third principle, phenomenology refrains from doing something that we are so used to in most approaches to research: *reducing* phenomena to research objects that become "fileable" entities and abstracting them from the uniqueness of subjective experience. Theory describes the world from a "third perspective," a kind of impersonal position that is neither yours nor mine. In phenomenology, the phenomenon is *primary*, and theorizing and analyzing phenomena – whether systematically in medical education research, or in the way that we analyze things "informally" throughout our day – is rooted in this primary experience. Phenomenology aims to understand phenomena on their own terms rather than in terms of categories that have been formulated from a third-person, "outside" perspective.

In our patient study, we were not striving for an understanding of what was said in terms of building theory on psychological or sociological processes as could, for instance, be the aim of constructivist grounded theory. Instead, we wanted to describe commonalities between people's pre-reflective experiences. As an example, some patients reported on the importance of a clear role division between resident and supervisor that should not be breached during DO. But we also found indications that role breaching was sometimes treated as consistent with DO. Moreover, many patients emphasized that the experience had been pleasant because the resident and supervisor seemed in harmony with each other.

In a non-phenomenological approach, we might have induced from these findings a theory on role division and harmony in DO situations. Instead we traced these patients' ideas back to a recurring pre-reflective structure of the experience: being the patient in a DO situation meant being in a room with two doctors, not knowing how they will interact with each other and with oneself. This resonated with patients' needs for calm and friendly interactions, and their passive role in securing these.

To identify recurring patterns in the experience, we were guided by the question of whether the phenomenon would still be the phenomenon without this element (imaginative variation).[7] We had, for example, many codes about eye contact between the patient and the supervisor, which therefore seemed an essential element of the experience. However, we reasoned that without this eye contact, being the patient in a DO situation would still be the same phenomenon. Eye contact did not seem essential for DO. What seemed essential was the presence of a second, more senior doctor that the patient could relate to and be reassured by, in which eye contact often played a role.

Phenomenological practices in HPE research

Readers with a background in qualitative research might recognize aspects of many of the principles discussed above in their own methods, and wonder what constitutes the difference between phenomenology and (other forms of) qualitative research. Indeed, this is one of the challenges for HPE researchers in grasping what phenomenology is: it is often not immediately distinguishable from qualitative research in general.

There are historical and philosophical reasons for this. For instance, it is misleading to contrast phenomenology with social constructivist approaches, since social constructivism has been developed against the background of and in dialogue with phenomenologists like Husserl, Heidegger, and Merleau-Ponty. Foucault, one of the thinkers who has been influential in HPE research[24] (and the subject of a previous installment in this series[25]), is often categorized as a post-structuralist and associated with constructivism and constructionism. However, Foucault listed Heidegger as one of the most important influences on his thinking.[26] In historical terms, our modern versions of ethnography, constructivism, discourse analysis, and so on, are all to some extent dependent on the existence of the historical and philosophical movement of phenomenology. Studying phenomenology will therefore also lead to a better understanding of approaches that are often contrasted with it, but that actually depend on it.

The philosophical reason concerns the relationship between broad approaches to conducting research and concrete research methods. Without bracketing the natural attitude in the way we have described, one can apply Interpretive Phenomenological Analysis (IPA)[27] in a non-phenomenological way, just as one can take a phenomenological approach to ethnography with a deep commitment to being open to describe cultural phenomena on their own terms rather than from the perspective of one's own interpretive frameworks. Phenomenology is an *approach* to science, and not a particular scientific method. Not only does it provide answers, it also stimulates asking certain *questions* related to the concrete practice of doing research.

There are four questions we suggest all researchers, but especially those committed to conducting research from a phenomenological perspective, could ask themselves:

1. What immediate access do I have to the phenomenon I want to study, and what implications do different data collection methods have for access? For instance, through interviews I have a more direct access to what it was like for that person to be in that situation, but because the situation is in the past, there is always some extent of interpretation and reflection. Through video recordings of the situation I do have immediate access to what the situation is like in terms of what each participant says and does, but I do not have access to what they think or feel, or what their intentions are.

2. Related to the question of what my data gives me immediate access to, what are the limits to what I can know and assert about the phenomenon in my research? To conduct research means to be precise about what we are studying, what our relation is to that which we are studying, and what kind of statements we can or cannot make about it. We have to be clear what our data is (for instance, "audio recordings of people being interviewed about emotions," instead of "emotions") and what this research data allows us to say. In recordings of interviews, we do not observe "thoughts," but social actions such as descriptions, interactions, and so on. So, we do not say "patients think", but "participants report that...".

3. What is my natural attitude toward the situation I examine and what would it take for the phenomenon to show itself to me on its own terms? In contrast to reflexivity as it pertains to research in general (thus, including phenomenological research), this type of reflection is less about how my cultural background and assumptions would bias my perception of the (otherwise objective) phenomenon, but rather about assumptions regarding relationships, such as my relationship to the interviewee, or the relationship of the interviewee to the DO situation they are speaking about. The term "bias" refers to the natural (objectivist) attitude that says that there is a state of affairs out there that a subjective researcher has a perspective on. In other words, subjectivity is seen as a filter that we should disable as much as possible. Within phenomenology, however, subjectivity is not something bad or added on to phenomena, but rather it is an integral part of phenomena and a requirement to understand them. In Discursive Psychology,[28] for instance, we confine ourselves to only describing what is visible and audible in the recordings of the situation, and refrain from referring to interaction-external categories such as the institutional role that a participant is expected to fulfill or whether they are male or female – unless, of course, the participants themselves observably make these categories part of the interaction and therefore of the phenomenon.

4. How does my research apparatus factor into the phenomenon I am investigating? As this question suggests, the research apparatus – the whole constellation of the university I work in, whether I interview live or via Zoom, the way I code the interviews, the way I write up the paper – is considered part of the phenomenon rather than an outside perspective on it.[29] Research is a practice like other practices. It is contingent on the people who conduct it and the circumstances in which they conduct it. This means that we can never treat the research apparatus as neutral. It includes everything from one's work environment to methodological choices and questions asked during an interview. The researcher is not outside the research, but is "embodied," i.e., an integral part of it. We have to do justice to this insight in some way in every research project. One practical implication of this is to write in the active voice, so as not to give the impression that an analysis "was made" and themes "have emerged" from the data.

Magic at the end of the tunnel

What have I, Chris, learned while digging this tunnel over the last two years? First and foremost, that phenomenology is not a method but an approach to science. And that it calls for a radically different way of looking, suspending the natural attitude.

Second, as a practical researcher, I now know what kind of results I am looking for in a phenomenological interview study, and how these differ from results of other approaches that make use of interview data: we are not interested in people's thoughts, feelings, or opinions per se, but rather in the recurring structures of experience that underlie these ideas, opinions, and feelings. To me, that is the phenomenological magic: it is in the so-called "eidetic reduction"[8,30] of data, in bringing the data back to what it reveals about these recurring structures of experience. The magic, to me, is in the simplicity of its results that structure numerous accounts into a small number of meaningful characteristics of the phenomenon. The practical relevance of this is that taking this manageable number of characteristics into account may help resolve persistent problems.

To give one last example to illustrate this, in our investigation of patients' experiences with DO situations in general practice residency, patients experienced the presence of two doctors, a junior and a senior. This simple, recurring structure was responsible for all kinds of thoughts and behaviors of patients toward the senior.[1] For instance, patients often looked for signs of approval from the senior of the treatment plan. This finding made us question the appropriateness of a fly-on-the-wall approach by supervisors during DO; supervisors, by being there, completely change the situation that they intend to observe. This self-evident but often overlooked finding may have consequences for how we can best behave in these situations and how best to use them for purposes of learning and assessment.

Conclusion

Conducting HPE research from a phenomenological perspective is complex but valuable. Its complexity is not due to technical considerations, but to acquiring a basic attitude that is different from what many researchers, especially those with a medical science background, are used to. To achieve this, HPE researchers must make the effort to step back and contemplate some of the philosophical "biases"[31] that underpin our daily research practice. Without some basic idea of the fundamentally different approach that phenomenology takes, phenomenological "methods" may be phenomenological in name only.

Phenomenology is a logical start for investigating topics in HPE. Research is limited in advance by the degree to which it has apprehended the phenomenon even before the research starts. Most research in medical education starts with delineating the research object. Often, this is done by providing a definition of the research object. For instance, "reflection is a metacognitive process that...". From the perspective of phenomenology, this is reductionism: reducing the research object in advance to a specific interpretive framework that makes assumptions about the phenomenon in question. Anything that does not fit the interpretive framework is not seen at all or is dismissed as irrelevant to the research. Phenomenologists counter that, if the goal of our research is to understand a phenomenon, then we should start with trying to *understand* what the phenomenon is by letting it show itself on its own terms, instead of claiming to already *know* what it is. A phenomenologist brackets interpretive frameworks and assumes a "beginner's mind"[32] to the phenomenon. In the course of the phenomenological analysis it may become clear that a phenomenon like reflection can be further understood through the lens of cognition, the lens of emotion, the educational lens in which reflection should lead to a specific result, and so on. The initial attempt to understand a research object on its own terms fits closely with the ambition of HPE research to do justice to patient-centeredness, student-centeredness, and context sensitivity. In HPE research, we want to understand phenomena in *their* context, not *ours*.

Acknowledgment

The authors thank Marilyn Hedges for her feedback on English grammar and style.

Previous philosophy in medical education installments

Mario Veen & Anna T. Cianciolo (2020) Problems No One Looked For: Philosophical Expeditions into Medical Education, Teaching and Learning in Medicine, 32:3, 337-344, DOI: 10.1080/10401334.2020.1748634
Gert J. J. Biesta & Marije van Braak (2020) Beyond the Medical Model: Thinking Differently about Medical Education and Medical Education Research, Teaching and Learning in Medicine, 32:4, 449-456, DOI: 10.1080/10401334.2020.1798240
Mark R. Tonelli & Robyn Bluhm (2021) Teaching Medical Epistemology within an Evidence-Based Medicine Curriculum, Teaching and Learning in Medicine, 33:1, 98-105, DOI: 10.1080/10401334.2020.1835666
John R. Skelton (2021) Language, Philosophy, and Medical Education, Teaching and Learning in Medicine, 33:2, 210-216, DOI: 10.1080/10401334.2021.1877712
Zareen Zaidi, Ian M. Partman, Cynthia R. Whitehead, Ayelet Kuper & Tasha R. Wyatt (2021) Contending with Our Racial Past in Medical Education: A Foucauldian Perspective, Teaching and Learning in Medicine, DOI: 10.1080/10401334.2021.1945929

Associated Podcast

Let Me Ask You Something (iTunes, Spotify, Google Podcasts and https://marioveen.com/letmeaskyousomething/)

ORCID

Mario Veen (iD) http://orcid.org/0000-0003-2550-7193

References

1. Rietmeijer CBT, Deves M, van Esch SCM, et al. A phenomenological investigation of patients' experiences during direct observation in residency: busting the myth of the fly on the wall. *Adv Health Sci Educ Theory Pract.* 2021. doi:10.1007/s10459-021-10044-z. Epub ahead of print. PMID: 33765197.
2. Rietmeijer CBT, Blankenstein AH, Huisman D, et al. What happens under the flag of direct observation, and how that matters: a qualitative study in general practice residency. *Med Teach.* 2021:1–8. doi: 10.1080/0142159X.2021.1898572. Epub ahead of print. PMID: 33765396.
3. Rietmeijer CBT, Huisman D, Blankenstein AH, et al. Patterns of direct observation and their impact during residency: general practice supervisors' views. *Med Educ.* 2018;52(9):981–991. doi:10.1111/medu.13631.
4. Dowling M. From Husserl to van Manen. A review of different phenomenological approaches. *Int J Nurs Stud.* 2007;44(1):131–142. doi:10.1016/j.ijnurstu.2005.11.026.
5. Bynum W, Varpio L. When I say ... hermeneutic phenomenology. *Med Educ.* 2018;52(3):252–253. doi:10.1111/medu.13414.
6. Neubauer BE, Witkop CT, Varpio L. How phenomenology can help us learn from the experiences of others. *Perspect Med Educ.* 2019;8(2):90–97. doi:10.1007/s40037-019-0509-2.
7. Van Manen M. *Researching Lived Experience: Human Science for an Action Sensitive Pedagogy.* Taylor and Francis group, London and New York: Routledge; 2016.
8. Zahavi D. *Phenomenology: The Basics.* Taylor and Francis group, London and New York: Routledge; 2018.
9. van Manen M. But is it phenomenology?*Qual Health Res.* 2017;27(6):775–779. doi:10.1177/1049732317699570.
10. Zahavi D. Getting it quite wrong: Van Manen and Smith on phenomenology. *Qual Health Res.* 2019;29(6):900–907. doi:10.1177/1049732318817547.
11. Ajjawi R, Higgs J. Using hermeneutic phenomenology to investigate how experienced practitioners learn to communicate clinical reasoning. *Qual Rep.* 2007;12(4):612–638.
12. Bynum WE, Artino AR, Uijtdehaage S, Webb AMB, Varpio L. Sentinel emotional events: the nature, triggers, and effects of shame experiences in medical residents. *Acad Med.* 2019;94(1):85–93. doi:10.1097/ACM.0000000000002479.
13. McLachlan E, King N, Wenger E, Dornan T. Phenomenological analysis of patient experiences of medical student teaching encounters. *Med Educ.* 2012;46(10):963–973. doi:10.1111/j.1365-2923.2012.04332.x.
14. van der Meide H, Teunissen T, Collard P, Visse M, Visser LH. The mindful body: a phenomenology of the body with multiple sclerosis. *Qual Health Res.* 2018;28(14):2239–2249. doi:10.1177/1049732318796831.
15. Eskilsson C, Carlsson G, Ekebergh M, Hörberg U. The experiences of patients receiving care from nursing students at a Dedicated Education Unit: a phenomenological study. *Nurse Educ Pract.* 2015;15(5):353–358. doi:10.1016/j.nepr.2015.04.001.
16. Butler J. Performative acts and gender constitution: an essay in phenomenology and feminist theory. *Theatre J.* 1988;40(4):519–531. doi:10.2307/3207893.
17. Sd B. *The Second Sex.* Vol. 732. New York: A. A. Knopf; 1968:xiv.
18. Husserl E. *Logical Investigations.* 2nd ed. In: Moran D, ed. Taylor and Francis group: London and New York: Routledge; 2001:1900–1901.
19. Heidegger M. *Being and Time.* London: SCM Press; 1962/1927.
20. Høffding S, Martiny K. Framing a phenomenological interview: what, why and how. *Phenom Cogn Sci.* 2016;15(4):539–564. doi:10.1007/s11097-015-9433-z.
21. Dalkin SM, Greenhalgh J, Jones D, Cunningham B, Lhussier M. What's in a mechanism? Development of a key concept in realist evaluation. *Implement Sci.* 2015;10:49.
22. Husserl E. *Ideas: General Introduction to Pure Phenomenology.* Taylor and Francis group, London and New York: Routledge; 2012.
23. Veen M, Cianciolo AT. Problems no one looked for: philosophical expeditions into medical education. *Teach Learn Med.* 2020;32(3):337–344. doi:10.1080/10401334.2020.1748634.
24. Hodges BD, Martimianakis MA, McNaughton N, Whitehead C. Medical education... meet Michel Foucault. *Med Educ.* 2014;48(6):563–571. doi:10.1111/medu.12411.
25. Zaidi Z, Partman IM, Whitehead CR, Kuper A, Wyatt TR. Contending with our racial past in medical education: a foucauldian perspective. *Teach Learn Med.* 2021:1–10. doi:10.1080/10401334.2021.1945929.
26. Foucault M. Final Interview [Thomas Y. Levin & Isabelle Lorenz, trans.]. In: Barbadette G, ed. Raritan Review V1 (1985): 1-13; 1985.
27. Biggerstaff D, Thompson AR. Interpretative phenomenological analysis (IPA): a qualitative methodology of choice in healthcare research. *Qual Res Psychol.* 2008;5(3):214–224. doi:10.1080/14780880802314304.
28. Potter J, Wetherell M. *Discourse and Social Psychology.* London: Paul Chapman Publishing Ltd; 1987.
29. Tamboukou M. Archival research: unravelling space/time/matter entanglements and fragments. *Qual Res.* 2014;14(5):617–633. doi:10.1177/1468794113490719.
30. What is Phenomenology? The Philosophy of Husserl and Heidegger https://youtu.be/IvA9FxsM9G8.
31. Andersen F, Anjum RL, Rocca E. Philosophical bias is the one bias that science cannot avoid. *Elife.* 2019;8:e44929. doi:10.7554/eLife.44929.
32. Varpio L, MacLeod A. Philosophy of science series: Harnessing the multidisciplinary edge effect by exploring paradigms, ontologies, epistemologies, axiologies, and methodologies. *Acad Med.* 2020;95(5):686–689. doi:10.1097/ACM.0000000000003142.

8 OPEN ACCESS

Black, White and Gray: Student Perspectives on Medical Humanities and Medical Education

Madeleine Noelle Olding (ID), Freya Rhodes (ID), John Humm (ID), Phoebe Ross (ID) and Catherine McGarry (ID)

ABSTRACT

Issue: In recent years, the value and relevance of humanities-based teaching in medical education have become more widely acknowledged. In many medical schools this has prompted additions to curricula that allow students to explore the gray—as opposed to the black and white—areas of medicine through arts, humanities, and social sciences. As curricula have expanded and diversified in this way, both medical educators and students have begun to ask: what is the best way to teach medical humanities? *Evidence:* In this article, five current medical students reflect on their experiences of medical humanities teaching through intercalated BSc programmes in the UK. What follows is a broad exploration of how the incorporation of medical humanities into students' time at university can improve clinical practice where the more rigid, objective-driven, model of medicine falls short. *Implications:* This article reinforces the merit of moving beyond a purely biomedical model of medical education. Using the student voice as a vector for critique and discussion, we provide a starting point for uncovering the path toward true integration of humanities-style teaching into medical school curricula.

Introduction

It is possible, and easy enough, to view medicine entirely from a scientific, biomedical perspective. A patient presents with a series of symptoms. The doctor takes a history and elicits signs on examination. Investigations may follow; a diagnosis is made. A management plan, based on a scientific understanding of the underlying pathology, is prescribed to the patient. When phrased like this with no nuance, no humanity, and no wider factors considered, medicine is easily framed as a black and white exercise. However, neither the patient's nor clinician's experience exist in black and white. In each clinical encounter, the gray areas of humanity are brought to the forefront and shape the complex relationships between patient and doctor. Symptoms, signs, investigations, and management are shrouded in undefined areas of gray.

An increasing focus on humanities within medical education has generated opportunities for students to delve into these gray areas; simultaneously broadening and deepening their knowledge outside of the core curriculum. But *how* exactly does one delve into the gray? How can we best teach medical humanities (MH) to students?

The value of MH teaching - not only for future clinicians, but also for patients whose demographics and disease experience have so far been neglected by traditional biomedical models - is well documented.[1–3] Arno Kumagai describes how MH assist students in: dismantling assumptions and attitudes upheld in medicine; encouraging reflection on our experiences; broadening perspectives and prompting analysis of medical care through different lenses; providing outlets for expressing and understanding our experiences; and driving empathy in clinical encounters.[2] Kumagai argues that the arts and humanities "lead us to a knowledge of a thing through the organ of sight instead of through recognition":[3(p6)] in essence, through questioning ideas that are held to be true, we engage

---

This is an Open Access article distributed under the terms of the Creative Commons Attribution-NonCommercial-NoDerivatives License (http://creativecommons.org/licenses/by-nc-nd/4.0/), which permits non-commercial re-use, distribution, and reproduction in any medium, provided the original work is properly cited, and is not altered, transformed, or built upon in any way.

more deeply with the information presented to us and as such better our understanding.

Despite their demonstrable value, the optimal approach to teaching MH is less clear cut. In order to elucidate how best to optimize the value of MH teaching, this piece discusses its integration in medical school curricula. Building upon ideas put forth in the Association of American Medical Colleges' (AAMC) 2020 report *The Fundamental Role of the Arts and Humanities in Medical Education*, we explore attitudes toward MH from a medical student perspective and the impact of a reluctance to step away from objective, positivist thinking amongst educators and learners alike.[4]

The AAMC proposes a working definition of MH in medical education as "content or pedagogy derived from arts and humanities and integrated into the teaching and learning of medical students, trainees, and practicing physicians."[4(p.4)] Importantly, the AAMC discusses some of the barriers to integrating MH into curricula, including the belief that the syllabus is already "full" and there is no room nor funding available. As such, where MH are included in the curricula, they are often added on for those who are interested, rather than built into the foundations of the course.

This phenomenon demonstrates Alan Bleakley and Robert Marshall's concept of "weak inclusion:"[5(p.129)]

"The weak version of inclusion of the medical humanities in the curriculum appears as optional study, a bolt on, usually advertised as a compensation for science. The strong version, however, involves a core, integrated curriculum component as a complement to science, creating a more nuanced educational culture".[5(p129)]

"Weak inclusion"[5(p129)] encompasses many of the approaches to MH we have experienced at our respective medical schools in the UK. However, the teaching we have received through undertaking an optional year of study - a so-called intercalated Bachelors degree[6] - in MH, has shown that strong inclusion is both possible and desirable. "Strong inclusion" of MH in curricula advocates for the development of an interdisciplinary approach to these interventions whereby medicine and MH are not seen as distinct entities but rather symbiotic approaches to understanding human problems.

Thus far, the student perspective has remained relatively absent in this discussion. There are numerous examples of students contributing to MH literature but explicit acknowledgement of student perspectives on teaching approaches is currently lacking.[7,8] We believe that the barriers to integration can be explored further by showcasing the student perspective. As current medical students who have recently completed intercalated Bachelors of Science (intercalated BSc or iBSc) in MH, the evidence we present is largely anecdotal. Imbuing personal experience into the methodologies of medical education is a relatively new approach that has gained traction in recent years, most particularly within the realms of MH.[9]

To organize our reflections of the gray areas of medicine and medical education, we have isolated five themes relating to specific domains of MH. These include history, narrative medicine, anthropology, and philosophy and ethics. We also comment on a variety of practical considerations to contextualize the delivery of MH teaching in the UK and beyond. Through these reflections, we provide a starting point for a critical discussion of learning experience, aiming to improve the synergy of MH teaching in medical education.

The medical student perspective

Medical education does not end at graduation. Students should be supported and empowered to critique, challenge, and advocate for changes in their experience at medical school in preparation for continued learning as a doctor.

In an earlier installment in this series, Gert Biesta and Marije Van Braak[10] highlight the need for increased engagement in the purposes of medical education, as opposed to just focusing on the processes. In this piece, they discuss socialization (becoming a member of the professional group) and subjectification (becoming a thoughtful, independent, responsible professional) as important goals of medical education. We believe that we can better achieve these purposes by including MH and the student perspective in the discourse surrounding medical education.

Using the medical student perspective in academic research, we can better explore attitudes toward MH teaching amongst current learners. Student perspectives on current curricula provide detailed, nuanced learning points for educators and are often accompanied by practical real-world solutions from current students, for future students. A recent, excellent example of such a paper comes from Liu and colleagues[11] discussing shortcomings in medical ethics teaching and assessment. Another recent paper looking at health systems and scientific education was conducted more traditionally by a team of researchers who analyzed student questionnaire responses and did not probe student perspectives directly.[12] Reading these two papers one after another, the power and precision of the student perspective for medical educational research becomes abundantly clear. Educational research using questionnaires or focus groups made up of medical students and then interpreted by academics is, of course, not without merit and the paper in question makes several important conclusions with which we do not disagree. However, in our reading, it becomes weighed down by data collection, methodology, and terminology. Whereas student perspective research papers can be more reflective and critical, resonating with current students and potentially resulting in better, more directed, changes in educational approaches.

Understanding student attitudes toward learning MH is crucial in recognizing the pitfalls of MH teaching. Amongst medical students, there exists a rhetoric that MH are "tick box exercises" that function purely to coax out empathy and soft skills, such as teamwork, leadership, and problem solving. This has been recognized previously as a significant barrier to integration of MH.[2] Hunter Birden and Tim Usherwood comment on similar attitudes toward professionalism teaching whereby students are able to anticipate the desired outcomes and game the system[13(p408)] as opposed to exercising reflective abilities. We have seen this played out in our own experiences, where reluctant students feel MH are being unnecessarily forced onto them by educators. Students resist participating in activities prescribed by the medical school unless they directly ascertain the benefit before engaging in the process. Often, there is a correlation drawn between what students know is examinable content and whether they are motivated to engage with it. Of course, MH educators will promote their subject; they have already demonstrated a degree of passion by choosing to teach it. Students, by contrast, have no such vested interest in promoting MH and therefore positive perspectives on the learning experience are more authentically received by peers. As such, students can play a pivotal role in encouraging MH engagement; by communicating the benefits of MH teaching, their contemporaries are more amenable to participating themselves. Furthermore, learning from student perspectives opens opportunities for peer teaching that allows a longitudinal flow of knowledge beyond a perceived hierarchy of teacher-student relationships.

Not everything of value in medical education is taught through the formal curriculum. Consciously and subconsciously, medical students learn from clinical experiences with patients and other healthcare professionals. With regards to medical education and MH, it is important to create an informal space in which students can autonomously explore and reflect on their experiences. A consideration of this so-called hidden curriculum allows for more well-rounded research in medical education.[45] In essence, learning within the hidden curriculum is centered in student experience and, as such, exploring these perspectives offers an inlet for understanding. MH must be both accessible and ubiquitous within curricula such that all students are comfortable contributing to the field and the wider discussions it opens up, without fear of making mistakes or getting things wrong. In providing MH opportunities to all medical students, as opposed to the self-selecting few, we broaden the scope for their impact on future practice.

Intercalating in the UK

The AAMC report comprehensively outlines the benefits of MH within the American medical school model, however this differs greatly in structure to the UK system. In the UK, there is an opportunity to undertake an intercalation: students interrupt their five-year undergraduate medical degree to spend an extra year studying a topic related to medicine. These courses need not be taken at a student's home university and are either crafted specifically for intercalators or allow students to join a cohort of undergraduates from beyond medicine. Intercalated courses are offered in a range of subjects and, from our own experience, popular choices include anatomy, neuroscience, and women's health. A prevailing misconception that intercalation is reserved for the most academically minded students, combined with the propensity toward electing "traditional" science-based courses mean that the uptake for MH intercalated courses is still relatively low, although this is not well documented aside from university-specific websites. For example, in the 2020/2021 uptake at University College London, just nine internal students undertook an MH intercalation (in either Medical Anthropology or History and Philosophy of Science & Medicine) compared with 37, 34, and 24 students for Cardiovascular Science, Neuroscience, and Pediatrics and Child Health respectively.[14]

Intercalators gain an extra degree qualification in the form of a BSc, MSc, MRes, BMedSci, etc. Intercalation in this format is unique to UK medical schools but similar programmes are run in Ireland, Australia, New Zealand, the West Indies, Hong Kong, South Africa, and Canada.[15] Despite the patchy uptake from students and schools alike, MH's intercalated courses have certainly become more popular.

Developing from a tiny minority, we have seen an international interest beginning to rise and an increase in uptake of humanities-based courses in medical schools in the UK and the US.[4]

Our experience that the majority of intercalating students come to value their BSc year and develop skills beyond the scope of the core medical curriculum is confirmed by the literature.[16] Students see this as an opportunity to develop how they think, write, and communicate as well as a chance to work within interdisciplinary teams, contribute to research, and maximize their future career options. A great deal of the literature on motivations to intercalate highlight the benefits in terms of future employability; the transferable skills of critical appraisal, statistical analysis, and in-depth research are highly sought after in students choosing a BSc.[17] In terms of MH, an intercalated degree is arguably a stronger version of inclusion than a one-off assignment or workshop. Reflections on how strong inclusion has been achieved in our experiences of MH intercalation are explored in the Gray Areas section of this piece.

However, we represent a self-selected group of students, brought together by our interest in MH. This highlights one of the pitfalls of intercalation as a stronger form of inclusion: it is voluntary and, as such, attracts only those with prior interest or belief in MH as a facet of becoming a good doctor. Furthermore, despite being a year-long course, intercalation is still condensed and sporadic in terms of its relation to the broader medical curriculum. An isolated one-year engagement with MH has the propensity to perpetuate the goal-oriented, objective success measures of medical education as it facilitates medical students' belief that the breadth of skills amassed through engagement in the humanities can be reduced down to focused but intermittent study. This is demonstrably untrue: one does not become proficient in history, art, anthropology, or any of the other academic fields encompassed by studying humanities overnight, or over a series of lectures. Similarly, as many students intercalate having undergone two or three years of their medical degree, much of the early part of the course requires an un-learning of the notion that clinical medicine is derived from pure science, devoid of the gray areas MH seeks to understand.[18]

An isolated day, or even year, of engagement with MH by no means makes a student an expert. A developed comparison between MH and the more traditional areas of medical education (such as anatomy or physiology) is required in order to manage expectations. One would not expect to gain a wholly comprehensive understanding of neuroscience from one year studying the subject as a BSc – application of this expectation to humanities courses is only accepted among medical educators because the end goal is less well-defined compared with clinical medicine. As students, we can work toward refining this goal.

Gray areas

In this section, we organize our reflections across five domains from within the MH. We focus on how teaching in these areas has allowed for exploration beyond the black and white biomedical model and whether or not learning outcomes were provided by strong or weak inclusion of MH.

History

A great deal of medical education is centered around case studies, illustrated by the global rise in interest of "problem-based-learning".[19] Encouraging students to build their approach to modern practice around contextual criticism of historical events mirrors this method of learning. Today's medical schools employ teaching strategies that have been around for centuries. However, the sociological impact of these strategies is rarely explored within medical education. Foucault's *The Birth of the Clinic* delineates how dissection, one example of a teaching strategy that has prevailed through the ages, fundamentally changed the practice of medicine through its development of the medical gaze.[20] The medical gaze presents a broad lens for understanding the objectification of patients.

More specifically we can consider an item all medical students are familiar with, the stethoscope. The stethoscope made previously inaccessible bodily processes audible to the doctor, through which the doctor came to know more about the patient's condition than themselves. Slowly, these 'signs' began to take precedence over the patient's symptoms.[21] As medical students, we can recall being sent by our seniors to examine a patient with an interesting heart murmur or breath sounds, listening to the chest and returning to report our findings: the patients' internal intonations taking precedence over their personal story. Not dissimilarly, students and doctors alike are often presented with radiographic images, ECGs, or blood results to interpret without ever having seen the patient from whose body they were derived. We have found that understanding how medicine has changed since the advent of dissection, the stethoscope, and other historical developments installs a sensitivity to the ethics and biases of modern practice.

Learning from history allows a greater reflection and awareness of ethical practice, how to act and – perhaps more importantly – how not to act in clinical settings and within research. This is a point of deviation between weak and strong inclusion of history within medical education. In our experiences, weak inclusion tends to be hagiographic focusing on "successes and achievements" of our predecessors, while missing out "follies, omissions, and failures of the past".[22(p.629)] The over-glorification of the past paints medicine as an institution and practice never in the wrong, only doing good. Well-rounded teaching in history shows this to be a false and potentially dangerous idea to present to medical students. Understanding both its successes and failures is essential to the history of medicine.

The Tuskegee syphilis study is a poignant example of the importance of ethics and equipoise in medical research.[23] Without an understanding of where these values come from, it becomes difficult to appreciate their monumental importance in future research. In the Tuskegee study, black male participants who had contracted syphilis were observed over a 40-year period to study the natural history of the disease. Over this time, treatment for syphilis became available but was not given to the participants such that their condition could be researched: this led to a significant number of unnecessary deaths (for more information on this study, see 'The Tuskegee Timeline'[23]). Since this trial, a number of studies have revealed a tangible, lasting impact in the therapeutic relationship between African Americans and medical institutions and research.[24,25] Work from historian Susan Reverby suggests that the reasons for this distrust goes back much further than the trial in Tuskegee.[26] There is evidence of slaveholders instilling fears of 'night riders' who would steal slaves for medical experimentation and, later in the 19th century grave robbers selling black bodies to medical schools for dissection. The Tuskegee study may have added to the sense of mistrust that we see today, but this is built on centuries of pain and suffering inflicted on black individuals at the hands of the medical community. For us, in the contemporary context, where enduring structural inequalities between ethnic groups have manifested in dire outcomes and significant variation in vaccination uptake throughout the Covid-19 pandemic, an understanding of the racialised history of medicine is ever more pressing.[27,28]

The manner in which we look back on and approach historic events in the field is important for the public face of medicine. In 2019, protesters in Central Park, New York demanded the removal of a statue depicting Dr J Marion Simms, a gynecologist who experimented on black female slaves without their consent or analgesia. This brutal manipulation of power eventually culminated in the development of a number of pioneering gynaecological surgical techniques and the eponymous Sims speculum, an instrument still in use today.[29] In our experience integration of historical context into curricula is vital to produce healthcare professionals informed about the origins of Western healthcare practice, sensitive to the implications of that history, and therefore have the tools to speak out against the injustices that still exist within medicine.

In an earlier installment, Zareen Zaidi et al. consider the idea of 'normalization' within medicine and medical education.[30] This links to the examples discussed in this section as we can see how socially constructed ideas bring about an idea of what is normal, and alongside this, what is abnormal. We can see from these examples that the white perspective and experience is dominant and therefore normalized, resulting in the black perspective becoming the abnormal or othered perspective.

A detailed knowledge of the history of medicine, as would be fostered through a stronger inclusion of MH in curricula, trains a critical lens on damaging presentist and hagiographic views of our past, which remain rife through current medical education and healthcare.[31]

Literature

In contrast to the sciences, the humanities utilize qualitative data over quantitative. The investigation and analysis of written, literary evidence allows for nuanced evaluation of gray areas, otherwise missed by scientific methods. That is not to say that MH are without distinct methods or fields of study, nor are its conclusions without concrete evidence. For medical education, these methodologies not only provide valuable academic research; they also provide frameworks for understanding medicine beyond black and white scientific binaries.

In our experience, educators spending time to teach MH methodologies carefully and from the ground up equips students with the vocabulary for understanding not only patient experiences, but our own experiences and wider structural problems with medicine. For example, auto-ethnography, a research methodology based on the reflexivity of the researcher, allows medical students to study and question "the interrelationships between self and culture", moving beyond commonly used simple reflective exercises.[32(p 975)] The importance of studying language in order to improve clinical communication is discussed in depth by John Skelton in his paper, 'Language, Philosophy, and Medical Education.' In this piece, he argues that there does not exist one singular method of communication which is effective in all patient scenarios, and it is, therefore, only the awareness and knowledge to select from a range of linguist approaches that can lead to success in these scenarios.[33]

One such source for qualitative evidence is patient narratives. When considered fully, these stories allow for a richer holistic understanding of the patient experience. Studying literary examples such as Tolstoy's *The Death of Ivan Illych* and *Wit* by Margaet Edson offers medical students an opportunity to develop a diverse set of tools for analyzing and contextualizing patient narratives.[34,35] Case histories and summaries encourage students to condense the complexities of patient experience into a short, often one-minute, summary. In our experience, this results in a specific way of talking and thinking about patients and introduces the opportunity to neglect a holistic appreciation of the many ways in which illness can affect a person's life. For example, as a medical student reporting the most damaging impact of a patient's condition as the inability to walk their dog, rather than their chronic pain, could result in a disillusioned response from senior colleagues. This causes significant changes in clinical behavior over time. Students become conditioned to forget their initial enthusiasm for approaching patients as whole people and instead learn, through observing doctors, that clinical signs and symptoms are more important. In our own experience, leading with information about the patient's life and social factors when presenting a patient to a senior doctor is often met with 'but did you find out what is actually wrong with them?'. These interactions reinforce the idea that patient stories are unimportant in clinical medicine.

Rita Charon argues that narrative understanding is a key skill for healthcare professionals.[36] Medical students should develop "narrative competency"[36(p1897)] and learn to "absorb, interpret and respond to stories".[36(p1897)] Narrative belongs to the "intersubjective domains of human knowledge"[36(p1898)] and thus require two subjects: "a teller and a listener, a writer and a reader",[36(p1898)] student and teacher, doctor and patient. Hence narrative understanding leads to an enrichment of clinical communication. In contrast is the detached, 'objective' observer of "logico scientific knowledge".[36(p1898)] In this way, narrative medicine brings both the experiences of doctor and patient into view, and promotes a medical practice built around "empathy, reflection, professionalism and trustworthiness".[36(p1897)]

Philosophy and ethics

For us, the value of philosophy to medical education lies in the provision of new angles of understanding; examining existing assumptions, leading to answers for "problems no one looked for"[37(p343)] and enlightening us to new, better ways to do medicine.[37] In the same vein, addressing ontological questions, such as what medicine *is*, can provide insight and guidance to what medicine ought to be and consequently be used to shape medical education.

Phenomenology is a philosophical methodology that has had a profound effect on our clinical placements. Most recently and thoroughly explored by Havi Carel in *Phenomenology of Illness* (2016); phenomenology can be used in tandem with other humanities methodologies in its focus on the careful examination of experience as it pertains to the individual.[38] Through so doing, phenomenology explores illness as firstly a lived experience, that is distinct biomedicine focus on biological disease. For medical education, phenomenology provides a new perspective onto what illness, healthcare, and medicine mean for individual patients and necessarily promotes a pluralistic approach. We can apply this to our experience to patients with illness that lacks a clearly understood biological pathway. These include psychiatric illnesses and "medically-unexplained" syndromes like fibromyalgia. Phenomenology's emphasis on patients' lived-experience *a priori* to the biological phenomena adds validity to the illness experience of these patients and it aids understanding of these experiences for the healthcare professional.[39] Furthermore, understanding the epistemic bias of biomedicine toward disease over illness as a lived-experience can explain why these groups of patients can be side-lined in modern healthcare and often struggle to receive a diagnosis. The phenomenological approach is discussed in more depth in Veen and Rietmeijer (2021).[40]

In her paper on changing the medical curriculum, Sundeep Mishra explains that it is important to maintain medical students' orientation with the external environment, that is the one outside the world of medicine, as well as keeping us "grounded to reality".[41(p187)] Philosophy and ethics facilitate the conversations that keep medicine in perspective by questioning concepts that are otherwise taken as assumptions and accepted to be true. As students studying MH, we have explored what is meant by disease, what the purpose of medicine is - reducing pain, prolonging life, curing disease, etc. - and what the reasonable means to achieving these ends are. Even if we never arrive at a definitive answer, we have found value in navigating the grays of difficult arguments, understanding the perspectives of others, and deepening our own reflections on clinical practice.

Asking some of these big questions may seem like the opposite of keeping medicine "grounded to reality"; [41(p.187)] however, this approach provides a wide-angle lens with which to view society and allows us to assess the bigger implications of medical decisions. Medicine is affected by economics, politics, culture, media, and public opinion and in turn it has effects on these sects of society. Yet, as medical students, we can become more and more detached from the outside world as we continue our studies. With different demands than other students, different term times, more years of study, even clubs and societies exclusively for medical students, it is no wonder we risk forgetting to orientate ourselves in the external environment. It is important that we engage medical students with MH to create a group of empathetic and broad-minded future clinicians so that they might engage and propagate this understanding of medicine as inextricably grounded in society.

Two recent popular memoirs from surgeons Henry Marsh and Paul Kalannithi in *Do No Harm* (2014)[42] and *When Breath Becomes Air* (2016)[43] respectively offer a powerful insight into the challenges, possible benefits, and effect of patient objectification described by Foucault.[20,44] Resonating with our experiences, in both Marsh's and Kalanithi's work, we see patients reduced to objects-containing-disease which enable the surgeons to disconnect and carry out their work. However, this is arguably at the expense of empathy as patients are viewed as less than whole individuals.

David Rothman's *Strangers at the Bedside* details the history of medical decision making, and the subsequent rise of bioethics, in the second half of the 20th century.[45] He expertly draws out how medicine has changed and become disconnected from the world and its patients. Through the medical profession's quest for ever more knowledge and techniques it became more scientific, more specialized and less personal. Rothman's work is a poignant example of how factors outside of clinical medicine, that is to say beyond the bedside, can influence medical decision making and the patient-doctor relationship.[45] For us as medical students, understanding the history of medical ethics, rather than rote learning the principles and laws, shows what is considered to be good, or ethical, medical practice is always situated in history and, to a certain extent, dictated by the historical period. Notably, Rothman goes so far as to suggest that MH may be able to close the gap between doctor and patient that modern biomedical models and specialization opened up.[45]

When teaching and learning aspects of medicine, perhaps especially ethics, we must consider the role and importance of the hidden curriculum. Educators and students must be aware of both the advantages and disadvantages of learning within the hidden curriculum such that its potential benefits are maximized.[46] MH teaching has been found to mitigate some of these disadvantages. Jack Coulehan and Peter Williams explore how students are immunised[47(p.598)] from the negative consequences of the hidden curriculum through teaching on ethics and MH. We can confirm the findings of this paper and know the skills of reflection, critique, and empathy that are cultivated through MH allow students to sift through their experiences on placement, picking out the things they wish to emulate, and others that they hope to avoid.[48] Furthermore, reflections are enabled and promoted by MH, especially the arts by the process of "making strange".[3] This involves a novel presentation and consequentially new perspectives on our "normal", automatic, everyday behavior. For example, one can make the process of surgery strange to an experienced surgeon by presenting aspects in artwork, film, and narratives. This forces analysis and reflection upon previously unexamined biases and ideas, leading to new insights and approaches to clinical care.

Anthropology

Posited as both the most social of the sciences and the most scientific of the humanities, anthropology traverses traditional academic disciplines in both content, context, and the competencies it develops. Ethnographic data, the mainstay of research for anthropologists, shares a lot of the principles of medical research in its scope for teasing apart the human experiences of particular cultural phenomena. Ultimately, medicine is a service profession. As clinicians, our work is indelibly influenced by the nuance and variation in the human condition. An anthropological framework with which to think on medicine allows future doctors to understand the origins and implications of western biomedicine. Much unlike the rigid schema of biomedicine would have us believe, it is not the only viable method of treating disease and ill-health. For students who, ultimately, will go on to uphold the hegemony of biomedicine, it is crucial to think critically of its origins and to be open to the possibilities of alternative healing practices.

For medical students and healthcare workers alike, studying anthropology offers an insight into methodologies for better understanding how medicine is contingent on culture, and culture is contingent on medicine. Medical schools attempt to address this interplay through teaching "cultural competence", a fashionable yet nebulous subject that seeks to equip students with enough knowledge about culture in order to treat patients equitably regardless of the social determinants of health they are impacted by. Much like the manner in which MH education often involves the adoption of techniques from different fields and ill-fittingly superimposes them onto a biologically focused model of teaching, cultural competence teaching inadvertently assumes that culture is a static phenomenon that can be digested and acted upon accordingly. Clearly, as Arthur Kleinman argues in *Anthropology in the Clinic*, this is not the case.[49]

Workshops and teaching in cultural competence, in our experience, seek to highlight patients' protected characteristics yet do little to dismantle the structures through which these characteristics prevent access to appropriate care. For example, it is important to consider that the transgender male patient may have the same contraceptive requirements as a cisgender female: it is even more important to consider how this may be a dysphoric experience for our patient and devise solutions through which our healthcare systems can mitigate this harm. In our experiences, students who are members of, or allies for, the transgender community are more likely to take the time to learn about the clinical impact of being transgender. In the absence of teaching on transgender health in the curriculum, these students perform better in exams. We strongly advocate for more teaching on the barriers to healthcare that marginalized groups face, such as contraception for transgender patients. However, going beyond and teaching students the clinical guidelines and adding anthropological understandings of the structural and political barriers to healthcare. We believe this adds poignancy and an importance to these topics. On reflection, we find this results in better student engagement with this material and better student advocacy for marginalized groups.

What studying anthropology, and MH more generally, provides is a methodology through which to think on the social and cultural pressures faced by patients and clinicians alike. Anthropology has a critical role in the clinic, in its capacity to develop empathy, understanding, and humanism beyond the boundaries of traditional clinical competence.

Practical considerations

The value of a strong inclusion of MH is well demonstrated by teaching that seeks to conceptualize and promote holistic approaches. However, there are significant barriers to integration of MH which we will discuss here.

As well as the sheer breadth of content to cover, financial pressures encourage students to prioritize what they perceive to be important outcomes (for example, building a clinically-focused resume). Given that intercalation adds an additional year of study, financial planning is certainly important when considering the "worth" of exploring a new subject, particularly for students from widening participation backgrounds. The economic constraints of intercalation, by extension, impact engagement in MH. Addressing misapprehensions about the employability of students that have intercalated in MH is vital, such that students, who are capable of and want to invest their money in intercalation, know they are getting value in terms of research *and* clinical competency.

Another such area is the matter of assessment. Rather than assessments which encourage flexibility and creativity, UK medical students are repeatedly presented with multiple-choice, single-best-answer examinations in which marks are broadly reduced to correct vs. incorrect. Furthermore, theoretical frameworks from humanities and the arts can provide critiques and insights into assessment itself for medical education to improve itself.[50]

MH are more difficult to mold to a proforma through which medical schools traditionally mark their students. Written work is useful to educators in determining the accreditation of a student's degree, yet students often interpret these tasks as an extension of "tick-box exercise" medical education, whereby one must demonstrate proficiency in a particular skill in order to move onto the next phase. Students will perform what is expected of them, rather than truly engaging with the task, if the benefit is unclear or assessment unimportant.[51] This teaching model often fails to captivate potential students and, once again, demonstrates how MH teaching is often shoehorned into the predetermined methodologies and administrative structures of current medical schools. Engaging with MH teaching, and the conversations one has with peers in order to consolidate new areas or patterns of thought have been shown, through our experience, to offer equally tangible learning outcomes.

At one UK medical school, all second year students were offered a day dedicated to small group teaching around interpreting Katsushika Hokusai's woodblock print *The Great Wave off Kanagawa* (circa 1829–1833). These workshops were spread over two days for the entire cohort of students to receive teaching. On the second day, workshop attendance was low; having heard from peers that there was no register or formal assessment, many decided it was not worth their time. This particular approach - a day long workshop - falls short of captivating the interests of those who cannot immediately see the value. When MH is added *on top of*, rather than built *into* the foundations to the curriculum, students are able, and willing, to disengage provided it does not affect their grade.

In our opinion, to encourage engagement, formal assessment must embrace the gray areas of medicine without separation from the core curriculum. As such, we must avoid the urge to quantify the value of MH teaching and embrace its epistemological origins. Educators might better engage students with the process by adopting techniques nascent to the academic field they are exploring; in fully integrating the strategies of academic humanities, students are offered a more authentic experience. Furthermore, adopting these techniques through strong inclusion best demonstrates the financial worth of MH to students and institutions.

Further work

There are of course considerations we have not covered; for example, is it better to join other medical students in a learning space, or do students learn more effectively when they join courses outside of the medical department? In positing our own relatively narrow range of experiences as evidence, it is important to recognize their limitations. Each of us studies at UK universities and as such cannot account for a global student perspective on how MH are weakly or strongly integrated in curricula: we invite further reflections on this topic, particularly from those which incorporate the student voice. The student perspective provides a novel lens for considering issues in medical education as we believe students are invaluable, not just as research participants but as researchers and authors themselves. This is significantly important in issues where we see a generation gap such as racism, LGBTQ+, climate change, and technology and innovation.

Similarly, as we represent a self-selected few who have reflected on and advocated for the value of MH in our curricula, our position is biased toward its benefits. Those who have poor experiences with MH or aspersions that present a counter-argument to what we have said; those who have witnessed particularly weak or strong inclusion, those with further reflections on the academic fields we have discussed, and those within realms of study we have missed are, too, invited to submit their observations. In order to best interweave MH into curricula and begin to make sense of the gray areas of medicine we must cultivate a well-rounded debate.

Conclusion

In this piece we have provided a broad overview of just some of the domains of MH and their value in medicine and medical education from the student perspective. As former intercalators in MH, our introduction to learning from within these disciplines has given us a renewed and nuanced way of viewing every aspect of medicine.

We have discussed the strengths and shortcomings of intercalation as a stronger method of inclusion for MH. While our discussion does not aim to define a single best method for integration, we have demonstrated how MH ought to be viewed as far more than optional extras which may invoke a better bedside manner. Rather, the existence of the gray demands global MH education.

Even the most hardened humanities-sceptic medical educators cannot argue in good faith that medicine exists in a vacuum of objective, black and white, facts, separated from the grays of society, its people and their problems. For us, MH provide an opportunity to look at these gray areas, and a framework for studying them carefully. Medicine can be changed for the better by the people within it, especially when they are given the tools to analyze its shortcomings. Utilizing the student perspective allows a deeper dive not just into *what* works well in MH, but *why* it works well and how we might develop education moving forwards. Students offer novel insights which contribute meaningfully to pedagogical discussions that ultimately help to shape medical education and practice. For an institution so consistently in flux, who better to envisage its future than the students at its core?

Previous Philosophy in Medical Education Installments

Mario Veen & Anna T. Cianciolo (2020) Problems No One Looked For: Philosophical Expeditions into Medical Education, Teaching and Learning in Medicine, 32:3, 337-344, DOI: 10.1080/10401334.2020.1748634

Gert J. J. Biesta & Marije van Braak (2020) Beyond the Medical Model: Thinking Differently about Medical Education and Medical Education Research, Teaching and Learning in Medicine, 32:4, 449-456, DOI: 10.1080/10401334.2020.1798240

Mark R. Tonelli & Robyn Bluhm (2021) Teaching Medical Epistemology within an Evidence-Based Medicine Curriculum, Teaching and Learning in Medicine, 33:1, 98-105, DOI: 10.1080/10401334.2020.1835666

John R. Skelton (2021) Language, Philosophy, and Medical Education, Teaching and Learning in Medicine, 33:2, 210-216, DOI: 10.1080/10401334.2021.1877712

Zareen Zaidi, Ian M. Partman, Cynthia R. Whitehead, Ayelet Kuper & Tasha R. Wyatt (2021) Contending with Our Racial Past in Medical Education: A Foucauldian Perspective, Teaching and Learning in Medicine, DOI: 10.1080/10401334.2021.1945929

Chris Rietmeijer & Mario Veen (2021) Phenomenological Research in Health Professions Education: Tunneling from Both Ends, Teaching and Learning in Medicine, DOI: 10.1080/10401334.2021.1971989

Associated Podcast

Let Me Ask You Something (iTunes, Spotify, Google Podcasts and https://marioveen.com/letmeaskyousomething/)

Funding

The author(s) reported there is no funding associated with the work featured in this article.

ORCID

Madeleine Noelle Olding (iD) http://orcid.org/0000-0001-8020-7068
Freya Rhodes (iD) http://orcid.org/0000-0001-8630-1709
John Humm (iD) http://orcid.org/0000-0002-6888-8988
Phoebe Ross (iD) http://orcid.org/0000-0001-9021-6881
Catherine McGarry (iD) http://orcid.org/0000-0003-1338-558X

References

1. Cole TR, Carlin NS, Carson RA. *Medical Humanities: An Introduction.* New York, US: Cambridge University Press; 2015.
2. Kumagai A . Beyond "Dr. feel-good": a role for the humanities in medical Education. *Acad Med.* 2017;92(12):1659–1660. doi:10.1097/ACM.0000000000001957.
3. Kumagai AK, Wear D . "Making strange": a role for the humanities in medical education":. *Acad Med.* 2014;89(7):973–977. doi:10.1097/ACM.0000000000000269.
4. Howley L, Gaufberg E, King B. *The Fundamental Role of the Arts and Humanities in Medical Education.* Washington, DC: AAMC; 2020.
5. Bleakley A, Marshall R. Can the science of communication inform the art of the medical humanities? *Med Educ.* 2013;47(2):126–133. doi:10.1111/medu.12056.
6. McManus I, Richards P, Winder B. Intercalated degrees, learning styles, and career preferences: prospective longitudinal study of UK medical students. *BMJ.* 1999;319(7209):542–546. doi:10.1136/bmj.319.7209.542.
7. Potash J, Chen J, Tsang J. Medical student mandala making for holistic well-being. *Med Humanit.* 2016;42(1):17–25. doi:10.1136/medhum-2015-010717.
8. Olding M, Moore J. Society, sexuality, and medicine in Hogarth's Marriage A-la-Mode. *Br J Gen Pract.* 2019;69(681):192–193. doi:10.3399/bjgp19X701969.
9. Millard C. Using personal experience in the academic medical humanities: a genealogy. *Soc Theory Health.* 2020;18(2):184–198. doi:10.1057/s41285-019-00089-x.
10. Biesta G, van Braak M. Beyond the medical model: thinking differently about medical education and medical education research. *Teach Learn Med.* 2020;32(4):449–456. doi:10.1080/10401334.2020.1798240.
11. Liu Y, Erath A, Salwi S, Sherry A, Mitchell MB. Alignment of ethics curricula in medical education: a student perspective. *Teach Learn Med.* 2020;32(3):345–351. doi:10.1080/10401334.2020.1717959.
12. Gonzalo JD, Davis C, Thompson BM, Haidet P . Unpacking medical students' mixed engagement in health systems science education. *Teach Learn Med.* 2020;32(3):250–258. doi:10.1080/10401334.2019.1704765.
13. Birden H, Usherwood T . "They liked it if you said you cried": how medical students perceive the teaching of professionalism. *Med J Aust.* 2013;199(6):406–409. doi:10.5694/mja12.11827.
14. UCL Medical School. iBSc Statistics. University College London. https://www.ucl.ac.uk/medical-school/sites/medical-school/files/allocation_figures_last_three_years.pdf. Updated 2021. Accessed March 15, 2021.
15. Jones M, Hutt P, Eastwood S, Singh S. Impact of an intercalated BSc on medical student performance and careers: A BEME systematic review: BEME Guide No. 28. *Med Teach.* 2013;35(10):e1493–e1510. doi:10.3109/0142159X.2013.806983.
16. Agha R, Fowler A, Whitehurst K, Rajmohan S, Gundogan B, Koshy K. Why apply for an intercalated research degree? *Int J Surg Oncol (N Y)).* 2017;2(6):e27 doi:10.1097/IJ9.0000000000000027.
17. Agha R, Howell S. Intercalated BSc degrees – Why do students do them? *Clinical Teacher.* 2005;2(2):72–76. doi:10.1111/j.1743-498X.2005.00059.x.
18. Jamall O, Iqbal S, Rizvi A, Nayeem O, Rashid S, Khan A. When should undergraduate medical students do an intercalated BSc? *Med Educ Online.* 2015;20(1):30599 doi:10.3402/meo.v20.30599.
19. Pfeiffer S, Chen Y, Tsai D. Progress integrating medical humanities into medical education: a global overview.

Curr Opin Psychiatry. 2016;29(5):298–301. doi:10.1097/YCO.0000000000000265.

20. Foucault M. *The birth of the clinic.* 3rd ed. London, UK: Routledge; 2003.

21. Baron R. An introduction to medical phenomenology: I can't hear you while I'm listening. *Ann Intern Med.* 1985;103(4):606–611. doi:10.7326/0003-4819-103-4-606.

22. Jones DS, Greene JA, Duffin J, Harley Warner J. Making the case for history in medical education. *J Hist Med Allied Sci.* 2015;70(4):623–652. 2015doi:10.1093/jhmas/jru026.

23. Centers for Disease Control and Prevention. U.S. Public Health Service Syphilis Study at Tuskegee. U.S. Department of Health & Human Services. https://www.cdc.gov/tuskegee/timeline.htm. Updated March 02, 2020. Accessed January 28 2021.

24. Shavers V, Lynch C, Burmeister L. Knowledge of the Tuskegee study and its impact of willingness to participate in medical research studies. *J Natl Med Assoc.* 2000;92(12):563–572. PMID: 11202759.

25. Corbie-Smith G. The continuing legacy of the Tuskegee syphilis study: considerations for clinical investigation. *Am J Med Sci.* 1999;317 (1):5–8. doi:10.1016/S0002-9629(15)40464-1.

26. MacKenna B, Curtis H, Morton C, Inglesby P, Walker A, Morley J. Trends, regional variation, and clinical characteristics of COVID-19 vaccine recipients: a retrospective cohort study in 23.4 million patients using OpenSAFELY. https://www.medrxiv.org/content/10.1101/2021.01.25.21250356v2. Updated January 27, 2021. Accessed February 14, 2021.

27. Reverby S. More than fact and fiction: Cultural memory and the Tuskegee syphilis study. *Hastings Cent Rep.* 2001;31(5):22–28. doi:10.2307/3527701.

28. Khunti K, Platt L, Routen A, Abbasi K. Covid-19 and ethnic minorities: an urgent agenda for overdue action. *BMJ.* 2020;369:m2503. doi:10.1136/bmj.m2503.

29. Cooter R, Stein C. *Writing History in the Age of Biomedicine.* 1st ed. New Haven; USA: Yale University Press; 2013.

30. Zaidi Z, Partman I, Whitehead C, Kuper A, Wyatt T. Contending with our racial past in medical education: a foucauldian perspective. *Teach Learn Med.* 2021;33(4):453–462. doi: 10.1080/104014.2021.1945929

31. Ojanuga D . The medical ethics of the 'father of gynaecology', Dr J Marion Sims. *J Med Ethics.* 1993;19(1):28–31. doi:10.1136/jme.19.1.28.

32. Farrell L, Bourgeois-Law G, Regehr G, Ajjawi R . Autoethnography: introducing 'I' into medical education research. *Med Educ.* 2015; 49(10):974–982. doi:10.1111/medu.12761.

33. Skelton J. Language, philosophy, and medical education. *Teach Learn Med.* 2021;33(2):210–216. doi:10.1080/10401334.2021.1877712.

34. Tolstoy L. *The Death of Ivan Ilych and Other Stories.* London, UK: Wordsworth Editions; 2004.

35. Edson M. *Wit.* 1st ed. New York, US: Faber and Faber; 2007.

36. Charon R . The patient-physician relationship. Narrative medicine: a model for empathy, reflection, profession, and trust. *JAMA.* 2001;286(15):1897–1902. doi:10.1001/jama.286.15.1897.

37. Veen M, Cianciolo A. Problems no one looked for: philosophical expeditions into medical education. *Teach Learn Med.* 2020;32(3):337–344. doi:10.1080/10401334.2020.1748634.

38. Tonelli MR, Bluhm R. Teaching medical epistemology within an evidence-based medicine curriculum. *Teach Learn Med.* 2021 Jan-Mar;33(1):98–105. 2020doi:10.1080/10401334.2020.1835666.

39. Carel H. *Phenomenology of Illness.* 1st ed. Oxford, UK: Oxford University Press; 2016.

40. Veen M, Rietmeijer C. Phenomenological research in health professions education: tunneling from both ends. *Teach Learn Med.* 2021.

41. Mishra S. Do we need to change the medical curriculum: regarding the pain of others. *Indian Heart J.* 2015;67(3):187–191. doi:10.1016/j.ihj.2015.05.015.

42. Marsh H. *Do No Harm.* 1st ed. London, UK: Orion Publishing Co; 2015.

43. Kalanithi P. *When Breath Becomes Air.* 1st ed. London, UK: Random House; 2016.

44. Foucault M. *Madness and Civilization.* London, UK: Routledge. 2008.

45. Rothman D. *Strangers at the Bedside.* 3rd ed. New York, US: Routledge; 2017.

46. Ozolins I, Hall H, Peterson R. The student voice: recognising the hidden and informal curriculum in medicine. *Med Teach.* 2008;30(6):606–611. doi:10.1080/01421590801949933.

47. Coulehan J, Williams P. Vanquishing virtue: the impact of medical education. *Acad Med.* 2001;76(6):598–605. doi:10.1097/00001888-200106000-00008.

48. Mahood S. Medical education. Beware the hidden curriculum. *Can Fam Physician.* 2011;57(9):983–985. PMID: 21918135.

49. Kleinman A, Benson P. Anthropology in the clinic: The problem of cultural competency and how to fix it. *PLoS Med.* 2006;3(10):e294 doi:10.1371/journal.pmed.0030294.

50. Gormley GJ, Johnston JL, Cullen KM, Corrigan M. Scenes, symbols and social roles: raising the curtain on OSCE performances. *Perspect Med Educ.* 2021;10(1):14–22. doi:10.1007/s40037-020-00593-1.

51. de la Croix A, Veen M. The reflective zombie: problematizing the conceptual framework of reflection in medical education. *Perspect Med Educ.* 2018;7(6):394–400. doi:10.1007/s40037-018-0479-9.

Because We Care: A Philosophical Investigation into the Spirit of Medical Education

Camillo Coccia ⓘ and Mario Veen ⓘ

ABSTRACT

Issue: Although in health care education we encounter the word care at every turn, the concept is hardly ever defined or subjected to scrutiny. Care is a foundational concept of health care education, and if we do not take control of our basic concepts, their meaning can be subject to other influences. We take a philosophical approach to care and ask what care *is*, to connect different conceptions of care in health care education to their common root. We do this by first examining how the concept is used in health care education, how it features in Martin Heidegger's *Being and Time*, and finally, how these philosophical implications may be applied to medical education. *Evidence*: The use of care in medical education suggests that it is foundational to understanding health care education. However, presently the concept is ambiguous and risks being a 'container concept' that becomes meaningless because it is used generally. In publications that feature the concept, it is usually in service of another aspect that is under investigation, and not care itself. For instance, publications on teaching patient-centred care focus on the meaning of 'patient-centeredness' rather than care. In 'health care', there are debates about what 'health' means, but not care. The concept is also used in different and sometimes contradictory meanings: care as the organizational structure of health care that safeguards (health *care* system), care as empathy or careful attention of medical trainees for patients (caring about one's patients, treating them carefully), and, finally, care as motivation and focus toward a goal (caring about graduating, making a contribution). We turn to the philosophy of Heidegger to integrate these different appearances of care into a unified structure. Heidegger's *Being and Time* describes care as the basic ontological structure of human existence. This turns out to be a structure of *time*: in the familiar structure of past present and future. Anticipating a future end, which determines our attitude toward the people, objects, and physical structures we are with now, and in the light of which we orient ourselves to what is already there. *Implications*: By describing the ontological (foundational) structure of care, we argue that care is the spirit of health care education. This unifying structure can be used to integrate phenomena that are recognized as important in health care education but are usually seen as separate. We use an example to illustrate how empathy, health protocols, and educational goals can be connected in one situation. Just as *health* provides a framework for patient management, *care* can provide this framework for education. This fundamental concept of care can be used in practice for reflection on anticipated ends in situations in which different modes of care seemingly conflict. Beyond our focus on care, we also illustrate how one can take an important concept in health care education and use philosophy to root it in a foundational understanding of that concept.

Introduction

In our daily experiences with health care education, care is a theme that arises constantly. Trainees are educated within a health care system where they are

supposed to care about and for their patients. To enroll in this education, we demand that they are sufficiently motivated to, that is, care about becoming competent health care professionals, to put in years of dedicated training. The many instances of 'care' in our professional lives as a community of educators, students, and health care professionals may lead us to believe we know exactly what 'care' means. But that which is closest to us and all around us is often most difficult to define. In this paper, we will try to go beyond particular instances of care to ask a philosophical question: What *is* care?

The concept of 'health' is widely discussed in medicine. What *is* health and what *is* illness? For instance, the WHO's definition of health states: "Health is a state of complete physical, mental and social well-being and not merely the absence of disease or infirmity."[1] This definition is subject to ongoing debate and many medical curricula include it as part of medical training. These take the form of programs where trainees examine definitions of health and wellness, and what it means to make distinctions between disease and illness, where one should draw the line between being healthy and unhealthy, what counts as evidence in which case, how to deal with uncertainty.[2–4]

A similar debate is lacking when it comes to care. While the need for detailed investigation is articulated,[5] there is little addressing what care *is*. The literature tends to focus on particular themes like compassion, patient-centred care, caring relationships, professionalism and how to show due consideration to others to explore how compassion relates to ethical behavior.[6–9] While these are crucial themes to explore and investigate, these approaches presuppose that the underlying principle of care is already understood, and only needs proper application. But while we agree that everyone has an 'everyday' understanding of care, which may seem so obvious that it does not warrant making explicit, we argue it is necessary to make this tacit understanding of care explicit. A central insight from Immanuel Kant's philosophy is that the concepts through which we experience and reflect on our practices are often not objects of experience and reflection.[10] These are concepts that shape our practices but are themselves not usually subject to investigation.

We argue that care can best be seen as the *spirit* of health care education. If health care education is a cake, care is not just one of its ingredients, but the laws of chemistry that guide the baking process. It permeates everything else that happens there; it is essential rather than peripheral, and therefore a fundamental concept. The question of what unites these different and legitimate meanings is not a theoretical question, but an ontological philosophical question. Since we all have a pre-reflective, embodied understanding of care, care is not something we have to 'learn' and then 'apply'. But to authentically understand what care means we have to make this pre-reflective understanding explicit, which is the task of phenomenology.[11]

If we do not take ownership of our fundamental concepts, they can be subject to political and economic interests, or whatever our cultural beliefs and habits happen to be. In this paper we treat care as a traveling concept that is flexible and open to change.[12,13] To be clear, our intention is not to define care finally, but rather to draw attention to care as something that should be subject to reflection. In order to do this, we need to also develop new modes of understanding a variety of philosophical avenues of inquiry in order to fully address foundational concepts like care.

Widely recognized as one of the major philosophical works of the 20th century, *Being and Time*[14] was central to the development of phenomenology and existentialism. The work focuses on the question of being, particularly of human being. Though it was published in 1927 and we need to acknowledge its author's later problematic personal and political choices in fascist Germany,[15] the work warrants further exploration if only because Heidegger concludes that care is the ontological structure of human existence. In the following, we will explore how the meaning of care as it occurs in the reality of health care education can be opened up for deeper reflection by examining it from the perspective of Heidegger's concept of care.

We will draw on Heidegger's ontological method[14] to relate the everyday use of care to its deeper meaning. Heidegger's philosophy, while highly influential, is notoriously difficult. We will limit ourselves to only one 'Heideggerian' notion: the difference between the ontic and the ontological. 'Ontic' (literally: being) refers to concrete, factual existence, while 'ontological' (literally: study of being) refers to the being of that being with due attention to its relations to other beings. For instance, ontically I may be alone in a room, while ontologically I am an inherently social being. *As this concrete, particular being* I may be either alone or with others, and might describe myself as having a more social or more introverted person. But ontologically, being-with-others is always at the heart of our being, no matter what else we do in life. For instance, avoiding the company of others is relating to others but in a negative way. While I remain ontically alone, I am still relating to others ontologically. In *Being and Time*,[14] Heidegger showed that doing ontology, in the sense of examining ways of being, can yield a more conscious and free relationship to beings ontically. Thus our analysis of ontic care in health care education in relation to ontological care will not tell us what to do, or which type of care is best, but rather open up the concept to a deeper reflection and exploration.

In philosophical terms, we will attempt to relate the *ontic* meaning of care with its *ontological* meaning. First, we will examine the meaning that care already has in the way that it is being used in health care education. From this analysis emerge some clashes between its different meanings, which we illustrate with a working example. Then, we will investigate Heidegger's perspective of existential analytic on Care and ask how it can shed light on how 'care' is used in health care education today. Finally, we will attempt to show that an examination of health care education in terms of care reveals that becoming a doctor is not a mechanical, formulaic process but rather an immersive and reflective one.

The everyday meaning of care

Care in everyday life

In everyday life, the word 'care' conjures up images of a mother nursing a child, or memories of ourselves being nurtured by our loved ones when we are sick. Tenderness and intimacy are commonplace in advertising as representations of care. These are often representations of something important to us, igniting the catchphrase: "Because we Care". On a larger scale, we find a less intimate and more assertive version of care, in the sense of protection against harm. We may view care as advocacy: those who are unable to have a voice may be supported and spoken for by those who can. But this meaning also indicates importance: one defends, protects or advocates for that which one cares about.[16] In a more neutral sense, care is also used to imply the provision of whatever is necessary on a personal or institutional level (daycare, financial care, veteran care, legal care), or even on an (inter) national level, of which health care is a prime example.

Care in health care education

In health care education we can find variations on everyday meanings of care. This is logical as health care education is itself part of a 'care system' that concerns itself with providing training that forms willing and able prospective physicians into competent medical professionals. Health care professionals work within a system that requires them to ask a system to distribute medical funding toward their patients.

Within this system, people have access to a collective body of knowledge about how to care for health, and the skills to apply this knowledge in practice, in the sense of the Hippocratic Oath: "I will follow that system of regimen which, according to my ability and judgment, I consider for the benefit of my patients, and abstain from whatever is deleterious and mischievous."[17]

Care as protection has a multitude of practical ways of showing itself. We may think of safety mechanisms and ethical boundaries which protect patients from overzealous doctors, and of institutional protocols that guide doctors toward safer methods when they deal with situations with which they are unfamiliar. We can imagine this as care in the way that what matters to the treating physician is the well-being of their patient. As they care about their patient's well-being, they protect them against harm (firstly against the harm they themselves could do by making a medical or ethical mistake), and nurse them, that is, give them the medical attention they need to alleviate what ails them. In the same way, we can think about the structure of health care education, where educational professionals are expected to care for and about medical trainees by setting up a system that provides them with what they need to become competent professionals.

There are other ways in which care is addressed in health care education. The first is expressed by the concept of 'patient-centred care'. Why would this concept exist if there were no alternatives for what to center care around? The fact that the concept of patient-centred care exists implies that it is not a given that the patient's health needs and wishes drive health care. By agendizing patient-centeredness in relation to care, the word care emerges as pointing to what is important. Institutions can have this in their mottos to indicate that it is what they care about. In this sense, care is also a commitment: if one cares about someone or something, this is a promise that one will take care of their needs.

Care is also addressed in discussing reflection in health care education. It is a concept that is closely related to protection: reflective practitioners are lifelong learners who examine their past experiences and mistakes in the present in order to inform their actions in the future.[18]

The meaning of care as importance is closely related to care as intimacy: we can imagine waiting rooms of hospitals with families waiting for news on loved ones' medical conditions. In listening to a patient presentation, or delivering bad news, or in any other interaction with patients and their families, doctors have been taught not to just apply their medical knowledge to diseased bodies, but to care about the patient as a human being. This is discussed in health care education literature under headings such as empathy or compassion, and the concept of professionalism is also included. Care, in this sense, is often described as an emotion or an attitude,[6] and conceptualized as a cognitive process within individual trainees. There are discussions about whether we can reasonably expect trainees to care about every patient an intimate way, or if it is too exhausting and perhaps even impossible to expect that they would care about people who are different from them in some respect to the point where it is difficult for them to imagine what something is like for the other person. There are also debates on whether, in addition to the technical and empirically verifiable use of care outlined above, care as intimacy can be subjected to the same types of measurement as the quality and effectiveness of, for instance, emergency care protocols or educational programs.[19-21] For instance, trainees report a feeling of dissonance when they are expected to say "I'm sorry to hear that" when they do not authentically experience empathy.[22]

In addition to empathy with other people, care as emotion and importance (what matters to a person) are also linked in studies under the header of motivation. Studies about motivation examine what factors indicate whether a medical student is *motivated*,[23] and distinguish between intrinsic and external motivation.[24] The goal is to distinguish what is required for a trainee to, for instance, study health protocols or do other things that are necessary to become competent. Do they already care about this enough, or should they be made to care, for instance, by coupling tests to assessment? In relation to reflection and empathy it has been said that the culture of examination may clash with the culture of reflection[20] and empathy[21], which can be rephrased as a clash between two meanings of care: care as anticipation versus care as emotion. Opponents of psychometric assessment of phenomena like empathy and reflection argue that assessment brings out performances of behavior that is associated with them, but demanding performance interferes with the authentic and emotional experience of caring that makes it valuable. Proponents counter that if we would no longer assess these competencies, trainees might not care enough to learn them.

In these meanings, the temporal aspect of care becomes visible: care as anticipation, but also of awareness of the past and present. The family members in the hospital waiting room are worried *in anticipation* of what news they might receive.

Reflective practitioners analyze their past actions in the present, *in order to* learn from it in future situations. Empathy in communication has a lot to do with anticipating what another person might feel if one were to say this, or what one should say in order to elicit this response that would provide one with medically relevant information about a patient. But it can also be a sign of care if one remembers the personal details that a patient shared in a previous consultation.

Caring in practice

So far we have focused on the plurality of meanings associated with the word 'care' in health care education, and how a few common qualities bind different modes of caring. The risk with such a broad analysis is that the word becomes a container concept that can be taken to mean anything and thereby loses its conceptual power. This does not mean that we should all mean exactly the same thing by a concept, but that there is enough intersubjectivity to "meaningfully disagree".[12(p. 13)] Concepts can become more clearly distinguished in a concrete situation in which its different meanings can be seen to clash. We will now look at a practical example and examine how this example looks in the light of the everyday meaning of care.

Imagine a junior resident in internal medicine has seen a patient after-hours as a referral from the ER. Upon admission, the resident notices a blood test is required as a routine investigation prior to admission. Upon consulting with the patient, the resident notices that multiple attempts had been made to draw blood and that the patient's arms were bruised, making the patient restless and uncomfortable. On the morning ward round the attending requests the blood results and, naturally, the resident is at a loss. The attending at this point is annoyed that no decision can be made without the results of a blood test. It also may seem to the attending that the resident did not care to do the blood tests at all.

There are a multitude of elements at work in this example. Care in the intimate sense of not wanting to do harm to someone that one feels compassion for may be conflicted with the safeguarding of the patient's well-being. Anticipation is also at work here. The resident does not actually attempt to draw blood but worries that even confronting the patient with the question may bring about an unpleasant environment or that she somehow would undermine their trust.

Paradoxically, care shows itself even in what is perceived by the attending as carelessness. We can understand the residents' care about the patient's well-being, as well as the attending's view of the resident not following protocols. They might be annoyed that the resident did not see the importance of the routine blood tests for the decision that was to be made on the morning round and that a delay in decision-making may affect the health of the patient. From another perspective, however, we see that the resident did care. The resident cared that the patient may feel upset and experience physical pain for what the resident sees as a minor procedure. It might be seen as a way of caring that the resident prioritized these concerns over procedural demands.

Three objects of care are competing for realization within the resident's decision as well as the attending's assessment of the situation: the role of the resident as a trainee who is assessed and not yet entrusted fully with patient care, as a health care professional who treats patients, and as an employee of the hospital who is expected to follow protocols. From the perspective of patient-centered care, the resident may be seen as fully caring. From the perspective of an employee, her actions conflict with the care structure that all employees are supposed to follow in the hospital. From the perspective of being a trainee, the attending may see the resident as failing at having learned something that they are supposed to learn.

Care is so fundamental that it is impossible to imagine the example without the resident caring about *something*. Whether that *something* is the junior doctor's career, the hospital's protocols, financial benefits or moral integrity, care is present. Since even in encounters with carelessness, care is always at work, the question is not '*do they care?*', but 'what form has care taken in this particular case?' The fundamental relationship of care to health care education is why we argue that care is not just a practical, educational or psychological matter, but a deeply philosophical one.

Philosophical encounters with care

In *Being and Time*,[14] Heidegger writes from the beginning of the 20th Century during an explosion of knowledge in the modern world. During this time, Heidegger asks philosophy to return to the most fundamental question: what does it mean to be? In contrast to earlier philosophers, he does not approach human beings as isolated entities, but as beings that are completely immersed in daily life with all its befuddlements, ambivalence, joys, and difficulties. In this setting a person may ask, "what am I doing here?" Heidegger's response is care. Heidegger does not see care as an attitude or technique but as a response to the question: "What does it mean *to be?*"

From the perspective of *Being and Time*, all our daily activities are structured around care. In this context, health is only one of the objects of care that human beings are concerned with: we care for our health not for its own sake, but because we want to feel well, to spend time with our family, to live a long life, to be able to work and put a roof over our heads, and so on. Being healthy allows us to direct our attention to other matters such as work, family, or living a long life. For Heidegger, health care is about postponing death. It is precisely because we are mortal that care exists. Put differently, in health care education, the most fundamental of these three terms is care. Both the reason that hospitals exist and that the resident in our example feels guilt and resignation at her apparent failure indicate care at their origin.

We can see in simple examples there is always an underlying direction to which these needs align. Heidegger identifies this with the structure of time. One might need something now in the present, but it is only because we imagine a future arising from the current state of affairs. Heidegger introduces his idea of care with three elements that are intertwined with time: past present and future, which he calls already-there, being-with and not-yet.

Already-there: "into this house we're born. Into this world we're thrown" – the doors 1967

Heidegger primarily acknowledges the fact that we arrive in a world which has been in existence long before us. The resident is in a hospital that was already there before they started medical training. A multitude of systems and equipment serve to assist them in doing their duty. Even the simple act of taking a routine blood sample is contingent on a coordinated structure of global manufacturing supply chains, stock ordering, and management, training in clinical skills etc. In medical training, the resident is 'thrown' into a world that was already there and has been constructed because care is already present.

Being-with: "the environment of the human being is fellow human being." – Jules Deelder

Our resident encounters the patient primarily as someone who is scared, vulnerable, and perhaps overwhelmed. Their attention is drawn away from the practical reason that brought them to hospital (both in the sense of a reason for the visit that was already there and the future goal that needs to be accomplished) and instead to something else in the present. At this moment, the patient is no longer simply an object for investigation but a human being whose presence demands good communication, openness, and for the resident to acknowledge them as a person. This appeal is the beginning of forming a relationship which colors the resident's attitude or mood toward everything else. For instance, in light of the patient's appeal to her humanity, the resident may be annoyed that they cannot follow the procedure they need to but are bound to the processes of her department or supervisor.

The resident's situation is not a collection of things that are merely objectively *present* (the patient, the syringe, the room they are in). It is a constellation of elements that the resident is *with in* a particular way. In our example, the resident's relationship with the situation is frustration as a response to the conflict of two competing objects of care. It is not any distinct individual element that is frustrating. Everything occurs in the light of being frustrated, just as a person who is in love or bored experiences everything in the light of being in love or of boredom.

Not-yet: "the future enters us, to change itself in us, long before it happens." Rilke, letters to a young poet, letter 10

The final dimension of care is the most important for Heidegger. Even though all three are one unity, this is the one that gives care its meaning and direction. The reason the resident is sitting there in the first place, *being with* a patient within a structure that was *already there*, is that they are in medical training: they want to become a physician. In our example, the attending may point out that this routine blood sample is important to do for patient safety but most importantly it is crucial that the resident understands why the test is important for her own professional growth.

In this example, we see these anticipatory facets at work. The patient must be protected from the possibility of harm and the resident must learn the importance of these routine tests for them to show her growth and learning. The conflict arises when the resident is concerned and scared of hurting the patient for what may possibly be an unnecessary test. This conflict is between possible events, not actual events, and yet they decisively shape the situation.

For Heidegger, this is the crux of the matter. The medical trainee is not yet a doctor but is in the process of becoming one. This asks a medical trainee to reflect on what is significant to them and how they see themselves being in the future. The resident in this example is ambivalent: she cares about the suffering her patient will experience but also cares what her attending will think of her and the effect this may have on her assessment. In this conflict of objects of care it is obvious that the resident is confronted by a difficult choice. In fact, this conflict cuts to the very core of the different commitments a doctor makes to their patients. It brings into view the need to closely examine what these objects of care really are and how they function. This is where we discover that a fundamental focus of education is helping trainees identify and comprehend the important considerations when navigating these difficulties in clinical or ethical decision-making.

How can philosophy help us navigate these complicated conflicts? Care in *Being and Time* can be described as follows: anticipating an end that shapes our attitude to being with others, things, and equipment, that illuminate our current moment. This is not a technical model that we utilize for maximizing effectiveness of our teaching programmes but a reflective paradigm that can help us bring the human elements of health care education into full focus.

Implications: Care in medical education

In our philosophical analysis of care in health care education, we have attempted to explore how the concept of Care as it appears in *Being and Time* can open up a deep reflection on care as the spirit of health care education. We have consciously limited ourselves to *one* concept in *one* philosophical work to explore this, rather than, taking 'the philosopher Heidegger' or a comparison of different philosophical perspectives as a starting point.

For further avenues of exploration, we could look at other interpretations of care beyond *Being and Time*. Heidegger himself further developed his philosophy after this work; for instance, the *Zollikon Seminars*[25] is a series of lectures he gave for medical professionals. But there are other philosophers who critically built on Heidegger's existential analytic who could be used to point us to neglected modes of care in health care education. Levinas places emphasis on the Other in acting compassionately in the ethical encounters of life.[26] Foucault, who named Heidegger and Nietzsche as his two major influences, showed that 'ontically', care is never neutral but it happens in a network of power/knowledge relations.[27] Following De Beauvoir's work,[28] health care education's sexist past could be seen as highlighting a mode of care that privileges some over others. While caring was seen as the duty of a woman, the work of nursing was seen to be the work of caring, the duty of the (presumably male) doctor was seen as a cold detached and scientific understanding of disease. We argue that both of these are modes of care and thus should be expected of all health care professionals, regardless of role or gender. Finally, Stiegler points us to the fact that technology is also a mode of care, but that its double-sided nature can also threaten care.[29,30]

We reflect on our choice to stay within the boundaries of *Being and Time*. The purpose of the series in which this paper appears is to explore how philosophy can be helpful for health care education. Previous installments have explored how the work of a philosopher[31] or even an entire philosophical tradition[11] or philosophical field[4] can elucidate an issue as a whole.

If we examine care as an ethic, we find it already present in health care education literature. The models of health care education currently view making a medical student by adding together anatomy, physiology, pharmacology clinical skills and ensure that the doctor knows how to apply these in a caring manner. However, while we are trying to teach empathy, medical students are becoming less empathetic through their education.[32] But if, ontologically, care is ubiquitous, the question changes from "why do students care less?" to "why are students taught to privilege one mode of care over others?"

The practical value of understanding care on an ontological level emerges through reflective learning. While reflection is a slippery subject,[33] the goal of reflection is to expand learning and to better understand a work environment. Of course, we want medical students to reflect on the material circumstances of the patients' medical condition, their general physical health, and the nature of the causal agents that brought the patient to where they are today. But in doing this they must also notice the facial expression or the pointed silence which can invite questions like "what does this diagnosis mean for me?"

Heidegger draws this into the domain of philosophical enquiry as it is the practicalities of everyday life that prevent us asking difficult questions about our existence. However, Heidegger also notices that these practical distractions are always directed at some deeper structure of care. For instance, I might well be putting up an IV line as part of my checklist, but I am also playing a role in a patient's first dose of chemotherapy. The aim of a care-based analytic is to be able to bring to light the underlying temporal structure of these everyday technical processes. These underlying structures are not necessarily causal agents but are rather the commitments that underlie the being of a Health Care Professional. If we were to continue to look at the ontic manifestations of care, we might only be able to judge whether a HCP acted correctly or incorrectly in a given situation. But if can look beyond these manifestations of care we see that the underlying structure is completely open for philosophical investigation.

Our claim is that a reflective practitioner ought to do both. They should be able to pause and reflect on whether an investigation is appropriate or whether some more attention should be paid to better understanding pathology or treatment modalities. However, they should also be able to investigate how these technical processes are ultimately aimed at the various commitments that constitute being a doctor. We argue that this is the place of philosophy in health care education, not to teach categorical determinations of what action should or should not be taken, but rather to help us to ask the right questions. Ultimately this is the challenge to health care education. Are we able to look past the technical processes of education and teaching and start asking: What does it mean to be a doctor?

Previous Philosophy in Medical Education Installments

Mario Veen & Anna T. Cianciolo (2020) Problems No One Looked For: Philosophical Expeditions into Medical Education, Teaching and Learning in Medicine, 32:3, 337-344, DOI: 10.1080/10401334.2020.1748634

Gert J. J. Biesta & Marije van Braak (2020) Beyond the Medical Model: Thinking Differently about Medical Education and Medical Education Research, Teaching and Learning in Medicine, 32:4, 449-456, DOI: 10.1080/10401334.2020.1798240

Mark R. Tonelli & Robyn Bluhm (2021) Teaching Medical Epistemology within an Evidence-Based Medicine Curriculum, Teaching and Learning in Medicine, 33:1, 98-105, DOI: 10.1080/10401334.2020.1835666

John R. Skelton (2021) Language, Philosophy, and Medical Education, Teaching and Learning in Medicine, 33:2, 210-216, DOI: 10.1080/10401334.2021.1877712

Zareen Zaidi, Ian M. Partman, Cynthia R. Whitehead, Ayelet Kuper & Tasha R. Wyatt (2021) Contending with Our Racial Past in Medical Education: A Foucauldian Perspective, Teaching and Learning in Medicine, DOI: 10.1080/10401334.2021.1945929

Chris Rietmeijer & Mario Veen (2021) Phenomenological Research in Health Professions Education: Tunneling from Both Ends, Teaching and

Learning in Medicine, DOI: 10.1080/10401334. 2021.1971989

Madeleine Noelle Olding, Freya Rhodes, John Humm, Phoebe Ross & Catherine McGarry (2022) Black, White and Gray: Student Perspectives on Medical Humanities and Medical Education, Teaching and Learning in Medicine, 34:2, 223-233, DOI: 10.1080/10401334.2021.1982717

Associated Podcast

Let Me Ask You Something (iTunes, Spotify, Google Podcasts and https://marioveen.com/letmeaskyou something/)

Funding

The author(s) reported there is no funding associated with the work featured in this article.

ORCID

Camillo Coccia (iD) http://orcid.org/0000-0002-0687-6703
Mario Veen (iD) http://orcid.org/0000-0003-2550-7193

References

1. Davids T. 2021. Constitution of the World Health Organisation. Retrieved 10 August, 2021, from WHO website: https://www.who.int/about/governance/constitution.
2. Anjum RL, Copeland S, Rocca E. Introduction: why is philosophy relevant for clinical practice?. In: Anjum RL, Copeland S, Rocca E, editors. *Rethinking Causality, Complexity and Evidence for the Unique Patient: A CauseHealth Resource for Healthcare Professionals and the Clinical Encounter.* Cham: Springer International Publishing; 2020, p. 3–11.
3. Tonelli MR, Upshur REG. A philosophical approach to addressing uncertainty in medical education. *Acad Med.* 2019;94(4):507–511. doi:10.1097/ACM.0000000000002512.
4. Tonelli MR, Bluhm R. Teaching medical epistemology within an evidence-based medicine curriculum. *Teach Learn Med.* 2021;33(1):98–105. doi:10.1080/10401334. 2020.1835666.
5. Veen M. Wrestling with (in)authenticity. *Perspect Med Educ.* 2021;10(3):141–144. doi:10.1007/s40037-021-00656-x. Epub 2021 Mar 16. PMID: 33725315; PMCID: PMC8187704.
6. Gelhaus P. The desired moral attitude of the physician: (III) care. *Med Health Care Philos.* 2013;16(2):125–139. doi:10.1007/s11019-012-9380-1.
7. Laughey WF, Brown MEL, Dueñas AN, et al. How medical school alters empathy: student love and break up letters to empathy for patients. *Med Educ.* 2021;55(3): 394–403. doi:10.1111/medu.14403.
8. Sinclair S, Norris JM, McConnell SJ, et al. Compassion: a scoping review of the healthcare literature. *BMC Palliat Care.* 2016;15:6. doi:10.1186/s12904-016-0080-0.

9. Zaidi Z, Razack S, Kumagai AK. Professionalism revisited during the pandemics of our time: COVID-19 and racism. *Perspect Med Educ.* 2021;10(4):238–244. doi:10.1007/s40037-021-00657-w. Epub 2021 Mar 18. PMID: 33738767; PMCID: PMC7971352.
10. Kant I. *Critique of Pure Reason.* Rev. ed. New York: Colonial Press; 1899.
11. Rietmeijer CBT, Veen M. Phenomenological research in health professions education: tunneling from both ends. *Teach Learn Med.* 2022;34(1):113–121. doi:10.1 080/10401334.2021.1971989.
12. Bal M. *Travelling Concepts in the Humanities: A Rough Guide.* Toronto: University of Toronto Press; 2002, p. xvi, 369p.
13. Veen M, van der Tuin I. When I say… travelling concepts. *Med Educ.* 2021;55(2):146–147. doi:10.1111/medu.14400.
14. Heidegger M. *Being and Time.* London: SCM Press; 1927, p. 1962.
15. Safranski R. *Martin Heidegger: Between Good and Evil.* Harvard: Harvard University Press; 2011.
16. Tomkins L, Eatough V. Meanings and manifestations of care: a celebration of hermeneutic multiplicity in Heidegger. *Human Psychol.* 2013;41 (1):4–24. doi:10.1 080/08873267.2012.694123.
17. Askitopoulou H, Vgontzas AN. The relevance of the Hippocratic Oath to the ethical and moral values of contemporary medicine. Part I: the Hippocratic Oath from antiquity to modern times. *Eur Spine J.* 2018;27(7):1481–1490. doi:10.1007/s00586-017-5348-4.
18. Sandars J. The use of reflection in medical education: AMEE Guide No. 44. *Med Teach.* 2009;31(8):685–695. doi:10.1080/01421590903050374.
19. Muller JZ. *The Tyranny of Metrics.* First paperback edition. ed. Princeton: Princeton University Press; 2019, p. xxiii. 220p.
20. Hodges BD. Sea monsters & whirlpools: navigating between examination and reflection in medical education. *Med Teach.* 2015;37(3):261–266. doi:10.3109/014 2159X.2014.993601.
21. Veen M, Skelton J, de la Croix A. Knowledge, skills and beetles: respecting the privacy of private experiences in medical education. *Perspect Med Educ.* 2020;9(2):111–116. doi:10.1007/s40037-020-00565-5.
22. Laughey WF, Brown MEL, Finn GM. I'm sorry to hear that'-empathy and empathic dissonance: the perspectives of PA students. *Med Sci Educ.* 2020;30:1–10.
23. Kunanitthaworn N, Wongpakaran T, Wongpakaran N, et al. Factors associated with motivation in medical education: a path analysis. *BMC Med Educ.* 2018;18(1): 140. doi:10.1186/s12909-018-1256-5.
24. Kusurkar RA. Autonomous motivation in medical education. *Med Teach.* 2019;41(9):1083–1084. doi:10.108 0/0142159X.2018.1545087.
25. Heidegger M, Boss M. *Zollikon Seminars: protocols, Conversations, Letters.* Evanston, Ill.: Northwestern University Press; 2001, p. xxxiii, 360p.
26. *Totality and Infinity: An Essay on Exteriority.* Alphonso Lingis (trans.), Pittsburgh: Duquesne University Press; 1969.
27. Ball SJ. *Foucault, Power, and Education.* New York, NY: Routledge; 2013.
28. de Beauvoir S. *The Second Sex.* New York, NY: Routledge; 1949, p. 2009.

29. Stiegler B. *Taking Care of Youth and the Generations*. Stanford, Calif.: Stanford University Press; 2010.

30. Stiegler B, Ross D. *What Makes Life Worth Living: On Pharmacology*. English edition. Cambridge, UK: Polity; 2013.

31. Zaidi Z, Partman IM, Whitehead CR, Kuper A, Wyatt TR. Contending with our racial past in medical education: a foucauldian perspective. *Teach Learn Med.* 2021;33(4):453–462. doi:10.1080/10401334.2021.1945929.

32. Neumann M, Edelhäuser F, Tauschel D, et al. Empathy decline and its reasons: a systematic review of studies with medical students and residents. *Acad Med.* 2011; 86(8):996–1009. doi:10.1097/ACM.0b013e318221e615. PMID: 21670661.

33. Schaepkens SPC, Veen M, de la Croix A. Is reflection like soap? a critical narrative umbrella review of approaches to reflection in medical education research. *Adv Health Sci Educ Theory Pract.* 2021; Nov 12. doi:10.1007/s10459-021-10082-7.

🔒 OPEN ACCESS

A Matter of Trust: Online Proctored Exams and the Integration of Technologies of Assessment in Medical Education

Tim Fawns Ⓙ and Sven P. C. Schaepkens Ⓙ

ABSTRACT

Issue: Technology is pervasive in medicine, but we too rarely examine how it shapes assessment, learning, knowledge, and performance. Cultures of assessment also shape identities, social relations, and the knowledge and behavior recognized as legitimate by a profession. Therefore, the combination of technology and assessment within medical education is worthy of review. Online proctoring services have become more prevalent during the Covid-19 pandemic, as a means of continuing high-stakes invigilated examinations online. With criticisms about increased surveillance, discrimination, and the outsourcing of control to commercial vendors, is this simply "moving exams online", or are there more serious implications? What can this extreme example tell us about how our technologies of assessment influence relationships between trainees and medical education institutions? *Evidence:* We combine postdigital and postphenomenology approaches to analyze the written component of the 2020 online proctored United Kingdom Royal College of Physicians (MRCP) membership exam. We examine the scripts, norms, and trust relations produced through this example of online proctoring, and then locate them in historical and economic contexts. We find that the proctoring service projects a false objectivity that is undermined by the tight script with which examinees must comply in an intensified norm of surveillance, and by the interpretation of digital data by unseen human proctors. Nonetheless, such proctoring services are promoted by an image of data-driven innovation, a rhetoric of necessity in response to a growing problem of online cheating, and an aversion, within medical education institutions, to changing assessment formats (and thus the need to accept different forms of knowledge as legitimate). *Implications:* The use of online proctoring technology by medical education institutions intensifies established norms, already present within examinations, of surveillance and distrust. Moreover, it exacerbates tensions between conflicting agendas of commercialization, accountability, and the education of trustworthy professionals. Our analysis provides an example of why it is important to stop and consider the holistic implications of introducing technological "solutions", and to interrogate the intersection of technology and assessment practices in relation to the wider goals of medical education.

Introduction: the technology of assessment

Technology is pervasive in medicine and medical education. Respiratory monitors, mobile phones, digital patient records, social media, and digital education platforms have all changed knowledge, practice, and relationships.[1-4] Technologies have reshaped professional roles and specialisms such as radiology and pharmacy.[5] Alongside the many benefits, there are also risks. Technology changes more than how we work and learn; it also influences our wider moral relations, beliefs, norms and values.[6,7] As educators negotiate new technologies, they are confronted not

only with technical challenges but also highly-complex, moral, and pedagogical ones.[5] Despite this, technology often goes unexamined by those who use it,[8] or our understanding is limited to questions about individual interactions, experiences, learning, and outcomes.[9]

Cultures of assessment also shape identities, social relations, and the legitimate knowledge and behavior recognized by a profession.[10-13] Assessment practice and culture have, in turn, been shaped over time by technologies such as rubrics, mark sheets, virtual learning environments, and plagiarism detection software.[14] Hodges,[15] speculating on future directions of

---

This is an Open Access article distributed under the terms of the Creative Commons Attribution-NonCommercial-NoDerivatives License (http://creativecommons.org/licenses/by-nc-nd/4.0/), which permits non-commercial re-use, distribution, and reproduction in any medium, provided the original work is properly cited, and is not altered, transformed, or built upon in any way.

technology in assessment, warns of an intensification of performativity in high stakes examinations through surveillance and automated judgements. Thus far, research on assessment technologies (and assessment more generally)[13] has focused on individual outcomes, framed around neutral and objective tools, rather than issues of equity, ethics, or values.[16]

One technology worth investigating is online proctoring—a service that creates invigilated examination conditions outside of the exam hall.[17] Such services existed before the Covid-19 pandemic, but their use increased significantly in 2020 as institutions sought continuity of secure assessment.[18] While exam halls still represent the standard to which it aspires, online proctoring has been positioned as an alternative to "not being able to run exams at all".[18(p8)] Across a variety of services,[19] a combination of regular software updates and data-driven approaches produces a sense of innovation[18,20] which, along with efficiency, is a key factor in technology adoption in assessment.[21] However, proctoring has been criticized as introducing new risks around learner privacy, foregrounding distrust,[18] discriminating against nonwhite and disabled people, and misusing data.[22]

Research on online proctoring is just emerging. Reviews of the field often rely on journalistic sources,[18,23,24] and few studies have adopted critical approaches. Coghlin et al.[24] raise concerns about increasing distrust toward institutions and an acceleration of surveillance and control. Lee and Fanguy[25] apply Foucault's "disciplinary governmentality"[26] to online proctoring at a South Korean university. They propose that surveillance constrains possibilities for thinking and behavior, and positions students as opponents in an atmosphere of competition. In Australia, Selwyn et al. analyze interviews, documents, and media to critically examine relations between universities, proctoring companies, and students.[18] Alongside surveillance, they question "the surrender of control to commercial providers", and the need for teachers to subvert the technology to maintain their educational values.

In medical education, online proctoring has not yet been subject to critical research. This is worrying, given medicine's emphasis on cultivating practitioners with integrity and professionalism. The technologized process of proctoring may reassure medical schools, employers, and the public that results are fair and objective.[25] However, while "all forms of examination are surveillance",[15(p3)] and while normative conceptions of trust, professionalism, and knowledge were already embedded within traditional assessment practice in medical education,[27,28] it is important to consider whether something more is going on than simply "moving exams online".

In this paper, we follow Veen and Ciancolo's[29] suggestion to slow down, consider context, and reflect on the interplay between assessment technology and culture in medical education, and the kinds of knowledge and professional identity they promote. We combine postdigital and postphenomenology approaches to analyze the 2020 online proctored United Kingdoml College of Physicians (MRCP) membership exam. We examine the scripts, norms, and trust relations produced through this example of online proctoring, and locate them in historical and economic contexts. Through this, we consider what is valued in terms of knowledge, professionalism, and relations between trainees and medical education institutions, before drawing out implications for the integration of technologies of assessment in medical education.

Theoretical framework: combining the postdigital and postphenomenological

While medical education research has been largely preoccupied with individualism, and the treatment of knowledge as "private capital",[30(p849)] some have employed more complex frameworks to examine technology within medical education. Body pedagogics[3] considers learning and practising as embodied processes that occur in interaction with the material environment (which includes technologies). Activity theory,[31,32] practice theory,[33] and other sociomaterial approaches[34] have helped us see how technology and people act together, in particular situations, such that neither can be understood in isolation. Such work focuses primarily on practice settings, and has not yet, to our knowledge, been used to examine assessment technology in medical education.

An emerging perspective for interrogating the complex entanglements of digital technology is that of the "postdigital".[35,36] Related to sociomaterial understandings of technology, it asserts that anything "digital" must be understood as embedded in a broader context. Outcomes of technology are contingent on the methods by which it is used, and the purposes, values, and contexts of multiple stakeholders.[37] Further, encounters with digital activity are embodied and emergent. Online exams take place in physical settings with physical bodies, and there can be no straightforward online *versions* of traditional educational practices.[35,38,39] Online proctored exams inevitably involve a different reality from the exam hall, albeit with some commonalities.[40] To augment this broader perspective, we first employ a postphenomenology of technology approach,[41–44] for a closer interrogation of the human-technology relations (behavioral scripts, social norms, and trust relations) promoted by an instance of proctoring technology. We then zoom out to consider how the assessment reality created by this technology is embedded in historical, political, pedagogical, and economic contexts, and what this means for relationships between trainees, institutions, and cultures of assessment technology.

Both postdigital and postphenomenological perspectives reject the idea that reality is based on human, subjective interpretation and action alone. We do not fully determine the world around us. On the other hand, both perspectives also criticize the view that reality is just "out there" and we can know it objectively. The world around us does not fully determine us. Conversely, both perspectives emphasize that "reality arises in relations, as do the humans who encounter it",[43(p568)] and technology has a role in shaping these relations.

Online proctored exams

Online proctoring creates a remote version of exam-hall conditions by monitoring and constraining possibilities for action and movement. The technology verifies each candidate's identity, and that they are alone and isolated from resources that could aid their performance. Wearing earplugs or handling textbooks or mobile devices may be considered a "serious breach of exam protocol".[45(p5)] Some services require exam-takers to install software on their device to block access to documents, applications, and websites. Authentication normally requires permission for the software to control webcams and microphones, which monitor the environment during the examination. Other data can include keyboard strokes, network traffic, and computer memory usage.[17] Monitoring can be live or retrospective via recordings, or both, and may involve an algorithm, or a human who is unknown to, and unseen by, the student. Before the exam, candidates must scan the examination space (often a bedroom, kitchen, or other private space within their home) with their webcams.

A recent example of high-stakes online proctoring is the United Kingdom's Royal College of Physicians (MRCP) membership exam. This two-part exam acts as a gateway into specialist training.[46] It is "the largest high stakes postgraduate clinical examination in the world" with "5000 candidates examined each year".[47(p2)] Part One is an introductory, written examination. Part Two is more advanced, consisting of two, three-hour written exams, both sat on the same day. Finally, there

is the Practical Assessment of Clinical Examination Skills (PACES). In 2020, MRCP offered the option of remote examination using different invigilation services for the different components. According to the MRCP guidance, proctoring would be performed "by a specialist provider" who would "be monitoring your activity throughout the exam, just as they would in a face to face exam encounter."[45(p5)]

In this paper, we limit our analysis to the written element in Part Two of the MRCP exam, excluding the practical component. While there are obvious concerns about the capacity for online proctoring to create equivalent assessment environments for demonstrating clinical skills, limiting our scope allows us to focus on how the technology creates constrained physical environments even for written assessments. In 2020, Part Two of the MRCP membership exam used the ProctorExam service. Examinees were required to choose a quiet location where they were "guaranteed" not be disturbed.[45] The exam space needed to be well lit and have reliable WiFi. Requirements included a laptop with webcam and microphone, Google Chrome browser, and a minimum Internet speed. ProctorExam did not measure eye movements or keystrokes, but prided itself as a "leader" in adding extra cameras (e.g. the candidate's smartphone) for additional "accuracy".[48] Screen and camera footage was recorded for "internal use" and not made available to candidates or examiners.[45]

Human proctors (either ProctorExam or institutional employees) watched the candidates, to ensure they started at the correct time and to provide assistance when needed (e.g. where candidates felt unwell or needed the bathroom). Moreover, they ensured that the exam environment was secure. This supportive framework underplayed the primary function, which was to flag abnormal behavior as potential cheating. In such cases, the medical education institution would have the final say on any action taken. Proctors were not visible to candidates; communication occurred via text chat. Candidates had to remain seated at their computer until the end of the allocated time, even if they had finished earlier.[45]

Postphenomology of proctoring: how technology creates reality

Postphenomenology, as developed by Ihde[41] and Verbeek,[42] challenges the idea that technology is an instrument designed with a certain purpose that simply does what we intend it to do.[49] Instead, technology mediates relations between human and world in non-neutral ways.[50] With this lens, we scrutinize how technology offers users particular scripts that shape how they can act in the world, and how technology presents the world to them.

Scripts and norms

Technological objects have a script, that is an "inclination or trajectory that shapes the ways in which they are used."[43(p569)] For example, fountain pens require us to think ahead and compose sentences before writing them down, while word processors invoke quick, flexible writing that mimics speech. One can write slowly and quickly with either, but each promotes a certain type of use while discouraging others.[43,51] Moreover, technologies are socially embedded and shape cultural norms. Early ballpoint pens were thought to impair children's quality of work by eliciting quicker, sloppy writing, whereas fountain pens were seen as producing neat and careful work.[43]

In online proctoring, examinees behavior is governed by the technology's surveillance function. ProctorExam claims to provide a *pure context,* with greater security and accuracy, through their multi-camera solution.[48] Purity of context is, however, undermined by the strict control of examinees' behavior, and by the inevitable interpretation by examiners.[51] In exam halls, candidates only need to purify their person (e.g. by excluding prohibited notes or devices); in online proctoring, they must purify their whole environment and range of bodily movement.

Thus, although exam hall invigilation also involves surveillance and interpretation of behavior (e.g. does looking toward a neighbor imply cheating or mind-wandering?), there are important differences. Firstly, whereas in the exam hall, (potential) cheating is framed as looking *at* prohibited resources, or speaking to other candidates, in online proctoring it is framed more widely: looking away from the screen, moving in an atypical fashion, unsanctioned use of the device being used for exam-taking, poor Internet connectivity, other technical issues, someone entering the room, etc. While many students do not seem to experience online proctoring as overly intrusive, and some forget about being watched or become apathetic to it,[18] strict monitoring of bodily movements, nonetheless, compels them to conform to an ideal model of an examinee.[22,27]

Secondly, in online proctoring, there is a variety of behavioral data (e.g. eye-movement, keystrokes, video feeds), and each represents a digitized slice of the test world. These data cannot directly confirm whether behavior is inappropriate. Proctors must "read" the benchmarks that indicate cheating, and examinees are encouraged by the technology to adapt to these standards. Thirdly, candidates cannot see online proctors, and neither they, nor their assessors, have access to how the software works, disrupting normal trust relations of exam hall invigilation.[24,25] Examinees are at a disadvantage, since their behavior is minutely recorded, while their understanding of what proctors do and observe is nearly absent.

Trust

Online proctoring technology intensifies norms of *surveillance over trust* by enforcing stricter protocols, while also conveying a false sense of objectivity. Technology becomes transparent to us when we use it (as with proctored examinees who forget they are watched).[18,43,50] We expect pens to write, Google to yield search results and proctor technology to identify cheaters. Nguyen applies the concept of trust, not only to relations between people, but also to those (technological) objects that we trust constantly.[52] To cope with an overwhelming world that poses demands beyond our physical and cognitive limitations, we outsource agency to human others, animals, and objects.[52] We may outsource our sight to a guide dog, the education of our children to teachers, and exam surveillance to proctor technologies. In each case, trust implies an unquestioning attitude to the technology's reliability. Consider a novice mountaineer, who requires training to forget their rope,[52] trusting it to stop them from falling, so that they can direct their precious attention elsewhere. The technology is no longer visible, or has become transparent. To work effectively with proctoring technology, examinees must learn to trust it not to flag them inappropriately, while examiners must trust it to appropriately detect cheating.

While multiple video feeds seemingly create objectivity for proctors, for examinees, the assessment is located in a highly-contrived reality in which their bodies are constrained, monitored, and controlled by external forces, in more detail than in exam halls. Breakdowns of transparency are provoked by notifications and warnings produced by the software when a candidate engages in potentially suspicious behavior (e.g. looking in the wrong place or moving in the wrong way). These forces are conveyed by proctoring companies as benevolent or neutral, but their primary function is enforcing constraint and reporting subversion through the minute technological scripting of movement and environment.

A postdigital view of online proctoring

We have argued that online proctoring involves a tighter script and more interpretation than exam hall invigilation. In this section, we broaden our postdigital view to zoom out and investigate the historical and economic contexts and assessment cultures in which the MRCP exam is located.

Historical context

Online proctoring is interpreted through a lens colored by the historical context of traditional examination settings. As Carless[53] argues, we trust exams, in part, due to their long tradition. They "represent continuity and stability, whilst other more innovative forms of assessment may be seen as risk-taking." [53(p82)] Further, equivalence between online and traditional exams is necessary for comparing candidates over time.

To reassure its customers, online proctoring mimics a preexisting distrust within the "established logics of university study" through which "students are placed in disempowered surveilled positions during any examination setting."[18(p13)] This mimicry of traditional invigilation practices is explicit in the MRCP guidance. It frames online proctors as working "just as they would in a face to face exam encounter".[45(p5)]

However, our case involved invisible online proctors, multiple cameras, control of shared environments, partnerships with 3rd party companies, and more. Further, while ProctorExam's datafication of behavior echoes the quantification of knowledge through exams, and a tradition of seeing numbers as more objective than other forms of information,[20,54] it is also part of an increasing trend of big data and algorithmically adjudicated truth.[20] With data-driven processes and constantly updating software, ProctorExam is imbued with a sense of relentless innovation,[18] while also being perceived as a lower-risk practice of continuity.

Economic context

As a commercial product, proctoring technology must create value. First, it frames medical schools as clients, inserting itself into the relationship between assessors and students.[18,48] Having spent considerable money, the medical school is invested in the system, and it is in its interests for the technology to be perceived as a success. Moreover, it would be expensive and complicated to change to a different assessment format that did not require proctoring.[18] This incentivises decision-makers to defend the technology against critiques, and to continue using it.

Second, proctoring technology frames students as potential cheaters and, therefore, as threats to the academic integrity of the medical school and the medical profession.[25] This is important for commercial sustainability, since the software is only necessary if people cheat.

Third, it also frames students as clients through its rhetoric of fairness and support. Online proctors are there to "assist you with any issues … They will not be visible on your screen but will be available should you need to alert them to a problem."[45(p13)] Hard-working, non-cheating students can be reassured that they are not disadvantaged by the cheating of others.[24,25] Finally, the technology's perceived effectiveness is also contingent on students as sources that generate data,[55] with no choice but to comply if they want to pass the exam.

Assessment culture

Assessment has a powerful influence over what and how students learn, and over what is valued within education systems[13] and professional disciplines.[10,56] Exams, for example, value "objective" knowledge, and constrain possibilities for demonstrating and validating other kinds of knowledge.[10] All invigilation is aimed at creating an environment for fair assessment of performance, based on standardization and equality of experience.[57] Yet preventing access to external resources and controlling bodily behavior prioritizes individualized, abstract, and propositional knowledge[58] at the expense of embodied, social, material and collective knowledge on which trust, relationships, and teamwork are founded.[59] It marginalizes critical or creative knowledge and inhibits the development of future autonomous practitioners.[10]

What was already a narrow view of knowledge is further tightened through online proctoring. In exam halls, all candidates perform in the same physical location, and are allowed only a highly-restricted set of materials. In online proctored exams, anyone not considered by the technology to conform to its model of how a student should behave, move, or look during an exam is associated with signifiers of a lack of integrity. The restriction of gaze and movement to a single digital interface is a strong commitment to the denial of material, non-cognitive knowledge and of diverse bodily characteristics and conditions. This is harder for some than others, and there are reports of online proctoring services discriminating against candidates in relation to gender, race, disability, language, culture, and more.[22,24,55] These, along with other circumstantial disadvantages (e.g. those with shared living spaces, caring responsibilities, limited technological resources, or physical challenges) are at odds with fair and objective assessment.

Discussion

Integrity, professionalism, and surveillance

In exams, definitive answers, the exclusion of resources, and behavioral control close down possibilities of being, thinking, knowing, and acting.[11] Further, "objective" assessment requires breaking ability down into standardized and decontextualized knowledge at the potential expense of collective, collaborative, and complex professional performance.[59-61] In online proctoring, the flexibility of enabling trainees to take exams from home increases the requirements of rules and surveillance. We have argued that this intensifies existing problematic framings of examinees, trust, and knowledge, in which more authentic or meaningful forms of assessment are sacrificed in the name of "fairness."[25]

In the 2020 MRCP exam, online proctoring may also have exacerbated existing forms of discrimination by heightening performativity, through which learners contort themselves to portray an imagined ideal candidate.[15] Surveillance in assessment is part of a broader process of normalization, through which "techniques of objectification... are constantly used to evaluate and control us because they exclude those who cannot conform to 'normal' categories."[27(p445)] Despite claims like the UK General Medical Council's that "equality, diversity and inclusion are integral to our work as a regulator,"[62(p3)] students may feel they need to amplify, sanitize, or suppress their ethnicity, "gender, sexuality, culture, religion, language or disability/ability."[15(p3)]

Further, surveillance may produce a kind of pseudo-integrity that is bound to conditions of being watched. This exacerbates a problem for exam assessment more generally, in how it prepares students to become part of and contribute to their disciplines,[10,63] since enforced integrity is likely to be counterproductive to the development of independent professionalism.[64-67] Technological surveillance promotes distrust between educators and students,[68] and the presence of cameras implies that students are potential cheaters who must be closely watched. Proctoring companies seek to normalize coercive and invasive measures in the homes of candidates, positioning surveillance as a "necessary evil" to protect the "academic integrity" of institutions and the rights of *trustworthy* students to a fair examination.[18]

It is in the commercial interest of proctoring companies to frame candidates as potential cheaters and cheating as a significant, growing, and dynamic problem,[69] with a technological solution.[18,22] MRCP's use of online proctoring as a "temporary emergency solution" follows a broader trend of technological automation and establishes "private and commercial providers as essential infrastructural intermediaries between students and their universities".[55(p2)]

Complex perspectives on technology in medical education

Philosophical approaches allow analyses to go beyond the usual forms of evidence, which are often limited in terms of how they address complexity.[11] Our broader postdigital perspective helps us see that there is no straightforward equivalence between exam halls and online proctoring. The "digital" technology of the 2020 MRCP exam was embedded in an assessment culture in ways that are entangled in a historical and economic context. The postphenomenological lens draws attention to scripts and how they shape the assessment reality. Combined, these two approaches "provide a convincing and defensible account of both the practice and its effects."[33(p219)] These or other complex frameworks can, and should, be applied to other applications of technology in medical education. For example, we might question the kinds of learning promoted via learning analytics,[35,70] or what it means for on campus teaching to "move online",[71] since the social and material context of online learning[72] is very different. In each case, the moral and ethical implications require looking beyond outcomes, terms, and conditions,[40] to *how* technology is embedded in particular cultures and practices.

Broader lessons for assessment technology in medical education

Nieminen and Lahdenperä call for research into how student agency in higher education assessment promotes or hinders future development.[10] Professional doctors must not only be competent but also trustworthy, and act with integrity without being monitored. Furthermore, they should be professional members of teams and wider systems. Conversely, in online proctored exams, trainees are constructed not only as potential cheaters, but also as objects of control who cannot think for themselves, take responsibility, or create new knowledge.[11]

It is unclear what will happen with online proctoring as the Covid-19 situation stabilizes. The challenge ahead is not simply to decide whether online proctoring tools are worthwhile,[73] or whether we need to soften their scripts and surveillance. While we acknowledge that exams might be effective under certain conditions, and we would not advocate letting candidates do whatever they want, we call for medical educators to ask questions about how we conduct high stakes assessment and why it is so reliant on invigilation. Our aim here is not to propose alternatives to invigilated examinations, nor that educators should avoid technology in assessment. Rather, we aim to provoke critical consideration of how the combination of technology and assessment promotes particular kinds of knowledge, identity, professionalism, and trust relations.[43] This is no simple task. It involves confronting a longstanding reluctance, across education more broadly, to ask fundamental questions about the purpose of assessment, how it affects educational relationships, or how it relates to "truth, fairness, trust, humanity or social justice".[74(p2)] A good starting point is to engage in honest dialogue around how we currently do assessment, and how we might reimagine our practices in ways that reinforce relations between trainees and medical education institutions, such that we no longer place trust in technology above trust in our students.

Conclusion

Assessment both reflects and shapes what is valued in medical education. Our analysis of the 2020 MRCP membership exam shows how online proctoring technology intensifies a norm of surveillance over trust that already exists in exam hall invigilation. This exacerbates some established tensions within the assessment culture of medical education, namely: a narrow conception of legitimate knowledge as standardized and decontextualized, a narrow model of the ideal, solitary exam candidate, and a default distrust of trainees. By examining the historical and economic contexts of the MRCP exam, we have showed how these tensions are reinforced by the commercial interests of proctoring companies that incentivise distrust and data-driven normative models of invigilation.

Veen and Cianciolo[29(pp337-338)] wrote, in the paper that launched this series, to slow down and consider context "to examine carefully what we are doing to care for learners and improve their performance, professionalism, and well-being." While we are confident that, *in general*, medical educators trust students, and work hard to support them to become trustworthy, we have argued that the assessment culture promoted by online proctoring technology,

and our employment of assessment technology more widely, are in need of review. If, as Bearman[75] suggests, the test world shapes the practice world, we must also ask: what kind of world do we generate through our use of assessment technology?

Acknowledgements

Thanks to Mario Veen for the invitation and for help along the way. Thanks also to Anna Cianciolo and two anonymous reviewers for their comments.

Previous Philosophy in Medical Education Installments

Mario Veen & Anna T. Cianciolo (2020) Problems No One Looked For: Philosophical Expeditions into Medical Education, Teaching and Learning in Medicine, 32:3, 337-344, DOI: 10.1080/10401334.2020.1748634

Gert J. J. Biesta & Marije van Braak (2020) Beyond the Medical Model: Thinking Differently about Medical Education and Medical Education Research, Teaching and Learning in Medicine, 32:4, 449-456, DOI: 10.1080/10401334.2020.1798240

Mark R. Tonelli & Robyn Bluhm (2021) Teaching Medical Epistemology within an Evidence-Based Medicine Curriculum, Teaching and Learning in Medicine, 33:1, 98-105, DOI: 10.1080/10401334.2020.1835666

John R. Skelton (2021) Language, Philosophy, and Medical Education, Teaching and Learning in Medicine, 33:2, 210-216, DOI: 10.1080/10401334.2021.1877712

Zareen Zaidi, Ian M. Partman, Cynthia R. Whitehead, Ayelet Kuper & Tasha R. Wyatt (2021) Contending with Our Racial Past in Medical Education: A Foucauldian Perspective, Teaching and Learning in Medicine, DOI: 10.1080/10401334.2021.1945929

Chris Rietmeijer & Mario Veen (2021) Phenomenological Research in Health Professions Education: Tunneling from Both Ends, Teaching and Learning in Medicine, DOI: 10.1080/10401334.2021.1971989

Madeleine Noelle Olding, Freya Rhodes, John Humm, Phoebe Ross & Catherine McGarry (2022) Black, White and Gray: Student Perspectives on Medical Humanities and Medical Education, Teaching and Learning in Medicine, 34:2, 223-233, DOI: 10.1080/10401334.2021.1982717

Camillo Coccia & Mario Veen (2022) Because We Care: A Philosophical Investigation into the Spirit of Medical Education, Teaching and Learning in Medicine, DOI: 10.1080/10401334.2022.2056744

Associated Podcast

Let Me Ask You Something (iTunes, Spotify, Google Podcasts and https://marioveen.com/letmeaskyousomething/)

Disclosure statement

No potential conflict of interest was reported by the authors.

Funding

The author(s) reported there is no funding associated with the work featured in this article.

ORCID

Tim Fawns http://orcid.org/0000-0001-5014-2662
Sven Schaepkens http://orcid.org/0000-0001-5513-3554

References

1. Ebeling MFE. Patient disempowerment through the commercial access to digital health records. *Health (London)*. 2019;23(4):385–400. doi:10.1177/1363459319848038.
2. Asan O, Smith PD, Montague E. More screen time, less face time - Implications for EHR design. *J Eval Clin Pract*. 2014;20(6):896–901. doi:10.1111/jep.12182.
3. Kelly M, Ellaway RH, Scherpbier A, King N, Dornan T. Body pedagogics: embodied learning for the health professions. *Med Educ*. 2019;53(10):967–977. doi:10.1111/medu.13916.
4. Greenhalgh T, Stones R, Swinglehurst D. Choose and Book: A sociological analysis of " 'resistance' to an expert system. *Soc Sci Med*. 2014;104:210–219. doi:10.1016/j.socscimed.2013.12.014.
5. Ellaway RH. Medical education and the war with the machines. *Med Teach*. 2014;36(10):917–918. doi:10.3109/0142159X.2014.955088.
6. Swierstra T. Identifying the normative challenges posed by technology's "soft" impacts. Etikk i praksis. *Nord J Appl Ethics*. 2015;9(1):5–20.
7. Kiran AH. Four dimensions of technological mediation. In: Rosenberger DI, Verbeek PP, eds. *Essays on Human–Technology Relations*. London: Lexington Books; 2015:123–140.
8. Hew KF, Lan M, Tang Y, Jia C, Lo CK. Where is the "theory" within the field of educational technology research? *Br J Educ Technol*. 2019;50(3):956–971. doi:10.1111/bjet.12770.
9. Lupton D. Critical perspectives on digital health technologies. *Sociol Compass*. 2014;8(12):1344–1359. doi:10.1111/soc4.12226.
10. Nieminen JH, Lahdenperä J. Assessment and epistemic (in)justice: how assessment produces knowledge and knowers. *Teach High Educ*. 2021. doi:10.1080/13562517.2021.1973413.
11. Biesta GJJ, van Braak M. Beyond the medical model: Thinking differently about medical education and medical education research. *Teach Learn Med*. 2020;32(4):449–456. doi:10.1080/10401334.2020.1798240.
12. Hodges BD. Validity and the OSCE. *Med Teach*. 2003;25(3):250–254. doi:10.1080/0142159031000102836.
13. Leathwood C. Assessment policy and practice in higher education: Purpose, standards and equity. *Assess Eval High Educ*. 2005;30(3):307–324. doi:10.1080/02602930500063876.
14. Schuwirth LWT, van der Vleuten CPM. A history of assessment in medical education. *Adv Health Sci Educ Theory Pract*. 2020;25(5):1045–1056. doi:10.1007/s10459-020-10003-0.

15. Hodges BD . Performance-based assessment in the 21st century: When the examiner is a machine. *Perspect Med Educ*. 2021;10(1):3–5. doi:10.1007/s40037-020-00647-4.
16. Thoma B, Turnquist A, Zaver F, Hall AK, Chan TM. Communication, learning and assessment: Exploring the dimensions of the digital learning environment. *Med Teach*. 2019;41(4):385–390. doi:10.1080/0142159X.2019.1567911.
17. Dawson P. *Defending Assessment Security in a Digital World*. London: Routledge; 2020. doi:10.4324/9780429324178.
18. Selwyn N, O'Neill C, Smith G, Andrejevic M, Gu X. A necessary evil? The rise of online exam proctoring in Australian universities. *Media Int Aust*. 2021. doi:10.1177/1329878X211005862.
19. Arnò S, Galassi A, Tommasi M, Saggino A, Vittorini P. State-of-the-art of commercial proctoring systems and their use in academic online exams. *Int J Distance Educ Technol*. 2021;19(2):41–62. doi:10.4018/IJDET.20210401.oa3.
20. Hodges BD. Ones and zeros: Medical education and theory in the age of intelligent machines. *Med Educ*. 2020;54(8):691–693. doi:10.1111/medu.14149.
21. Bennett S, Dawson P, Bearman M, Molloy E, Boud D. How technology shapes assessment design: Findings from a study of university teachers. *Br J Educ Technol*. 2017;48(2):672–682. doi:10.1111/bjet.12439.
22. Swauger S. Our Bodies Encoded: Algorithmic test proctoring in higher education. In: Stommel J, Friend C, Morris SM, eds. *Critical Digital Pedagogy*, 2020. Montreal, Quebec: Pressbooks. https://cdpcollection.pressbooks.com/. Accessed April 12, 2021.
23. Eaton SE, Turner KL. Exploring academic integrity and mental health during COVID-19: Rapid review. *J Contemp Educ Theory Res*. 2020;4:35–41. doi:10.5281/zenodo.4256825.
24. Coghlan S, Miller T, Paterson J. Good proctor or "big brother"? Ethics of online exam supervision technologies. *Philos Technol*. 2021;34(4):1581–1606. doi:10.1007/s13347-021-00476-1.
25. Lee K, Fanguy M. Online exam proctoring technologies: Educational innovation or deterioration? *Br J Educ Technol*. 2022. doi:10.1111/bjet.13182.
26. Foucault M. *Discipline and Punish: The Birth of the Prison/Michel Foucault; Translated from the French by Alan Sheridan*. Harmondsworth: Penguin; 1979.
27. Zaidi Z, Partman IM, Whitehead CR, Kuper A, Tasha R. Contending with our racial past in medical education: A foucauldian perspective. *Teach Learn Med*. 2021;33(4):453–462. doi:10.1080/10401334.2021.1945929.
28. Holtman MC. A theoretical sketch of medical professionalism as a normative complex. *Adv Health Sci Educ Theory Pract*. 2008;13(2):233–245. doi:10.1007/s10459-008-9099-1.
29. Veen M, Cianciolo AT. Problems no one looked for: Philosophical expeditions into medical education. *Teach Learn Med*. 2020;32(3):337–344. doi:10.1080/10401334.2020.1748634.
30. Bleakley A. Blunting Occam's razor: aligning medical education with studies of complexity. *J Eval Clin Pract*. 2010;16(4):849–855. doi:10.1111/j.1365-2753.2010.01498.x.

31. Engeström Y, Sannino A. Studies of expansive learning: Foundations, findings and future challenges. *Educ Res Rev.* 2010;5(1):1–24. doi:10.1016/j.edurev.2009.12.002.

32. Bleakley A. Broadening conceptions of learning in medical education: The message from teamworking. *Med Educ.* 2006;40(2):150–157. doi:10.1111/j.1365-2929.2005.02371.x.

33. Nicolini D. Bringing it all together: A toolkit to study and represent practice at work. In: *Practice Theory, Work, and Organization: An Introduction.* Oxford: Oxford University Press; 2013:213–242.

34. Fenwick T, Edwards R. Exploring the impact of digital technologies on professional responsibilities and education. *Eur Educ Res J.* 2016;15(1):117–131. doi:10.1177/1474904115608387.

35. Fawns T. Postdigital education in design and practice. *Postdigit Sci Educ.* 2019;1(1):132–145. doi:10.1007/s42438-018-0021-8.

36. Jandrić P, Knox J, Besley T, Ryberg T, Suoranta J, Hayes S. Postdigital science and education. *Educ Philos Theory.* 2018;50(10):893–899. doi:10.1080/00131857.2018.1454000.

37. Fawns T. An entangled pedagogy: Looking beyond the pedagogy – technology dichotomy. *Postdigital Sci Educ.* 2022. doi:10.1007/s42438-022-00302-7

38. Sinclair C, Macleod H. Literally Virtual: The reality of the online teacher. In: Jandrić P, Boras D, eds. *Critical Learning in Digital Networks. Research in Networked Learning.* Cham: Springer International Publishing; 2015:77–99. doi:10.1007/978-3-319-13752-0_5.

39. Gourlay L. There is no "Virtual Learning": The materiality of digital education. *NApprEdR.* 2021;10(1):57–66. doi:10.7821/naer.2021.1.649.

40. Adams C. TPACK's arc of technology transparency and teachers' ethical obligations: Understanding the digital as the new materia medica of pedagogy. In: Ochoa MN, Gibson D, eds. *Research Highlights in Technology and Teacher Education.* Fairmont: AACE;2020:49–58. doi:10.1016/B978-0-323-02998-8.50028-7.

41. Ihde D. Preface. Positioning postphenomenology. In: Rosenberger DI, Verbeek P-P, eds. *Essays on Human–Technology Relations.* London: Lexington Books; 2015.

42. Verbeek P-P. *Moralizing Technology. Understanding and Designing the Morality of Things.* Chicago: The University of Chicago Press; 2011.

43. Verbeek P-P. Postphenomenology and technology. In: Scharff RC, Dusek V, eds. *Philosophy of Technology.* Chichester: Wiley; 2014:561–572.

44. Rosenberger R, Verbeek P-P. A field guide to postphenomenology. In: Rosenberger DI, Verbeek P-P, eds. *Essays on Human–Technology Relations.* London: Lexington Books; 2015:9–42.

45. (MRCPUK) Membership of the Royal Colleges of Physicians of the United Kingdom. *Preparing for Your MRCP (UK) Part 2 Online Examination.* 2020. https://www.mrcpuk.org/sites/default/files/documents/PROCTOREXAMCandidateguide.pdf.

46. (MRCPUK) Membership of the Royal Colleges of Physicians UK. *MRCP(UK) examinations.* 2020. https://www.mrcpuk.org/mrcpuk-examinations.

47. Verma A, Griffin A, Dacre J, Elder A. Exploring cultural and linguistic influences on clinical communication skills: A qualitative study of International Medical Graduates. *BMC Med Educ.* 2016;16(1):1–10. doi:10.1186/s12909-016-0680-7.

48. Haven D, Portnaar D-P. Landelijke studentenvakbond op het matje bij ProctorExam. *Risk and Compliance.* 2021. https://www.riskcompliance.nl/news/landelijke-studentenvakbond-op-het-matje-bij-proctorexam/.

49. Visser G. *Heideggers Vraag Naar de Techniek.* Amsterdam: Vantilt; 2013.

50. Verbeek P-P. Moralizing technology: On the morality of technological artifacts and their design. In: Kaplan M, ed. *Readings in the Philosophy of Technology.* New York: Rowman & Littlefield; 2009:265–284.

51. Ihde DA. Phenomenology of technics. In: Scharff RC, Dusek V, eds. *Philosophy of Technology.* Chichester: Wiley; 2014:539–560.

52. Nguyen CT. Trust as an Unquestioning Attitude. In: *Oxford Studies in Epistemology.* Oxford: Oxford University Press; forthcoming.

53. Carless D. Trust, distrust and their impact on assessment reform. *Assess Eval High Educ.* 2009;34(1):79–89. doi:10.1080/02602930801895786.

54. Pacheco JA . The "new normal" in education. *Prospects (Paris).* 2021;51(1-3):3–14. doi:10.1007/s11125-020-09521-x.

55. Williamson B, Hogan A. *Pandemic Privatisation in Higher Education: Edtech & University Reform.* Brussels: Education International; 2021.

56. McArthur J. Assessment for social justice: the role of assessment in achieving social justice. *Assess Eval High Educ.* 2016;41(7):967–981. doi:10.1080/02602938.2015.1053429.

57. Kaposy C. Postphenomenology of the robot medical student. In: Rosenberger DI, Verbeek P-P, eds. *Essays on Human–Technology Relations.* London: Lexington Books; 2015:191–202.

58. Beckett D, Hager P. *Life, Work and Learning.* New York: Routledge; 2005.

59. Hager P, Beckett D. *The Emergence of Complexity: Rethinking Education as a Social Science.* Cham: Springer; 2019.

60. Hodges BD. Assessment in the post-psychometric era: Learning to love the subjective and collective. *Med Teach.* 2013;35(7):564–568. doi:10.3109/0142159X.2013.789134.

61. Bleakley A, Bligh J, Browne J. *Medical Education of the Future: Identity. Power and Location.* New York: Springer; 2011. doi:10.1016/S0140-6736(00)70457-0.

62. General Medical Council. *Outcomes for Graduates.* 2018. https://www.gmc-uk.org/education/undergraduate/undergrad_outcomes.asp.

63. Fawns T, Mulherin T, Hounsell D, Aitken G. Seamful learning and professional education. *Stud Contin Educ.* 2021;43(3):360–376. doi:10.1080/0158037X.2021.1920383.

64. Ross J, Macleod H. Surveillance, (dis)trust and teaching with plagiarism detection technology. In: Bajić M, Dohn N, de Laat M, Jandrić P, Ryberg T, eds. *11th International Conference on Networked Learning.* Zagreb: Zagreb University of Applied Sciences; 2018:235–242.

65. Ajjawi R, Molloy E, Bearman M, Rees CE. Scaling up assessment for learning in higher education. In: Carless D, ed. *The Enabling Power of Assessment*. Vol 5. Singapore: Springer; 2017:129–143. doi:10.1007/978-981-10-3045-1.

66. Carless D. Trust and its role in facilitating dialogic feedback. In: Boud D, Molloy E, eds. *Feedback in Higher and Professional Education*. London: Routledge; 2013:90–103.

67. Fawns T, Ross J. Spotlight on Alternative Assessment Methods: Alternatives to exams. *Teaching Matters*. 2020. https://www.teaching-matters-blog.ed.ac.uk/spotlight-on-alternative-assessment-methods-alternatives-to-exams/.

68. Darbyshire P, Thompson DR. Can nursing educators learn to trust the world's most trusted profession? *Nurs Inq*. 2021;28(2). doi:10.1111/nin.12412.

69. Rapanta C, Botturi L, Goodyear P, et al. Online university teaching during and after the Covid-19 crisis: Refocusing teacher presence and learning activity. *Postdigit Sci Educ*. 2020;2(3):923–945. doi:10.1007/s42438-020-00155-y.

70. Knox J, Williamson B, Bayne S. Machine behaviourism: future visions of 'learnification' and 'datafication' across humans and digital technologies. *Learn Media Technol*. 2020;45(1):31–45. doi:10.1080/17439884.2019.1623251.

71. Fawns T, Jones D, Aitken G. Challenging assumptions about "moving online" in response to COVID-19, and some practical advice. *MedEdPublish*. 2020;9(1):83. doi:10.15694/mep.2020.000083.1.

72. Fawns T, Aitken G, Jones D. Online learning as embodied, socially meaningful experience. *Postdigit Sci Educ*. 2019;1(2):293–297. doi:10.1007/s42438-019-00048-9.

73. Nigam A, Pasricha R, Singh T, Churi P. A systematic review on AI-based proctoring systems: Past, present and future. *Educ Inf Technol (Dordr)*. 2021;26(5):6421–6445. doi:10.1007/s10639-021-10597-x.

74. Rowntree D. *Assessing Students : How Shall We Know Them?* London: Kogan Page; 1987.

75. Bearman M. Bringing reality to assessment: lessons from clinical simulation. *Med Educ*. 2020;54(10):870–872. doi:10.1111/medu.14293.

Being-Opposite-Illness: Phenomenological Ontology in Medical Education and Clinical Practice

John Humm (iD)

ABSTRACT

Issue: Phenomenology has proven to be a very useful tool for medicine. Descriptive, first-person accounts of patient experiences can reveal new and unique insights. These insights can inform renewed approaches to medical education and practice. However, comparatively little research has been done on the other side of the clinical encounter. This leaves the lived experiences of doctors diagnosing and treating illness unaddressed and the ontological transformation of medical students through medical education unexplored. *Evidence*: This paper provides a phenomenological description of the clinical encounter and ontological transformation of the medical student into the doctor. I argue doctors have a unique ontology, rooted in the objectification of the patient, for which I use the term being-opposite-illness This is achieved, through phenomenological examination of my experiences as a medical student and through descriptions of three distinct types of face-to-face encounters: the basic encounter with the Other, the encounter with illness, and the clinical encounter, which I argue are all metaphysically distinct. Finally, textual analysis of popular first-person accounts from two doctors, Henry Marsh and Paul Kalanithi, provide an illustration of being-opposite-illness in clinical practice and how this ontological transformation occurs through medical education. *Implications*: Together, the phenomenology of the clinical encounter and textual analysis of Marsh and Kalanithi reveal clinical practice and medical education be an ontological transformative process. This paper attempts a new understanding of this experience of doctors by accounting for their unique ontology. In sum, I suggest being-opposite-illness can represent a new lens for analyzing the experience of doctors. Through this, I hope to promote new medical education and practice approaches.

Introduction

Illness is something that happens only to patients. This is an important lesson you learn early on as a medical student.

Henry Marsh1[(p215)]

Do No Harm

Phenomenology is a useful tool for medicine. Descriptive, detailed accounts of lived experiences of illness bring to light features that can be missed by quantitative scientific inquiry alone.[2] Phenomenology can reveal underlying aspects of human ontology.[3] Ontology' and 'ontological' in this work refer to Heidegger's study of being developed.[4] Different aspects of, or changes to, our ontology, or way-of-being, change the way we experience the world. To

use a simplified example for readers new to these concepts: de Beauvoir's study of being female is based on a phenomenological examination of her experience of being a woman.[5] De Beauvoir presents becoming a woman as an ontological transformation over time, "one is not born, but rather becomes, a woman," in part through her examination of her and other women's everyday experiences.[5(p295)] This work applies this approach to the experience of medical students. My intention is to provide a phenomenological description of my experience as a medical student interacting with patients, and how this has changed over time. By doing so, I intend to open a discussion on the ontology of the doctor.

Illness fundamentally affects one's way of experiencing the world.[2] To use Heidegger's term: it affects a patient's being-in-the-world. I suggest witnessing and treating illness can also have ontological effects.[4] I argue this results in a unique way of being for the doctor, for which I use the term being-opposite-illness. In brief, being-opposite-illness refers to the ontological result of objectifying patients, which appears to be required to reduce one's bodily response to seeing illness.

Phenomenology has also been shown to be a useful tool for Medical Education.[6,7] Specifically, phenomenology's careful examination of everyday experiences demonstrates how seemingly unremarkable occurrences can hide underlying structures of those experiences. Acknowledging and acting on these influences can help medical educators produce renewed approaches to educational practice. Furthermore, this work shows how learning and reading philosophy changed the way I, a medical student, see patients.

This work is split into three sections. In section one, I introduce phenomenology as a philosophical method and stress the differences between biomedical and phenomenological views of the body. In section two, I describe three types of experience to build up layers of phenomenological description: the basic encounter with the Other (how we interact with any other person), the encounter with illness (how we experience someone who is ill or injured), and the clinical encounter (how doctors interact with patients). Being-opposite-illness is a key difference between the clinical encounter and how the public may encounter illness. In section three, I explore first-person accounts from two doctors: Henry Marsh[1] and Paul Kalanithi.[8] I suggest both accounts provide powerful illustrations of being-opposite-illness and its effect on doctors and the doctor-patient relationship.

To define the terms and set out the limits of my description. The 'Other' is another person which we encounter.[9] 'Doctor' refers to the trained clinician of western contemporary conventional healthcare. 'Patient' refers to an individual with illness. Disease refers to "physiological dysfunction of the body."[2(p1)] This 'pathological anatomy' is the focus of the medical gaze.[10(p152)] Instead, illness denotes the subjective lived experience of "serious, chronic, and life-changing ill health."[2(p2)] We will see this be an important separation between the way patients and doctors interact with illness. By clinical encounter, I refer to the face-to-face meeting between doctor and patient. This includes the consultation and physical examination, as well as treatments conducted by doctors face-to-face, such as surgery. I also explore the general public's encounter with illness. By 'public' I refer to non-medically trained members of the general population. Lastly, this is not an examination of a single

clinical encounter and its ontological effects upon me or a specific doctor. Rather, I attempt generalization of the clinical encounter, doctor, and patient to identify essential features and support this with textual analysis in the final section.

As with any first-person phenomenology, my experience is dictated by my embodiment as a white, able-bodied, cis-gender male. The lived experience of those who do not identify with these categories will be different from my own. Thus, my description here intends to be only a starting point. Furthermore, my phenomenological analysis is rooted in, and spreads outwards from, my lived experience through medical school as an undergraduate. Medical education varies significantly at the international, institutional, and individual levels. Hence, I have attempted to draw on aspects of medical education and clinical practice common to all those who have trained in modern Western biomedicine.

Section 1: background

Descartes, biomedicine, and objectification

Descartes' designation of the body as *res extensa* was vital for the development of the western scientific approach to medicine. Descartes argued the soul was attached to the immaterial mind, not the body, making the body a non-religious object. This allowed the body to be studied by science through the dissection of cadavers, which was previously prohibited.[11] Foucault[10] recounts the resulting changes in medical practice following the development of dissection. He argues the scientific study of 'pathological anatomy' enabled a new understanding of disease which encouraged abstraction of the individual patient.[10(p152)] Through dissection, for the first time, "western man could constitute himself in his own eyes as an *object* of science."[10(p243)] Therefore, the development of Foucault's objectifying medical gaze depended on cartesian ontology.

Modern biopsychosocial clinical practice keeps the same ontological assumptions and focuses on the body-object.[11,12] Thus, objectification becomes an essential part of the clinical encounter explored in Sec. 2.3. Other works of philosophy have shown the clinical examination to have an objectifying touch, gaze, and auscultation.[10,13–15] Furthermore, Foucault[10] recounts changes in the language of the history-taking: moving away from symptoms (lived patient experiences) and toward identifiers of underlying disease of the body-object, largely bypassing the patient as an individual subject.

Phenomenology of the body and illness

Phenomenology is the careful study of experience *as it appears to us*. This emphasis results in significantly different attitudes to the body compared to Descartes.[2,16] When we carefully consider how we interact with objects, or *phenomena*, in the everyday, our mind and body are inseparable. They are part of one being which I understand to be myself. My body as it is for me each day, or the lived body, enables our experience of the world. I can touch and experience my own body as if it were an object, but I can only touch because I am first embodied.[16,17]

Heidegger[4] uses phenomenology to examine the underlying structures or ways of 'being' which make human existence possible. In German, he forms long new words intended to describe complete unified ways of being. These are hyphenated when translated to English to maintain this original meaning. Being-in-the-world describes human inseparability from the world itself and how we always already find ourselves within the world. This is an essential, unavoidable part of being.[4] Building on the work of Heidegger, Sartre[9] describes the body as normally passed-by-in-silence in my everyday experience in the world. My body is rarely the focus of my attention, instead, in the background, it enables me to complete whatever task I happen to be doing. In contrast, in illness, our projects are interrupted, and the body is no longer passed-by-in-silence, it reveals itself as an object within the world and draws our attention.[2,18,19] Illness also affects how we interact with the world and thus effects our being-in-the-world.[2,18] In the next section, I suggest witnessing illness in the Other, the body again reveals itself as an object, as it does in illness, however more faintly and subtly.

Toombs[18] makes observations about the different ways doctors and patients attend to illness within the clinical encounter. For Toombs, doctors focus upon certain aspects of illness and 'thematise' it into a diagnosis of disease. How we thematise any experience is ultimately dependent upon habits of mind, which are dictated by our biographical situation.[18] Therefore, the way in which doctors focus on disease and the body-object is dependent on, and results from, their being-a-doctor, and thus their medical education. Crucially, Toombs does not provide a detailed description of the embodied experience of the doctor. Therefore, I attempt to show the embodiment of the doctor influences the clinical encounter itself, and the clinical encounter influences the doctor's embodiment.

Section 2: the clinical encounter

The basic encounter

My experience of another person is different to my experience of objects. Through their behavior, as embodied consciousnesses, I see other individuals (or the Other) orientate themselves toward their goals and projects as I would.[17] By seeing the Other as *being like me* in their dynamic, complex, embodied behavior, I realize myself as *being like them*. Through their animated behavior, I see the Other does not behave like any other object, and neither do I. To be clear, this is not an intellectual judgment we make after carefully considering our own behavior and the behavior of the Other, rather it is the basic way in which we experience the Other.[16]

I suggest, our response to the illness of the other depends on this similar embodiment to the Other. My encounter with the table is not the same as my encounter with the Other. Therefore, my experience and reaction to breaking a table leg are fundamentally different to seeing someone break their leg. My immediate reaction to the Others illness, pain, and experience is rooted in my similar embodiment to them.

The encounter with illness

Each individual who becomes ill will have a unique experience. A person's experience up to the point of becoming ill, their current situation and the specific pathology make each instance of illness unique. However, philosophers suggest there are underlying features of this experience that are common to all.[2,18] This section aims to explore the similar underlying structures in the experience of encountering the Other who is, or becomes, ill.

In seeing the old man fall on the street, passersby will wince and recoil. In seeing someone injure themselves, our arms are brought to our chests as if protecting our own bodies. I see a child knock their teeth out and there is an uncomfortable sensation within my own teeth. I grasp my leg looking at an x-ray of a broken femur as the Orthopedic surgeon explains how the injury occurred to the patient. Before medical school the first time I saw surgery, aged seventeen, I was overwhelmed with nausea, unable to concentrate, and fainted. There is an immediate unconscious, bodily response to seeing someone with an illness, whether this is someone falling or someone on a ventilator. This response does not occur through conscious consideration of how the same illness could occur to me. Rather, the body reacts before I have a chance to consciously consider what has occurred. Previous research has also shown the presence of and stressed the educational importance of this emotional response in students through biomechanics simulation.[20] Möller and their colleagues concluded there is educational value for learners to "contextualize the visual representations [of injury] relative to one's own body."[20(p144)]

Stein's phenomenology of empathy has received recent attention in the cognitive sciences and provides an explanation for this bodily response. Stein describes a basic type of empathy as "felt experiences of other living bodies."[21(p746)] Stein suggests bodily responses to the experiences of another is a type of empathy. I suggest, when we see another person who is ill, or who injures themselves, it is this type of bodily response we experience. This occurs *before* we might imagine the same happening to us, not *because* we do. It is *pre-reflective*. Through this bodily response to illness in the Other, the focus of our attention may turn away from the person who is ill and onto our own bodies, as it does in illness itself. For instance, I found it (unsurprisingly) difficult to concentrate on the patient's surgical procedure while trying not to faint from the nausea in my stomach.

Importantly, Stein's empathy does not exclude other types of imaginative empathy, through which doctors may also relate to patient experiences.[21] Therefore, even in the absence of bodily reactions to the body-object of the patient, other forms of empathy are possible between doctor and patient. I can empathize with people whom I have never met face to face and share little common experience, such as refugees feeling war. I may achieve this by consciously imagining their experiences and replaying them in my head. Stein's phenomenology of empathy does not *exclude* this form of empathizing but rather provides an explanation for how we can empathize *pre*-consciously through a bodily reaction

Zaner in *The Context of Self* states "it would be an utter naivety" to assume the body-object only announces itself in times of our own illness, instead it is "present, however faintly, in the healthy body."[19(p56)] I suggest when we see the child knock their teeth out, we become aware of our own teeth as objects that could similarly be knocked out. Whereas, normally I am unaware of my teeth and their apparent fragility. Through seeing illness, the body is no longer passed-by-in-silence and is replaced, perhaps only briefly, by an awareness of my body-object as a fragile, vulnerable thing within the world.

Another example: if I see my mother cut herself while chopping the vegetables, I wince, and my stomach turns. I may even unconsciously grab my own finger. When I take over the cutting from her, I cut with more care than I would have if I had not seen her cut herself. Through my bodily reaction, I have become aware of my fingers as fragile objects within the world. Zaner alludes to the unique, uncomfortable nature of encountering illness in another:

> Indeed, what gives [illness] such peculiarly dramatic force—the hush, anxiety and awe engendered when the "normal" person encounters the ailing or the maimed—is precisely that illness and impairment affect us directly in what seems our unique humanity.[19(p159)]

Our recognition of ourselves in the Other and our awareness of our own body gives the encounter with illness its salience and strangeness. When confronted with illness face-to-face, the body is no longer passed-by-in-silence. I argue, this awareness made of one's own body presents a challenge to medical practice and education. If we flinch when we see someone cut themselves, how can we learn to cut straight with a scalpel? How am I now able to assist in surgery, aged twenty-five, and not faint? A certain level of detached objective thinking appears to be required from doctors, and doctors appear to have a reduced bodily response to seeing illness. As a result of medical education, an unnamed, unaddressed, and untaught ontological transformation appears to have already occurred within me. The result of this transformation is being-opposite-illness. With this in mind, we now come to the clinical encounter itself.

The clinical encounter

Unlike the public, through medical education, doctors possess extensive knowledge on anatomy and pathology and treatment options. As Toombs discussed, through medical education, the thematization of illness into disease becomes possible and is used to diagnose patients.[18] Medical students learn to look with an objectifying, medical gaze.[10] It is the presence of the doctor, their education, goals, and expertise which distinguishes the clinical encounter from the general public's encounter with illness. Next, I will focus on Sartre's phenomenology of 'the look' to link patient objectification to the doctor's reduced bodily response to illness.[9(p276–326)] I suggest the doctor as the objectifier and the patient as objectified forms the ontological axis of opposition for being-opposite-illness.

Sartre[9] provides an account of becoming aware of his body-as-object while looking through the keyhole. While previously he was focused on what was occurring on the other side of the door, when he hears someone coming, he becomes aware of his own body and how it appears to them. Through the shame brought about by the look of the Other, Sartre becomes aware of his body as an object in the world. Sartre's account of shame parallels directly with accounts of shame felt by patients within the clinical encounter, where one is objectified as their body-object is focused upon.[9,22]

One can escape this fear and "recover [oneself]" if we constitute the Other as an object. While looking through the keyhole, if we turn and realize what we thought was the Other looking at us is instead, say, the shadow of a tree, we realize we are no longer looked at and the body fades back into silence, since one cannot be an "object for an object."[9(p313)]

For the public's encounter with illness, one recognizes their body as a vulnerable object in the world, through their similar embodiment to the Other-with-illness. Patient objectification by the doctor constitutes the patient as an object. Since the doctor cannot be objectified by an object, this maintains the doctor's being-as-subject, limits their bodily response, and thus their focus remains beyond themselves and toward the patient. Being-*opposite*-illness specifically refers to this ontological polarity. The patient is reduced to an object as the doctor maintains themselves as a subject, tending to their goals, with their body passed-by-in-silence. In the clinical encounter, the patient tends to be considered as *only* their body, whereas the doctor's body is forgotten.

To use a prior example, in the extreme, if anatomy class allows me to experience a patient's leg as no different from a table leg, my nausea in the operating theater for a femur fixation would be significantly reduced. I could see the operation as nothing more than a procedure of academic craftsmanship. Furthermore, Kalanithi considers covering faces during dissection. This is objectifying for the patient and limits his bodily response to the procedure.[8]

The patient undergoing surgery, inert under general anesthesia, is no doubt objectified more than the patient examined in the clinic. However, I maintain that complete objectification—constituting the patient's leg as no different from the anatomical model—is not possible. Even in death, our reaction to a cadaver is not the same as another object.[4] As one learns about the body at medical school, one's bodily response to patients and cadavers does reduce. However, doctors cannot remain completely unaffected by the experiences of patients showing complete objectification is not possible. This is shown in the well-documented phenomena of burnout and vicarious traumatization.[23,24] In fact, doctors distancing themselves through objectification may only be necessary because they can be affected by their patients. In my experience, even in surgery, the patient as body-object maintains their humanity and are not reduced entirely to an object. Despite this, objectification raises ethical concerns and debates. Patients and cadavers are not objects like a table, and should never be treated as such.

Let us explore a final example where the doctor may struggle to objectify the patient. General Medical Council guidance states doctors should be registered to a General Practitioner outside their family.[25] I suggest, in part, it is difficult for doctors to treat their family objectively precisely because it is difficult to objectify them. One imagines if a surgeon was to operate on a member of their family, they would struggle to focus. The lack of objectification stops the doctor from thinking objectively and results in a more emotional, bodily response to illness. It is difficult to constitute a person close to us as an *object* because we are aware of everything they are as a *subject*. We are aware of their likes, dislikes, hopes, and dreams. As I have argued, a lack of objectification results in an inability to maintain the body passed-by-in-silence. Thus, doctors are more able to think in a detached manner when they can objectify the patient in front of them and limit their bodily response, and this is harder to do with a family member.

In this section, I have attempted to show when seeing illness in the Other, our similar embodiment presents the experience of 'bodily fragility': an uncomfortable experience through which our body is realized as a vulnerable object within the world. I account for the reduction of bodily fragility in doctors within the clinical encounter through patient objectification. This maintains their body as passed-by-in-silence and directs their focus toward the body of the patient. This transformation occurs through medical education, as this enables students to look with an objectifying medical gaze and thematise illness into disease. Thus, medical education can be considered an ontological transformation, where a student's response to illness changes from one aligned with the publics to the doctor's in being-opposite-illness. Being-opposite-illness, as a result of medical education, is the unique ontology of the doctor, demonstrated by the diminished bodily response to seeing illness, rooted in objectification of the patient.

Section 3: being-opposite-illness

This section will look at two popular first-person accounts from Paul Kalanithi[8] and Henry Marsh.[1] My analysis focuses on their objectification of patients' bodies, and how this impacts their way of being. Furthermore, the impact of being-opposite-illness upon lived experience can be seen when the authors fall ill themselves. This section does not intend to provide a comprehensive review of this type of literature. Instead, I focus on textual analysis to provide illustrations of the arguments put forward above.

Kalanithi's[8] *When Breath Becomes Air* is a heart-breaking candid account of the author's fight with cancer. During medical school, Kalanithi discusses learning to "objectify the dead, literally reducing them to organs, tissues, nerves and muscles."[8(p49)] However, for Kalanithi, on a medical student's first day, "you simply [cannot] deny the humanity of the corpse."[8(p49)] As Kalanithi increasingly objectifies the cadavers, his experience changes from one dominated by bodily feelings of "revulsion, exhilaration, [and] nausea" to an experience of merely "academic exercise."[8(p44)] Kalanithi adds "pretending" cadavers are "fake" and covering their faces "makes work easier."[8(p45)] Here we see both the impact and usefulness of being-opposite-illness to the medical student who needs to learn the anatomy and is limited by the distraction of bodily reactions. The salience and peculiarity of interacting with cadavers has been explored in more recent research and echoes Kalanithi's experiences.[3]

Kalanithi[8] continues his objectification into his career as a surgeon. He describes being in theater, not with patients but, with "cases" such as "giant aneurysms, intracerebral arterial bypasses, arteriovenous malformations."[8(p10–11)] It is only when illness, and death, strikes someone close to the author, he realizes his detachment from patients and how he "neatly packages" them into "various diagnoses," comparing himself to Ivan Ilych's doctor.[8(p85),26] I suggest, the author's familiarity with his friend and resulting inability to objectify them, drives the uncomfortable bodily reaction he has to the thought of conducting surgery on her.

We can see the impact of his objectification of patients on Kalanithi's embodiment when he becomes ill. In his own words, he transforms "from doctor to patient, from actor to acted upon, from subject to direct object" and its effect on him.[8(p180)] Echoing the epigraph quote from Marsh, Kalanithi chooses to describe his illness as if it were happening to a patient:

> thirty-five-year-old with unexplained weight loss and new-onset back pain—the obvious answer would be (C) Cancer.[8(p5)]

Kalanithi chooses to abstract himself from his own illness. He thematises his *illness* into the *disease* of an imaginary patient. Through this, Kalanithi can very easily provide a diagnosis but struggles to come to terms with the illness being his own. Later, Kalanithi doubts whether he has cancer, despite his ease when diagnosing the body-as-object:

> I knew a lot about back pain—its anatomy, its physiology, the different words patients used to describe different kinds of pain—but I didn't know what it *felt* like. Maybe that's all this was.[8(p12)]

It is clear from these passages Kalanithi finds it easier to deal with his illness by thematising it into disease. For Kalanithi, disease is an event in the objectified body and thus not his own as it is usually passed-by-in-silence and *un*felt. Kalanithi readily understands illness as it occurs to the cartesian body-object, but not the lived phenomenological body.

After ceasing to practice, Kalanithi describes a fast-physical decline and is stunned how he spent "nearly thirty-six hours" operating less than week before. Kalanithi concludes "without [the] duty to care for the ill pushing [him] forward, [he] became an invalid."[8(p125)] Being-opposite-illness in the operating theater, Kalanithi's body remained passed-by-in-silence by focusing on that of the patients. Once removed from clinical practice, Kalanithi's body becomes unmuted, he becomes far more aware of his symptoms.

Kalanithi's oncologist, Emily, respects him as another doctor and they often make decisions about his care together, as two clinicians would about a third patient.[7] However, Emily suggests he could abdicate his responsibility and allow her to "just *be* the doctor" implying Kalanithi *just be a patient.*[8(p182)] However, the thought of "abdicating control" is one Kalanithi finds "impossible." Instead, Kalanithi's "doctor-self [remained] responsible for [his] patient-self."[8(p183)] This passage highlights the powerful influence the medical profession has on an individual's ontology. For Kalanithi, the influence of his doctor-self extends far beyond the operating room and persists once he becomes ill. This shows being-opposite-illness is not something which is switched on and off as a professional persona.

Marsh's[1] experiences of medical school, surgery, and illness all bear similarities to Kalanithi's and mine. From the preface, Marsh[1(p.xi)] instructs: "You must learn to be objective about what you see, and yet not lose your humanity in the process." From the outset, Marsh focuses on the detachment required from doctors, which must be balanced with the emotional response to the suffering of others.

Later in the book lies the line which sparked my investigation. Marsh[1(p215)] notes the so-called hypochondria of "medical student syndrome" rarely persists as medical students learn about the "necessary detachment" required as a matter of "self-preservation." Marsh draws attention to how medical school changes one's relationship with their body. Through this changed relationship, students learn "illness is something that only happens to patients. That is something you learn early on a medical school."[1(p215)] Being-opposite-illness, then, allows an ontological separation from one's own body through patient objectification.

Marsh[1(p216)] remarks that doctors often "dismiss their initial symptoms" and are "slow to diagnose their own illnesses" all to escape becoming a "mere patient." All of which are behaviors Marsh finds in himself and are found in Kalanithi's account. Marsh describes breaking his leg and while waiting for his plaster to be changed, he describes a brief, remarkable encounter with a fellow consultant.

> 'Oh dear', he said in a very prim voice, as though he disapproved of the vulgar way in which, by allowing my leg to be broken, I had become a mere patient.[1(p229)]

The word choice of *allowing* infers an attitude that, as a doctor, Marsh breaking his leg was within his control. Of course, this is absurd, falling down the stairs, as Marsh did, could happen to anyone. A doctor's bones are no different to that of a patient. The bodies maintenance as passed-by-in-silence in being-opposite-illness promotes a false attitude of illness not occurring to doctors.

Marsh and Kalanithi's accounts demonstrate a unique ontology of the doctor and the transformation undergone throughout medical education. Patient objectification changes a doctor's ontology, distancing them from their own body. I suggest, this results in the lack of the doctor's bodily reaction being face-to-face with illness. However, by objectifying the Other I can direct my focus away from my own body.[9] By muting the body in this way, keeping it passed-by-in-silence, illness becomes "something that happens only to patients."[1(p215)] There is an ontological

separation between the patient's being-ill and the doctor's being-opposite-illness. As the patient is objectified, the medical gaze is not only a way of looking but becomes a way of being: the doctor looks without being looked at. The objectifying gaze denies the similar embodiment between doctor and patient. Being-*opposite*-illness denotes this ontological polarity between doctor and patient.

Limitations and conclusions

I am aware that I may be criticized as Merleau-Ponty, Heidegger, and Sartre all have been for providing accounts explaining only the experiences of white, cis-gendered, able-bodied, males.[2,5,27,28] This is an important critique and I hope further works can add to and correct mine. I have tried to focus on aspects of doctor's experiences common to all to identify features that apply beyond my own experiences. This investigation is built on my experiences of being a patient and seeing illness in other people both as an untrained member of the public as well as during my time as a medical student. At the time of writing, I am months from starting my first job as a doctor and I believe my years at medical school have given me enough experience to understand patient objectification. Additionally, this account concerns only western conventional contemporary medicine and attempts to describe only the face-to-face clinical encounter. It may or may not apply to nurses or other healthcare professionals. Finally, a limitation of this account is the psychiatric clinical encounter. Due to how psychiatric illness presents and the current academic understanding of psychiatric disease, I do not extend my account to the psychiatric clinical encounter and maintain the psychiatric clinical encounter warrants its own complete phenomenological analysis.

Further phenomena that I have excluded here I believe may affect the ontology of the doctor includes society's view of doctor and patient. As de Beauvoir[5] suggests and Young[28] builds upon, the way a society views an individual affects their being-in-the-world. Secondly, I have not explored the temporal element of the clinical encounter. On the ward round and in clinic, patients are encountered in series. Therefore, it may be that doctors detach themselves from each patient to focus on the next.

In conclusion, this analysis attempts to present a new way of exploring the experiences of doctors by accounting for their embodied lived experience. This account would not be possible without acknowledging the medical student experience and my medical humanities intercalation. As argued previously, this work illustrates the value of teaching philosophy to medical students.[7] The discussion of the clinical encounter as being between *two* embodied individuals may promote renewed approaches to the doctor-patient relationship and clinical skills education. Specifically, by accounting for the ontological transition of medical students. I hope as medical educators we can take a fresh look at phenomena like empathy and compassion, exploring how these are developed but also lost. Furthermore, future work may look at the impact of the ontological transition of medical students on medical ethics, perhaps exploring the bodily response to illness as an ethical demand to do good. In sum, I have attempted to show that one undergoes an ontological transformation at medical school and through clinical practice. This ultimately results in a unique way of being for doctors: being-opposite-illness.

Acknowledgements

I would like to thank Gregory Artus and Dr Tina Williams for their guidance and support in completing this work.

Previous philosophy in medical education instalments

Mario Veen & Anna T. Cianciolo (2020) Problems No One Looked For: Philosophical Expeditions into Medical Education, Teaching and Learning in Medicine, 32:3, 337–344, DOI: 10.1080/10401334.2020.1748634.

Gert J. J. Biesta & Marije van Braak (2020) Beyond the Medical Model: Thinking Differently about Medical Education and Medical Education Research, Teaching and Learning in Medicine, 32:4, 449–456, DOI: 10.1080/10401334.2020.1798240.

Mark R. Tonelli & Robyn Bluhm (2021) Teaching Medical Epistemology within an Evidence-Based Medicine Curriculum, Teaching and Learning in Medicine, 33:1, 98–105, DOI: 10.1080/10401334.2020.1835666.

John R. Skelton (2021) Language, Philosophy, and Medical Education, Teaching and Learning in Medicine, 33:2, 210–216, DOI: 10.1080/10401334.2021.1877712.

Zareen Zaidi, Ian M. Partman, Cynthia R.Whitehead, Ayelet Kuper & Tasha R. Wyatt (2021) Contending with Our Racial Past in Medical Education: A Foucauldian Perspective, Teaching and Learning in Medicine, DOI: 10.1080/10401334.2021.1945929.

Chris Rietmeijer & Mario Veen (2021) Phenomenological Research in Health Professions.

Education: Tunneling from Both Ends, Teaching and Learning in Medicine, DOI:10.1080/10401334.2021.1971989.

Madeleine Noelle Olding, Freya Rhodes, John Humm, Phoebe Ross & Catherine McGarry (2022) Black, White and Gray: Student Perspectives on Medical Humanities and Medical Education, Teaching and Learning in Medicine, 34:2, 223–233, DOI: 10.1080/10401334.2021.1982717.

Camillo Coccia & Mario Veen (2022) Because We Care: A Philosophical Investigation into the Spirit of Medical Education, Teaching and Learning in Medicine, 10.1080/10401334.2022.2056744.

Tim Fawns & Sven Schaepkens (2022) A Matter of Trust: Online Proctored Exams and the Integration of Technologies of Assessment in Medical Education, Teaching and Learning in Medicine, DOI: 10.1080/10401334.2022.2048832.

Anna MacLeod, Victoria Luong, Paula Cameron, George Kovacs, Molly Fredeen, Lucy Patrick, Olga Kits & Jonathan Tummons (2022) The Lifecycle of a Clinical Cadaver: A Practice-Based Ethnography, Teaching and Learning in Medicine, DOI: 10.1080/10401334.2022.2092111.

Associated podcast

Let Me Ask You Something (iTunes, Spotify, Google Podcasts and https://marioveen.com/letmeaskyousomething/).

Funding

The author(s) reported there is no funding associated with the work featured in this article.

ORCID

John Humm http://orcid.org/0000-0002-6888-8988

References

1. Marsh H. *Do No Harm*. 1st ed. London, UK: Orion Publishing Co; 2015.
2. Carel H. *Phenomenology of Illness*. 1st ed. Oxford, UK: Oxford University Press; 2016.
3. MacLeod A, Luong V, Cameron P, et al. The lifecycle of a clinical cadaver: a practice-based ethnography. *Teach Learn Med.* 2022;34(4):1–17. doi:10.1080/10401334.2022.2092111.
4. Heidegger M. *Being and Time*. 1st ed. Macquarrie J, Robinson E, trans. Oxford, UK: Blackwell Publishing; 2016.
5. De Beauvoir S. *The Second Sex*. 1st ed. Parshley H, trans. London, UK: Vintage; 1997.
6. Rietmeijer C, Veen M. Phenomenological research in health professions. *Teach Learn Med.* 2021;34(1):113–121. doi:10.1080/10401334.2021.1971989.
7. Olding M, Rhodes F, Humm J, McGarry RP, Black C. White and gray: student perspectives on medical humanities and medical education. *Teach Learn Med.* 2021; 34(2):223–233. doi:10.1080/10401334.2021.1982717.
8. Kalanithi P. *When Breath Becomes Air*. 1st ed. London, UK: Random House; 2016.
9. Sartre J. *Being and Nothingness*. London, UK: Routledge; 2010.
10. Foucault M. *The Birth of the Clinic*. 3rd ed. London, UK: Routledge; 2003.

11. Mehta N. Mind-body dualism: a critique from a health perspective. *Mens Sana Monogr.* 2011;9(1):202–209. doi:10.4103/0973-1229.77436.

12. Engel G. The need for a new medical model: a challenge for biomedicine. *Science.* 1977;196(4286):129–136. doi:10.1126/science.847460.

13. Leder D, Krucoff M. The touch that heals: the uses and meanings of touch in the clinical encounter. *J Altern Complement Med.* 2008;14(3):321–327. doi:10.1089/acm.2007.0717.

14. Rice T. "Beautiful murmurs": stethoscopic listening and acoustic objectification. *The Senses and Society.* 2008;3(3):293–306. doi:10.2752/174589308X331332.

15. Baron R. An introduction to medical phenomenology: I can't hear you while I'm listening. *Ann Intern Med.* 1985;103(4):606–611. doi:10.7326/0003-4819-103-4-606.

16. Hass L. *Merleau-Ponty's Philosophy.* Bloomington: Indiana University Press; 2008.

17. Merleau-Ponty M. *Phenomenology of Perception.* Smith M, trans. London: Routledge Kegan Paul; 1974.

18. Toombs S. The meaning of illness: a phenomenological approach to the patient physician relationship. *J Med Philos.* 1987;12(3):219–240. doi:10.1093/jmp/12.3.219.

19. Zaner R. *The Context of Self.* 1st ed. Athens, OH: Ohio University Press; 1981.

20. Möller H, Creutzfeldt J, Valeskog K, et al. Technology-enhanced learning of human trauma bio-mechanics in an interprofessional student context. *Teach Learn Med.* 2021;34(2):135–144. doi:10.1080/10401334.2021.1893735.

21. Svenaeus F. Edith Stein's phenomenology of sensual and emotional empathy. *Phenom Cogn Sci.* 2017;17(4):741–760. doi:10.1007/s11097-017-9544-9.

22. Dolezal L. The phenomenology of shame in the clinical encounter. *Med Health Care Philos.* 2015;18(4):567–576. doi:10.1007/s11019-015-9654-5.

23. Dunkley J, Whelan T. Vicarious traumatisation: current status and future directions. *Br J Guid Couns.* 2006;34(1):107–116. doi:10.1080/03069880500483166.

24. Kumar S. Burnout and doctors: prevalence, prevention and intervention. *Healthcare.* 2016;4(3):37. doi:10.3390/healthcare4030037.

25. Good Medical Practice. General Medical Council. https://www.gmc-uk.org/ethical-guidance/ethical-guidance-for-doctors/good-medical-practice. Published 2021. Accessed December 29, 2021.

26. Tolstoy L. *The Death of Ivan Ilych and Other Stories.* Maude A, Duff J, trans. New York: Signet Classics; 2012:93–153.

27. Bakewell S. *At the Existentialist Café: Freedom, Being & Apricot Cocktails.* 1st ed. London: Penguin; 2017.

28. Young I. Throwing like a girl: a phenomenology of feminine body comportment motility and spatiality. *Hum Stud.* 1980;3(1):137–156. doi:10.1007/BF02331805.

The Lifecycle of a Clinical Cadaver: A Practice-Based Ethnography

Anna MacLeod (iD), Victoria Luong (iD), Paula Cameron (iD), George Kovacs, Molly Fredeen, Lucy Patrick, Olga Kits (iD) and Jonathan Tummons (iD)

ABSTRACT

Phenomenon: Cadavers have long played an important and complex role in medical education. While research on cadaver-based simulation has largely focused on exploring student attitudes and reactions or measuring improvements in procedural performance, the ethical, philosophical, and experiential aspects of teaching and learning with cadavers are rarely discussed. In this paper, we shed new light on the fascinating philosophical moves in which people engage each and every time they find themselves face to face with a cadaver. *Approach:* Over a two-year period (2018/19–2019/20), we applied ethnographic methods (137 hours of observation, 24 interviews, and the analysis of 22 documents) to shadow the educational cadaver through the practical stages involved in cadaver-based simulation: 1. cadaver preparation, 2. cadaver-based skill practice with physicians and residents, and 3. interment and memorial services. We used Deleuze and Guattari's concepts of becoming and acts of creation to trace the ontological "lifecycle" of an educational cadaver as embedded within everyday work practices. *Findings:* We delineated six sub-phases of the lifecycle, through which the cadaver transformed ontologically from person to donor, body, cadaver, educational cadaver, teacher, and loved one/legacy. These shifts involved a network of bureaucratic, technical, educational, and humanistic practices that shaped the way the cadaver was perceived and acted upon at different moments in the lifecycle. By highlighting, at each phase, 1) the ontological transitions of the cadaver, itself, and 2) the practices, events, settings, and people involved in each of these transitions, we explored questions of "being" as it related to the *ontological ambiguity* of the cadaver: its conceptualization as both person and tool, simultaneously representing life and death. *Insights:* Engaging deeply with the philosophical questions of cadaver-based simulation (CBS) helped us conceptualize the lifecycle as a series of meaningful and purposeful acts of becoming. Following the cadaver from program entry to interment allowed us to contemplate how its ontological ambiguity shapes every aspect of cadaver-based simulation. We found that in discussions of fidelity in medical simulation, beyond both the physical and functional, it is possible to conceive of a third type: *ontological*. The humanness of the cadaver makes CBS a unique, irreplaceable, and inherently philosophical, practice.

Introduction

Scholars have recently called for a more explicit philosophical turn in medical education inquiry, encouraging our community to engage with philosophies of science, and to explore "problems no one looked for."[1,2] Questions of *ontology*, the branch of philosophy that deals with *being*, have been raised as important considerations in the realm of medical education.[3] We responded to this call by both empirically and philosophically exploring

one of the most complex practices of medical education: cadaver-based simulation (CBS). In this paper, we shed new light on the fascinating philosophical moves in which people engage each time they find themselves face to face with a cadaver.

Cadavers are an important element in many medical education programs, traditionally in the realm of anatomy education.[4,5] The literature on traditional cadavers in medical education has explored not only their effectiveness for teaching anatomy,[6] but also some of the ethical[7,8] and professional[9-11] complexities associated with their use. Many have reflected on the controversial history of cadaveric dissection, which has evolved from a once "dubiously moral and barely legal activity" [11(p3)] to one demanding the highest standards for respect, which are reflected in current ethical guidelines and legal regulations around cadaver-based education.[12] As well, recent authors have explored the various physical and psycho-emotional reactions medical trainees have in relation to cadaveric dissection—ranging from ocular irritation, to anxiety, surprise, and enthusiasm.[7,13-17] Generally speaking, these studies attest to the superiority of cadaver-based learning compared to other methods of anatomy education,[6] as well as the positive impacts cadavers may have on student empathy and humanstic care.[18,19]

Some scholars, however, such as McDonald[20] and Hallam,[21] have taken an anthropological and ethnographic approach to attend to the dynamic and unfolding character of cadavers. McDonald demonstrates how cadavers are "acquired" by students; in an "ever-active process of micro articulation," students learn to see, smell, handle, and hear in various ways over time.[20(p129)] For example, the author explains how students gradually learn to match diagrams illustrated in their manuals to the cadavers before them: a process McDonald describes as "acquir[ing] particular eyes...learn[ing] to see." Moreover, Hallam[21] considers the dissection of a body after death a "relational process"[21(p100)] whereby the cadaver is always understood in relation to the social and material elements involved in their procurement, use, and memorialization. In this manner, "bodies after death are valued as persons, as materials for the generation and communication of anatomical knowledge, and as gifts for the advancement of medical science"[21(p99)]

More recently, advancements in preservation techniques have led to new uses for cadavers, specifically in the realm of procedural skills teaching and simulation.[22-27] CBS, like any form of simulation, is based on the idea that learners practice skills and apply knowledge in lifelike contexts. Arguably, no manikin can offer more fidelity in reproducing the complexity, variability, and particularity of the human body than an *actual* human body; thus, CBS is emerging as a promising approach for teaching, particularly for practicing high-skill, low frequency procedures.[22-27] Because these preservation techniques are still relatively new, there is a paucity of research examining the use of clinical cadavers specifically. The limited existing literature on CBS has largely focused on measuring its validity and effectiveness for learning,[22-28] with a few notable exceptions. Douglas-Jones'[29] ethnographic account, for example, details the cultural

specificities of donation in the Taiwanese Tzu Chi Buddhist Silent Mentor program Medical Simulation Center, where people make a deliberate effort to acknowledge the identity of the donor, by positioning photographs and telling stories about the donor's life.

Arguably, the ethical and professional complexities of these cadavers could differ significantly from those of traditional cadavers. For example, compared to traditional cadavers, bodies prepared for CBS are undeniably more lifelike—both visually and tactilely. *Hard-fixed* (traditional) cadavers are embalmed using the chemical formaldehyde, which delays the decomposition of the body's tissues, but also renders them stiff and unpliable. These cadavers maintain the intricate form and location of bodily tissues but poorly resemble living bodies.[30] In contrast, *soft-preserved* (CBS) cadavers, such as those more recently developed by Thiel,[31] as well as scientists in Taiwan,[29,32] Baltimore, and Halifax,[27,33] maintain the look and feel of anesthetized patients. Medical learners across the continuum can use these more lifelike cadavers, termed *clinical cadavers* by Kovacs and colleagues,[27] to practice procedures with high degrees of fidelity.[34]

Scholars such as McDonald and Hallam have given us rich insights into some of the anthropological and relational dimensions of cadaveric dissection, hinting at the multiple values and roles that bodies take on during the process of "anatomisation."[20,21] However, scholars in the field have not yet fulsomely examined the underlying philosophical and ontological questions associated with using lifelike cadavers to engage in CBS. And, while some have described the cultural nuances of programs using cadavers that are differently preserved in order to facilitate surgical skills teaching,[29,32] these pieces have not yet addressed the conceptual work in which people involved with CBS must engage to accomplish the variety of tasks at hand—ranging from administrative to educational. In an effort to address this gap, we worked with Deleuze and Guattari's notion of *ontology as creation* to analyze how medical educators develop an evolving suite of concepts to make sense of cadavers as they go about their work.[35] In their classic work *What is Philosophy?*,[35] the authors distinguished three primary acts in which we engage as we try to make sense of the world: science, art, and philosophy. We argue that medical educators have long engaged with the science and art of CBS; however, we have not yet carefully attuned to the philosophical aspects of this work, and in particular to questions of *ontology*.

Through a two-year practice-based[36] ethnographic study of CBS, we learned that cadavers are ontologically complex, and in a process of constant conceptual re-creation. We describe herein a six-step lifecycle of an educational cadaver, delineating the **ontological transitions** that must occur at each stage to facilitate the work of teaching and learning through CBS. This paper expands our current understanding, probing the deeper, philosophical complexities of working with lifelike cadavers.

Method

Theoretical frame

Our study is theoretically framed in Practice Theory.[36] Practice theory can be said to present a view of the social world as "a vast array or assemblage of performances made durable by being inscribed in skilled human bodies and minds, objects and texts and knotted together in such a way that the results of one performance become the resource for another."[37(p20)] Practices are materially mediated and entangled with the social and relational.[36] This approach focuses on understanding the networks of everyday activities in which groups of people engage in their workplaces and other everyday settings.[37,38]

We considered multiple human and non-human actors associated with cadaver work, taking care to note both people (e.g., cadaver staff, administrators, teachers, learners) and things (tools, spaces, legal and educational documents), as well as the cadaver itself, which exists in a liminal space, and is somehow both human, and non-human.[39] We selected a practice-based approach because we were interested in studying, in fine detail, the everyday, taken for granted elements of CBS in order to fulsomely understand and describe its complexities. Cadavers are part of the human and non-human arrangement and are relevant actors in these networks and practices as "... things might authorize, allow, afford, encourage, permit, suggest, influence, block, render possible, forbid, and so on."[40(p72)] Focusing on the practices of cadaver work allowed us to articulate, and better understand, the complexities of day-to-day activities performed in these professional settings.

With respect to analysis and interpretation, we drew on Deleuze and Guattari's ideas about becoming and difference to understand how the concept of "cadaver" evolves. Deleuze and Guattari have been referred to as *differential ontologists,* meaning that they worked with the assumption that concepts are always constituted on the basis of *difference* (we identify things by what they are not). Folding this perspective into questions of ontology, then, requires a deliberate effort to unravel traditional ideas about being in order to offer new ways of thinking or understanding.

Deleuze and Guattari did not believe that the purpose of philosophy was to "discover" what the world is really like. To them, this was an impossible goal. Instead, they equated philosophy to the *creation of concepts*: philosophy is about creating frameworks that help us make sense of the infinite complexity of the world. Each act in which we engage in our everyday life has the potential to inspire new concepts. Being, then, is conceptualized as a process of creation rather than discovery. This means that there is no one story, or unified truth to be discovered. Rather, it is up to us to create the concepts that structure the world.

Specific to our case, we are interested in putting forth a series of concepts that help us better understand the profound complexity of the practices of human body donation and cadaver-based simulation. Linking these Deluezian ideas to our practice-based approach, we see that the everyday activities of human body donation and cadaver-based simulation can, in fact, be taken as acts of becoming. From this perspective, a cadaver has no fixed identity; it is constantly becoming something different each time we interact with, or do things to, it.

Setting

We conducted a practice-based ethnographic investigation of the Dalhousie Clinical Cadaver Program (CCP). The Dalhousie CCP provides newly deceased, soft-preserved, *clinical cadavers* that allow residents and physicians to practice highly specialized, often life-saving, procedural skills within a controlled setting. The Dalhousie CCP obtains their bodies from the Dalhousie University Human Body Donation Program (HBD), which accepts approximately 150 bodies per year. Administrators and staff from the CCP and HBD work in concert to ensure that both programs operate smoothly.

Methodology

Ethnographic immersion is consistent with a practice-based theoretical approach, allowing researchers to observe and document everyday activity. We therefore used a range of data collection strategies in order to develop a detailed understanding of everyday practices of cadaver work in medical education. In accordance with Nicolini's approach to practice theory, we "zoomed in" on specific facets of cadaver work, and then "zoomed out" to locate these practices in broader societal conversations about cadaver work and simulation in medical education, more broadly.[38] In order to do this, we iteratively collected and analyzed data from multiple sources over a two-year period (2018/19–2019/20).

Team composition and reflexivity

We are a team of researchers with expertise in various facets of medicine and medical education including educational ethnography (AM, PC, OK, VL, JT), practice theory (AM, PC, OK, VL, JT), clinical medicine (GK, VL, LP), and CBS (GK, LP). We brought our various areas of expertise together to ask new questions about procedural skills learning and simulation with clinical cadavers.

Throughout the process, we relied on insider knowledge of the CBS program from the Medical Director of the Clinical Cadaver Program (GK) and a learner experienced with CBS (LP) to guide our inquiry. These team members helped us identify key people to interview, as well as important educational endeavors to observe. They also facilitated connections with the workers of CBS, so that we might gain access to spaces in which cadaver work—everything from transportation to education—was taking place.

Reflexive conversations and refinement of our research processes and strategies were a regular part of our work. In other words, our process was not linear, and reflexivity was built into our emergent conversations. This was particularly important given the focus of the work, and the fact that encountering cadavers can be upsetting and unsettling.[16,20,41] We held regular analytical conversations to discuss and reflect upon our data. While these conversations served to advance our collaborative analysis of the data, they were also an exercise in reflexivity. One important exercise for our team was to reflect upon whether we, as individuals, would consider donating our bodies for educational purposes. We found that, depending on which scenario we had recently observed, or which person we had recently interviewed, the answer to that question changed.

Data collection

Ethnographic immersion

While we report below on the hours we spent *formally and informally* observing CBS related activities, our work is fundamentally ethnographic. This meant that we spent a significant amount of time "hanging around" the spaces and people of CBS and HBD. We read background materials and visited morgues, simulation suites, and cadaver preparation and teaching spaces. We worked hard to build trust and establish relationships with the people involved with HBD and CBS by sitting down to discuss our project with them, making time to answer their questions, and making ourselves available. This, in turn, provided us an opportunity to ask questions and spend time in the field in order to become comfortable and familiar with it.

Specifically, our field was the spaces and places of CBS at Dalhousie University in Halifax, Canada. Situated on the Atlantic Coast, Dalhousie Medical School is known as the Medical School of the Maritimes, and serves the communities of three Canadian Provinces: Nova Scotia, New Brunswick, and Prince Edward Island. Dalhousie Medical School is internationally recognized for our refinement of the Thiel Cadaver preparation technique, known as the Halifax Preparation[27] and our continuing professional development opportunities that make use of these clinical cadavers.

Despite years of working in medical education at this institution, many of these spaces were new to the non-clinician team members. Notably, much of the work of CBS takes place in underground spaces, connected by a series of tunnels that we had heard mentioned anecdotally, but had never had the opportunity to walk through. Thus, our ethnographic work was a strange process of discovering hidden spaces in familiar places, which we referred to in our informal conversations as "the underworld."

In contrast, the work of HBD, where donors are recruited, records are managed, and clinical cadavers are prepared for educational purposes, takes place on the highest floors of an office tower. The space includes small offices, as well as cadaver preparation spaces and teaching labs. Here, the space is bright, pristine, and hygienic. There were few clues about the cadaver preparation that happens here, except for the presence of washing machines and saws and other types of tools.

Some team members were able to participate, to some degree, in the activities of CBS, by joining a cohort of learners participating in a continuing professional development course. Rather than simply shadowing, we were engaged in the lectures, and even our participation was a sensory experience, as we were able see, smell, and touch the materials of CBS.

Observations

Our research team formally observed various facets of educational cadaver use including four continuing professional development airway management courses (40 hours of observations × 2–3 observers/session = 90 hours), four emergency resident teaching sessions (8 hours × 1–2 observers/session = 10 hours), as well as one interment and two memorial services honoring donors (5 hours × 2 observers = 10 hours) for a total of 110 hours of formal observation. We identified educational activities and other significant events/locations to observe based on consultation with expert team members, and on advice that emerged from participants during subsequent interviews. Field notes were guided by an observation guide (Appendix A), these recorded notes and reflections surrounding spaces, actors, activities, objects, acts, events, times, and goals.[42] We also engaged in multisensory participation,[38] documenting the sounds, smells, and emotions involved in CBS.

We also completed unstructured observations. These were observational sessions which were documented retrospectively rather than in vivo to reduce reactivity effects[43] and then discussed amongst the research team. They informed our overall knowledge of the program and the scope of the cadaver program. This included visits to the HBD main office (0.5 hours × 2 researchers = 1 hour), the university morgue (2 hours × 3 researchers = 6 hours), the cadaver preparation space (2 hours × 3 researchers = 6 hours), various hospital-based simulation spaces (3 hours × 2 researchers = 6 hours), and the local anatomy museum (2 hours × 4 researchers = 8 hours). This led to a total of 27 hours of unstructured observations.

In total, we gathered 137 hours of formal observational data.

Interviews

Alongside observations, we conducted 24 semi-structured interviews with learners (continuing professional development learners n = 5 & emergency medicine residents n = 4), clinical teachers (n = 4), as well as family members of past donors (n = 5). As well, human body donation staff (n = 6) included those involved in the administrative (e.g., contacting donors, record keeping), legal (e.g., accepting and managing bodies), and technical (e.g., preparing cadavers) tasks of the CCP program. We identified individuals to interview based on consultation with expert team members. We purposively recruited 24 people and interviewed all who accepted the invitation. Our interview guides were conversational in nature and were tailored to each participant's role (see Appendix B for an example); they were developed by multiple members of the research team. We continuously revised the guides according to evolving themes.

Document analysis

Documents related to the Human Body Donation program and cadaver-based education were also reviewed [n = 22]. This included legal acts and reports related to the process of body donation and burial; documents related to the human body donation program; educational material such as curriculum materials and advertisements; and media coverage. We refined our previously developed document review form to structure this piece of the analysis (Appendix C).[44]

Data analysis

Our analysis aligned with Wolcott's[45] three-step approach to the analysis of ethnographic data: description, analysis, and interpretation. This approach uses a combination of pure description (staying close to the data), systematic analysis (identifying key factors and relationships), and interpretation (extending beyond the data, making sense of what is happening). Although Wolcott distinguishes three ways to transform qualitative data, he emphasizes that they overlap and occur simultaneously. Accordingly, we followed an iterative approach to analysis, attuning to how the *concept* of the cadaver changed across the lifecycle, as well as the actors and materials contributing to its progression and transitions.

Broadly speaking, the descriptive phase involved reviewing each data set separately, including by source (document, observation, interview) and by type (observation of emergency residents or continuing professional development course participants; interview with student, teacher, staff, or donor/donor's family), and then reconsidering these insights as part of a broader whole. Three researchers (MF, PC, VL) independently reviewed and coded each data source using qualitative data analysis software (ATLAS.ti) which also assisted with secure data management and sharing.

At the analytic phase, ideas borne from our field work, interviews, and document review were actively translated, discussed as a group, and represented in written form. As we searched for patterns, consistencies, and inconsistencies, we became intrigued by the way in which participants were engaging in philosophical work as they managed the ambiguity of clinical cadavers. In particular, we noted that the ways in which donors/bodies/cadavers were conceived evolved significantly, depending on how they were being used. At this point, we identified the six stages of what we began to refer to as a "lifecycle," and specifically attuned to different language patterns and tasks which in turn allowed us to identify ontological transitions.

As we then engaged in interpretive work, we considered our practice-generated insights from a Deleuzian perspective, focusing on how the conceptual shifts allowed the cadaver to move through the lifecycle. This interpretive work involved exploring how the cadaver was in a constant state of becoming, and delineating how, at each stage, participants actively created new concepts to make sense of the body in front of them, as they engaged in various types of work.

Ethical considerations

The Nova Scotia Health Research Ethics Board approved this study (REB FILE#: 1023958). No identifying photographs, videos, or audio-recordings of observations were taken in order to preserve the confidentiality of human donors.

Results

Through Human Body Donation (HBD) and CBS, a deceased person participated in a "life after death" where their body "stood in" for a living patient. We describe herein this cycle, from donor enrollment to eventual interment, and the associated ontological transitions at each stage (Table 1). While the elements we describe are specific to the HBD program we studied, we believe the transitions, themselves, are transferable to other contexts.

Ontology focuses on questions of "being"—in other words, "what is." With respect to educational cadavers, the ontological questions were significant: Is this a person? Is this an educational tool? What makes something human? We noted that as a donor's body progressed through the HBD program, the ways in which study participants conceptualized the body changed significantly, and we refer to these changing concepts as ontological transitions. These transitions were apparent in the way participants used language. For example, staff, teachers, learners, and researchers alike interchangeably referred to the cadaver as a person, a "not-a-person", a patient, a specimen, this/that "guy", a body, a him/her, and an educational tool. These shifting ontologies were also apparent in the way participants handled the bodies. At times, they practiced on the body in ways that they would not on a living being; at others, they treated the body with a tenderness and respect that they likely would never show an inanimate object. In this manner, participants conceived of cadavers as not fully people, but also as much more than things.

The ontological complexity we observed in relation to the cadaver involved uncertain and shifting boundaries between person, human body, cadaver, and educational tool. How the cadaver was understood changed continuously over space and time, fluctuating and evolving in sometimes predictable, but sometimes, unpredictable ways. The following sections illustrate how this philosophical work brought about through

Table 1. The 6 stages of the LifeCycle of the clinical cadaver.

	Activities	People	Location
1. **Person to donor**	Developing program materials, interacting with potential donors, creating records Creating relationships, managing expectations, having awkward conversations	Human Body Donation (HBD) Program Administration	University-based, Human Body Donation program office
2. **Donor to body**	Declaring death, cleaning bodies Emotional work: getting used to dead bodies, deciding how to present a body to loved ones	Healthcare workers, HBD staff	Largely health care facilities
3. **Body to cadaver**	Bureaucratic work: notifying HBD staff, assessing eligibility; moving the bodies Creating professional, serious appearance; setting professional boundaries	HBD staff, Transport staff	Loading bays, vehicles
4. **Cadaver to educational cadaver**	Preparing the cadaver for education, suctioning, shaving, de-personalizing, cutting, anonymizing Deciding how human is human enough, recognizing and concealing signs of death, managing professional expectations	Anatomy Technicians (trained as funeral directors)	Morgue & Prep Space
5. **Educational cadaver to teacher**	Delivering the cadavers, laying out the cadavers, preparing them for specific skills/practices, priming learners for what they will experience Keeping the space clean, mopping up, encouraging learners, reducing discomfort, reminding learners of the cadaver's human-ness	Transportation staff, simulation technologists, medical teachers	Simulation space
6. **Teacher to loved one and legacy**	Cremating, memorializing donors, organizing service, reciting names Managing the cultural/religious element of death, finding the right tone	HBD staff, learners	Cemetery, church

professional practices drives the cadaver along its "life-cycle" from person to donor, body, cadaver, educational cadaver, teacher, and loved one/legacy.

We want to state clearly that the stages we describe are not "neat," nor are they discrete. We have simplified, in order to increase readability and clarify the ontological transitions, but in reality, these stages are not clearly defined nor are they static. Our perspective is that people/bodies/cadavers are in a perpetual state of becoming, and our description of the various stages are only "snapshots" representing points in time, when we zoomed in to focus on the practices associated with CBS and HBD at a given moment.

We did not set out to deliberately follow a cadaver from point of death to legacy, through the lifecycle we described. In fact, when we began this work, we had no concept of the lifecycle which we would eventually develop through collaborative description, analysis, and interpretation. Instead, we learned about the processes and activities of CBS and HBD through ethnographic immersion. In other words, by being present and building relationships with the people of HBD and CBS, we were able to identify and decide upon events/scenarios to formally observe.

Person to donor

A person became a *donor* after a (sometimes long) process of shared decision-making, bureaucratic work, and careful consideration of ethical concerns. According to the family members we interviewed, most people wished to become donors for altruistic reasons. As many suffered from illnesses that were poorly understood, an overarching wish to contribute "to science"—as in, to help future generations benefit from a greater understanding of their illness— permeated our conversations. This wish of donors and family members, we observed, presented a tension for some workers in the HBD program. HBD workers noted that participants often have the idea that their donation will be targeted. One person noted

'You know, my husband died of Parkinson's disease, so whatever I can do to help Parkinson's research.' I think [our program] is very honest. We [tell donors and families that we] don't really use the bodies for that, we use them for teaching. [Most donors say] 'oh, well, you know, that's fine too.' But, I always worry that there's a little disconnect. (HBD Staff)

Others clearly articulated that they wanted to help medical students gain "hands-on learning" that they simply "can't learn in a book" or, as one donor noted,

"we just thought it was a good idea if we could further somebody's studies." After finding out about the program (usually through family or friends who knew about the program), these individuals or their loved ones reached out to the program and initiated the paperwork involved in providing consent.

After this initial contact, HBD staff needed to accomplish several tasks in order for donation to occur. Much of this work was bound up in the production of texts: developing program materials (e.g., website, information pamphlets, consent forms) and recording-keeping. Our field noting[46] formed a key practice in documenting the evolving nature of administrative work associated with the transition from person to donor. Our ethnographic immersion provided the opportunity for us to review original ledgers, dating back to the early 1900s, listing the names of donors in handwriting. The documents designed to provide information for potential donors used carefully chosen language, that we described as "calm." Through our analysis of program documents, we noted that "the donation program is easily accessible, respectful, gentle, but firm on its regulations. The language used implies respect and ongoing remembrance (i.e. "lasting legacy")."

More informally, staff also needed to create trusting relationships with donors and their families, manage expectations around donation, and give them the confidence that the body would be treated with respect.

Further, staff grappled with the ethical challenges associated with body donation, such as informed consent. Chiefly, the HBD program considered informed consent "the pillar stone of everything [they] ever do". But what if the donor consented 30 years prior to their death and had not contacted the program since? What if the family was opposed? These are questions the program took seriously:

Because you don't want to put someone in that situation where they're just horrified by the fact that, you know, their father, mother, brother or sister or whatever would be here. And I think...that that should play a part in whether or not the person... because at the end of the day—it's hard to say this to a family and I never would—but at the end of the day, the person who's dead is not going to know. (Cadaver staff)

A person thus became a donor only after multiple people—including the donors themselves, their families, and staff from the HBD program—made important decisions, engaged in administrative work and record keeping, took concrete actions, and engaged in inevitable negotiations.

Donor to body

Death is the most obvious marker of the transition from donor to *body*. As one learner illustrated, the difference between a living, breathing person (a *somebody*) and a still, lifeless body (a *something*) felt unambiguous:

There's a huge difference between the 89-year-old who's under the covers asleep, breathing shallowly, and you're just looking in from the door. But there's something there that you just know they're alive. And when they die, it's gone. And I don't know what it is. But bodies just become furniture. You know, it's like there's a bed, a chair, a TV, and a dead person. Which is much different than there's a bed, a TV, a chair, and there's somebody sleeping in there. (Emergency Medicine Learner)

At the same time, the exact moment that the donor became a body was arguably not the moment the donor died. Rather, it was the moment those around them become *aware* of their death. This moment was up to the discretion of the doctor in charge who made the death "official" by examining the body for signs of life (e.g., pulse, pupil and tactile response, spontaneous respiration), declaring death, and signing a death certificate.

The declaration of death mobilized a routine set of events that eventually led to the creation of a clinical cadaver. Through our analysis of programmatic documentation designed to delineate what happens "at the time of death", we saw the conceptual shift beginning from a donor to a body. These materials focused on logistics, including instructions on how to proceed, depending on where the death occurred. These documents also included the first mention of the role of the "Inspector of Anatomy," who ultimately determined whether a body would be accepted into the program.

When a donor died in-hospital, nursing staff attended to removing heart and oxygen monitors, intubation tubes, central lines, IVs, body tape, and all other medical equipment from the body. They wiped blood and other substances from the skin, replaced blankets, and closed the eyes. These activities were especially important when a donor died outside of the hospital. In these cases, cleaning the body meant attenuating the horror of death because, in many cases, the appearance of newly dead bodies could be truly unsettling:

The first time you go and pick up a dead body. Their mouths' open, sometimes their eyes are open, there could be purge coming out of their mouth...you'll get people in a state where they're just, they're not clean.

And you're going to get some ulcers...if they soil themselves...they choke on their vomit... (Cadaver staff)

The purpose of these activities was to make the body look "presentable" to the outside world, transforming the way the family will perceive and react to the body, and serving to soften the blow for those who wish to view it.

Body to cadaver

After healthcare workers and HBD staff removed the most obvious signs of illness (e.g., oxygen monitors and intubation tubes) and death (e.g., blood, bodily secretions) from the body, it was ready to become a *cadaver*. A series of specialized, bureaucratic activities from the part of HBD staff served to complete this transition.

Regardless of where the donor died, healthcare workers would contact and inform the Inspector of Anatomy (IoA) as soon as they received the death certificate. Appointed by the Minister of Health, the IoA was the first point of contact to the HBD program. This individual would communicate with medical personnel in charge of their care, the family, and HBD staff in order to decide whether or not the body should be accepted into the program (i.e., to become a cadaver). Specifically, the IoA verified that the body lacked specific contraindications (e.g., risk of infectious disease, previous autopsy, morbid obesity, major amputations) and contacted the donor's family to ensure their ongoing consent. In circumstances of suspicious death, the medical examiner may have also been involved; need for an autopsy excluded the body from the program. Because the university morgue was only able to hold a certain number of cadavers and the HBD program required certain types of bodies for specific purposes at any given time, clinical cadaver staff aided the IoA in assessing how well the body met their current needs.

HBD workers involved at this stage were engaged in balancing the needs of the program with the needs of a family in distress. One participant described the challenges of managing the bureaucratic work involved in accepting a body into the program.

I can't act without a death certificate. ... So, if someone dies at home, I get a call... The person wishes to donate their body ...but without a death certificate, I can't do anything. And so, the body has to either stay at the place of death or at the family's expense, needs to be taken to a funeral home which has cold storage until a decision can be made about acceptance. (HBD Staff)

Once accepted by the program, the cadaver was often temporarily stored in the hospital or local public morgue. When space became available, the HBD program hired transportation staff to bring the cadavers to the university morgue. The importance of storage space was a key consideration throughout and pointed to a conception of the body as a *thing* to be managed. Participants from the HBD frequently described having "room" for a donor, and a need to operate within the physical capacity of the space. Through immersion and observation, the physical realities of the facilities, and related storage, challenges participants described were made plain. One researcher noted:

> [there were] buckets full of brains and a fridge full of bodies—stacked up on shelves. The hallways were lined with coffin-shaped cardboard boxes on their way to the crematorium. And in the middle of it all, there was a forklift. (Fieldnote)

Despite these physical and logistical storage challenges, in each of these locations, handling of the cadavers was taken seriously. Rather than the typical blue or white plastic bags of the university morgue, cadavers were transferred at this moment to bags of soft embroidered fabric. Despite being independent from the HBD program, transportation staff never failed to arrive fully dressed in formal suits to pick up and drop off the bodies.

Cadaver to educational cadaver

Once cadavers arrived at the university morgue, HBD staff began preparing them for their educational purposes. These individuals further cleaned the body of its secretions, suctioning the throat and stomach which had continued to build up fluids, and cleaned any further release of feces. They sometimes cut certain parts of the body, such as the trachea and esophagus, to halt further build-up of fluids. They then embalmed and froze the bodies. To make them as anonymous as possible, they shaved their heads; to identify each body thereafter, they attached tags to their toes with a number corresponding to one in a ledger book. Before each CBS session, staff unfroze these bodies, freshly cleaned and suctioned them, then covered their eyes with surgical caps and the rest of their bodies in blue surgical drapes. The covering of eyes and the top of the head were particularly significant, as one researcher noted:

> Once, though, a cadaver's face covering slipped, and I could see blank silver eyes, mouth agape and a broad gash roughly stitched across its skull. These details [bothered me]. Otherwise, strategic covering seemed

to do the trick to minimize the difference between a sleeping patient and cadaver. (Fieldnote)

The procedures described above, which HBD staff used to prepare an *educational cadaver,* differed markedly from those traditional embalmers and funeral professionals use to prepare bodies for a funeral service. For instance, bodies prepared for a funeral service are cleaned and dressed for purely esthetic purposes; there is no reason, in these cases, to sever the trachea and esophagus or cut open the chest to help visualize the lungs. Consequently, embalmers and funeral directors who were not involved in cadaver preparation often saw these acts as mutilation:

> In a funeral home, I mean everything is, there's a set kind of standard that funeral embalmers should adhere to. Whereas even the smallest diversion [is considered] doing something that you shouldn't. (HBD staff)

Participants described navigating this complexity by focusing on the work and keeping in mind that they were working toward a goal: using the cadaver to generate a meaningful educational experience.

> I find that the more I can concentrate on the task [the better]. ... If I do my job properly well that's going to help [learners]. ... Here again the same pride and the same attention is to create those teaching materials for the students. (HBD staff)

Hence, the specialized—and sometimes controversial—work of cadaver staff deviated from traditional funeral practices and transformed the cadaver into something different from a dead body: it was in the process of becoming a clinical tool.

Educational cadaver to teacher

In the simulation lab, dedicated staff placed cadavers on metal tables, covered in layers of moist, yellow-stained white sheets and clean, blue drapes. For short sessions, they often kept the cadavers in their body bags, ready to be zipped back up and returned to their refrigerators. They carefully arranged surgical instruments, machines, and screens throughout the room on side tables and mobile carts.

When the simulation sessions began, teachers and learners, dressed in yellow gowns and blue gloves, encircled the cadavers. The room would be busy as teachers, learners, and cadaver staff worked to provide an optimal learning environment. One researcher described the busyness of the space, noting,

> The way people have to duck around each other to get to different tools or spaces makes me think of

navigating a concert crowd – lots of shuffling and trying not to bump anything. (Fieldnote)

The sounds of suctioning and excited voices arose from huddles, and various smells—mostly embalming fluid mixed with bodily secretions—infiltrated all corners of the room. When one attended to it, irony was ripe in this environment. The surgical bonnets that covered the eyes of the cadavers were often decorated with colorful happy faces or teddy bears. On one occasion, a 3-wick candle burned slowly in the background, making the room smell of "sugared snicker doodle."

In these spaces, cadavers became things that were talked about, leaned on, touched, prodded, and cut. While the cadavers remained fully intact, they were conceptualized as a collection of isolated parts (a knee, a jaw, a chest window) that learners examined and manipulated. As they crowded around the body, each learner "claimed" a body part to work on for the time being, letting another learner take their place when they were finished. The affordances of the cadaver as an educational tool were clear, as teachers were able to demonstrate different techniques:

> The first group I stopped to observe: the teacher was describing an alternative head position to the "sniffing" position often advocated for in airway procedures. He encouraged participants to try the "sipping" position: how you might sip the top of a beer as you walk from the bar to your table. This description was met with gentle laughter in the cluster of participants gathered around him. (Fieldnote)

Equipment would begin piling up on the cadaver and between its legs. For many teachers and learners, the cadaver was, at this moment, a clinical tool:

> To me when they're there, they're just a…teaching tool. And I don't mean that in a disrespectful way. I mean they're there, I just don't think of them as what they *were*. (Teacher)

> I think part of it is like the, cognitively, we really separate the fact that… We really keep the fact that this was a person kind of separate. We treat them with respect, but we also… I don't think when we're in [the body preparation lab], I don't think very many of us are thinking like about who this person might have been when they were alive or something. I think that that's just sort of a cognitive separation thing that we all have. (Learner)

Both teachers and learners continuously replaced bonnets and drapes that slipped off the eyes and body during the course of the session. While keeping the body covered primarily aimed to preserve the patient's dignity, it also served to reinforce a "detachment" from viewing the cadaver as a person:

> We try to keep the cadaver as covered up as possible…I've seen over time, students describe like you know they get bothered by seeing—if you expose a cadaver's hands or feet. And I think…part of their comfort level in working with a cadaver as a teaching resource is that they may disconnect a little bit from saying this was a person. Where it's a little easier to do some invasive procedures over and over again if you can disconnect a little bit from that. (Teacher)

Despite accomplishing the important work of reducing learners' discomfort in the cadaver lab, teachers and senior learners also reinforced the idea that the cadaver was a (former) person, and reminded learners to treat the body with respect:

> We make a big point…to remind students that they are people. They are patients. We all have different speeches. Mine is basically about, you know, you treat the cadaver as if it's a patient who can hear you and their family members can hear you. And treat them as if they're any other patient. (Teacher)

> I'm still focusing on causing minimal damage…I wouldn't want to do something that I wouldn't do in real life with a real patient. (Senior learner)

Several learners conceptualized the cadaver teacher as an irreplicable resource, and even a lifesaver, or hero. One participant noted:

> I think that the biggest difference is going from what you're doing in [CBS] to the trauma room is so small because it's effectively the same thing … literally the next patient I was intubating like a week later was very similar in terms of their relaxation, the anatomy… you were just there. (Learner)

Teacher to loved one and legacy

Once the cadaver completed its intended role as an educational tool, the HBD program contacted the family and made arrangements to either return the body to them or to prepare it for cremation and/or burial in the university's dedicated cemetery. Family members of the donors were invited to an annual interment and memorial service in the Spring.

The interment ceremony happened at a cemetery. The ashes or urns of the donors were set out under a tent with plaques placed on top indicating their names. Attendees placed flowers and keepsakes beside them. A piper played, members of the clergy spoke, doves were released, and a representative from the HBD program read the names of more than 150 donors out loud. The event was both communal and deeply personal.

The memorial service happened in a grand Catholic church. HBD staff, faculty, and students—all formally dressed in funeral wear—joined the families of donors as they filled into the pews. Students contributed by handing out information booklets with forget-me-not seeds tucked neatly inside them. A number of people spoke: clergy, members of the HBD program, teachers, and learners. They spoke of gratitude, grief, generosity, and human connection:

> A number of learners from the various health professions come to the lectern to speak about how they've benefited from the program. For the most part, they're pretty textbook remarks. Thoughtful and kind enough, but the kind of thing you'd expect. But there's one guy who gives the most beautiful, meaningful speech. And, I've thought about this—I think the thing that made it so poignant was the fact that he focused on what connects us as humans. He talked about all the ways we can know someone, how learners come to intimately know the (former?) people they work on. How this is a bond that he shares with the people who were left behind. It's a subtle reorientation of the expected—a way to connect education, grief, and hopefulness. It was perfect. (Fieldnote)

The interment and memorial service was thus dedicated to thanking and commemorating the dead. In this manner, the cadaver-as-teaching-tool faded to the background. In its place, all celebrated the memory of the generous "hero" who donated their body and attendees appreciated them for all that they have offered, as illustrated in the following field note:

> There is an exceptional moment when one of the speakers asks first everyone who is here to celebrate their parent to stand, then those celebrating their sibling, then their loved one, then anyone who's benefitted from the loved ones' donation—everyone at the end of it was standing and the speaker said "this is the impact, this is the love, this is why we are here" and it was stunning. All of a sudden, the relatively small candle memorial makes sense—it's not just about the person's body but about the love they shared and the lives they've touched, all combined a massive and powerful energy that could never be captured by a display on a stage.

Discussion

Central to the complexity of cadaver work is what we refer to as its ontological ambiguity: the inability to qualify the cadaver as either a person or a thing; human or not human; or as a teacher or a tool. This distinction is becoming ever more ambiguous with the development of novel preservation techniques that render cadavers less and less distinguishable from the living. We recognize that some of the stages of the lifecycle we describe are not necessarily unique to clinical cadavers. Certainly, a traditional hard-fixed cadaver is transformed as it is used differently, in different contexts. We believe, however, that the philosophical work may be less troubling when the cadaver is rigid and gray—its humanity is perhaps easier to overlook. The ontological fidelity of *clinical* cadavers inspires specific practices at each stage of the lifecycle, which we identified in noting, and classifying, the ways in which people speak and act. These sayings and doings[36] are a product of the nebulous, but undeniable, humanness of clinical cadavers.

We observed that there is both an art, and a science, to CBS. With respect to art, the ways in which cadavers are prepared and presented was artful, with workers taking pride in presenting lifelike specimens that encouraged an interaction closer to a real clinical encounter. With respect to science, we noted the innovations in preservation techniques, the refined skill, the testing of tools and devices. The philosophy of cadaver-based simulation, however, was more nebulous to identify. Yet, once we attuned to it, it became clear that philosophical work was, in fact, foundational to CBS.

From a Deleuzian perspective, then, people engaged in CBS are *doing philosophy*.[47] This involves the conceptual, emotional, ethical, and technical work of managing ontological ambiguities as the cadaver passes through the lifecycle and is actively shaped by professional practices. While the making and remaking of teaching cadavers as anatomical objects is an important consideration[20] and the relational/social elements of cadaver-based pedagogy[21] have broadened our understanding of the complexity of educational cadaver work, attuning to the philosophical transitions across the lifecycle of a cadaver adds a nuanced element to the conversation. The transition from person to donor allowed participants to plan and organize for how a body will be used after death. The ontological transition from donor to body that occurred at death allowed the process to be set in motion for the actual hands-on work of cadaver-based education, which is intended to save future lives. The transition from body to cadaver meant that participants were able to make decisions about what to do with a particular body, in a particular set of circumstances. The transition from cadaver to educational cadaver allowed participants to depersonalize the cadaver as they focused on "the greater good": future, imagined patients who will need their care. The transition from educational cadaver to teacher allowed participants to do things to the cadaver, practicing clinical skills and procedures. Finally, the transition from teacher to legacy allowed participants to reflect on the complex work in which they engage, providing space to honor donors, and returning us to the start of the lifecycle where we remember the personhood of those who gave the gift of their body.

This philosophical work of ontological transitions is foundational to the tasks that must occur at each stage of the lifecycle. It is difficult to imagine, for example, cutting into a body to observe its anatomical structures had we never stopped thinking about that body as a person. We believe this philosophical work is, in fact, "pre-empirical."[35] This means that before we can engage in the art or science of cadaver-based education, we must first engage in philosophy, which Deleuze and Guattari defined as "forming, inventing, and fabricating concepts." [35(p2)] The concepts which participants created in order to make sense of the body before them are inseparable from the professional practices of CBS.

Ontological fidelity

The literature on CBS has primarily been focused on issues of simulator effectiveness. [22,27,34] In particular, CBS is appealing to medical educators because of its high *fidelity*, defined as the degree of realism, or exactness with which it reproduces reality.[48] Medical educators generally recognize two types of fidelity: physical (i.e., similarity in the look and feel of the simulator) and functional (i.e., similarity in how the simulator responds to manipulation or intervention).[49] Our study of CBS suggests, however, that there is more to fidelity than physical and functional. Specifically, we argue that there is a third relevant type of fidelity: *ontological fidelity*.

It is undeniable that ontological fidelity matters. In contrast to traditional, hard-fixed cadavers, there is something inherently unique to the clinical cadaver that makes it distinct from both the manikin simulator and the living body. The cadaver is human, and therefore needs to be treated with tenderness and respect. The cadaver is not, however, a living person, and therefore can be cut, prodded, and manipulated like an educational tool. The cadaver has a smell, a feel, and a story. The seriousness with which trainees approach CBS is incomparable to any other learning activity. Our study thus demonstrated that the question of being—what a cadaver *is*—matters to the practice of CBS, and makes it a unique and irreplaceable practice. Arguably, the most technologically advanced, *high-fidelity* manikin will never replace a real human body, because you simply cannot fake "human."

We believe ontological fidelity may be the missing piece related to Deleuze and Guattari's three modes of thought (art, science, and philosophy).[35] If art allows us to represent the sensory and perceptual aspects of a concept; science allows us to explain and manipulate its functions; then philosophy allows us to delineate and create new concepts. Conceptualizing fidelity as physical, functional, and *ontological* can help us represent CBS artistically, scientifically, and philosophically.

The concept of ontological fidelity of cadavers is a consequential one. Along with the emotional elements of working with "silent mentors" as described by Douglas-Jones,[29] it provides an important argument against eliminating in-person cadaver work. There has been some argument that cadavers are no longer necessary in the modern era. Particularly during the COVID-19 pandemic, there have been notable advancements in virtual technologies for anatomy learning that could eliminate the need for expensive and resource-intensive clinical cadaver programs.[50] However, our research suggests that the level of humanness of the cadaver—something much more difficult to convey through a screen—matters.[39]

Olejaz[41] describes the dissection lab as a *moral laboratory*, a space in which we may come to understand ethics training in practice, as well as a space where students are given a chance by donors to learn how to deal with the ambiguity of human bodies that are used for dissection. Similarly, the teaching spaces associated with CBS serve as a *moral pedagogy*. It is in this unique environment that learners across the continuum of medical education grapple with the material form of the cadaver in front of them, creating new concepts to facilitate the tasks that must be accomplished. While there are certainly other educational tools available in the form of manikins or other such simulators which enable the teaching of procedural skills, we believe that the ontological fidelity of cadavers, and the philosophical work associated with its use, are irreplicable.

Working with a real human body is inherently different from working with any other type of simulator in ways that influence what is, is not, or can be learned from simulation.

Limitations

In typical ethnographic tradition, our practice-based study provides an in-depth description of only one institution. The preparation of *clinical* cadavers, in particular, is unique to a limited number of institutions. While we believe the insights garnered herein translate to other contexts engaging in both human body donation and other types of cadaver-based education, we cannot guarantee the transferability of our work.

We drew on Deleuze and Guattari's *What is Philosophy* in order to demonstrate how philosophical principles can help us to reconsider important educational concepts. However, what we present here is simplified, focused, and intended to be instructive. We encourage readers who are motivated to engage in philosophical work in their own contexts to read the original contribution,[35] in order to understand the subtleties of Deleuze and Guattari's perspectives on art, science, and philosophy.

Conclusion

Cadaver-based simulation is a promising, and fascinating innovation within the long history of cadaver-based medical education. The educational cadaver, itself, exists in a space between life and death, and is in a cycle of "becoming" because of the practices performed by an interprofessional team both visible and behind the scenes. The "humanness" of the cadaver makes it a difficult material to categorize. However, this ambiguity also makes a powerful educational tool, inspiring not only procedural skills learning, but also conscious and unconscious reflection, made evident in the ways in which participants spoke about cadavers, and in the things they did, or did not do, to them. CBS, then, unsettles fixed ideas about the life/death binary, and about the practices required to establish educational relevance. We support Deleuze and Guattari's perspective that, when it comes to CBS, "what is real is the becoming, itself, the block of becoming, not the supposedly fixed terms through which that which becomes passes." [35(p238)]

Teachers, learners, and cadaver staff are actively *doing philosophy* as they manage the ontological malleability of cadavers. We believe this pre-empirical philosophical work is, in fact, the motor that drives CBS. Without conceptually managing and materially enacting these ontological transitions, the work of CBS would not be possible. We hope that in reflecting on the philosophical strategies invoked by our participants as they manage the cadaver across its educational lifecycle, this paper sheds new light on the complex world of cadaver work in medical education.

Previous philosophy in medical education installments

Mario Veen & Anna T. Cianciolo (2020) Problems No One Looked For: Philosophical Expeditions into Medical Education, Teaching and Learning in Medicine, 32:3, 337–344, DOI: 10.1080/10401334.2020.1748634

Gert J. J. Biesta & Marije van Braak (2020) Beyond the Medical Model: Thinking Differently about Medical Education and Medical Education Research, Teaching and Learning in Medicine, 32:4, 449–456, DOI: 10.1080/10401334.2020.1798240

Mark R. Tonelli & Robyn Bluhm (2021) Teaching Medical Epistemology within an Evidence-Based Medicine Curriculum, Teaching and Learning in Medicine, 33:1, 98–105, DOI: 10.1080/10401334.2020.1835666

John R. Skelton (2021) Language, Philosophy, and Medical Education, Teaching and Learning in Medicine, 33:2, 210–216, DOI: 10.1080/10401334.2021.1877712

Zareen Zaidi, Ian M. Partman, Cynthia R. Whitehead, Ayelet Kuper & Tasha R. Wyatt (2021) Contending with Our Racial Past in Medical Education: A Foucauldian Perspective, Teaching and Learning in Medicine, DOI: 10.1080/10401334.2021.1945929

Chris Rietmeijer & Mario Veen (2021) Phenomenological Research in Health Professions Education: Tunneling from Both Ends, Teaching and Learning in Medicine, DOI:10.1080/10401334.2021.1971989

Madeleine Noelle Olding, Freya Rhodes, John Humm, Phoebe Ross & Catherine McGarry (2022) Black, White and Gray: Student Perspectives on Medical Humanities and Medical Education, Teaching and Learning in Medicine, 34:2, 223–233, DOI: 10.1080/10401334.2021.1982717

Camillo Coccia & Mario Veen (2022) Because We Care: A Philosophical Investigation into the Spirit of Medical Education, Teaching and Learning in Medicine, 10.1080/10401334.2022.2056744

Tim Fawns & Sven Schaepkens (2022) A Matter of Trust: Online Proctored Exams and the Integration of Technologies of Assessment in Medical Education, Teaching and Learning in Medicine, DOI: 10.1080/10401334.2022.2048832

Associated podcast

Let Me Ask You Something (iTunes, Spotify, Google Podcasts and https://marioveen.com/letmeaskyousomething/)

Disclosure statement

The authors have no conflicts of interest to report in this work.

Ethical approval

This study was approved by the Research Ethics Board of the regional health authority.

Informed consent

We obtained informed consent from all the participants in this study. We followed standard procedures as outlined by the Tri-Council Policy Statement (TCPS-2): Ethical Conduct for Research Involving Humans Course on Research Ethics (CORE).

Presentations

Material from this manuscript was presented at the Canadian Conference for Medical Education on April 17, 2021 (oral presentation).

Funding

This study was funded by grants from the Social Sciences and Humanities Research Council [Grant number: 430-2018-00274] and the Royal College of Physicians and Surgeons of Canada [Grant number: A. MacLeod_2018 RC MERG].

ORCID

Anna MacLeod (iD) http://orcid.org/0000-0002-0939-7767
Victoria Luong (iD) http://orcid.org/0000-0001-9174-1207
Paula Cameron (iD) http://orcid.org/0000-0001-5621-6829
Olga Kits (iD) http://orcid.org/0000-0002-2444-7881
Jonathan Tummons (iD) http://orcid.org/0000-0002-1372-3799

References

1. Varpio L, Macleod A. Philosophy of science series: harnessing the multidisciplinary edge effect by exploring paradigms, ontologies, epistemologies, axiologies, and methodologies. *Acad Med.* 2020;95(5):686–689. doi:10.1097/ACM.0000000000003142.
2. Veen M, Cianciolo AT. Problems no one looked for: philosophical expeditions into medical education. *Teach Learn Med.* 2020;32(3):337–344. doi:10.1080/10 401334.2020.1748634.
3. MacLeod A, Ellaway RH, Paradis E, Park YS, Young M, Varpio L. Being edgy in health professions education: concluding the philosophy of science series. *Acad Med.* 2020;95(7):995–998. doi:10.1097/ACM.00000000 00003250.
4. Fountain TK. *Rhetoric in the Flesh: Trained Vision, Technical Expertise, and the Gross Anatomy Lab.* New York, NY: Routledge; 2014.
5. Hildebrandt S. The role of history and ethics of anatomy in medical education. *Anat Sci Educ.* 2019;12(4):425–431. doi:10.1002/ase.1852.
6. Streith L, Cadili L, Wiseman SM. Evolving anatomy education strategies for surgical residents: a scoping review. *Am J Surg.* 2022;2022. doi:10.1016/j.amjsurg.2022.02.005.
7. Arráez-Aybar LA, Bueno-López JL, Moxham BJ. Anatomists' views on human body dissection and donation: an international survey. *Ann Anat.* 2014;196(6):376–386. doi:10.1016/j.aanat.2014.06.004.
8. Comer AR. The evolving ethics of anatomy: dissecting an unethical past in order to prepare for a future of ethical anatomical practice. *Anat Rec.* 2022;305(4):818–826. doi:10.1002/ar.24868.
9. Ergano M, Gerbi A, Hamba N, et al. Assessment of the determinants of knowledge, attitude and practice (KAP) of Ethiopian medical students towards ethical cadaver dissection. *Transl Res Anat.* 2020;19:1–8. doi:10.1016/j.tria.2020.100067.
10. Jones DG. Using and respecting the dead human body: an anatomist's perspective. *Clin Anat.* 2014;27(6):839–843. doi:10.1002/ca.22405.
11. Jones DG. 2017. Human anatomy: a review of the science, ethics and culture of a discipline in transition. In: Sisu AM, ed. *Human Anatomy – Reviews and Medical Advances.* IntechOpen. https://www.intechopen.com/chapters/55062
12. American Association for Anatomy. Ethics and professionalism in teaching the anatomical sciences. https://www.anatomy.org/AAA/Resources/Anatomy-Ethics-Resources.aspx. Accessed November 3, 2021.
13. Prentice R. *Bodies in Formation: An Ethnography of Anatomy and Surgery Education.* Durham, NC: Duke University Press; 2013.
14. Bahşi İ, Topal Z, Çetkin M, et al. Evaluation of attitudes and opinions of medical faculty students against the use of cadaver in anatomy education and investigation of the factors affecting their emotional responses related thereto. *Surg Radiol Anat.* 2021;43(4):481–487. doi:10.1007/s00276-020-02567-8.
15. Boeckers A, Brinkmann A, Jerg-Bretzke L, Lamp C, Traue HC, Boeckers TM. How can we deal with mental distress in the dissection room? An evaluation of the need for psychological support. *Ann Anat.* 2010;192(6):366–372. doi:10.1016/j.aanat.2010.08.002.
16. Chang HJ, Kim HJ, Rhyu IJ, Lee YM, Uhm CS. Emotional experiences of medical students during cadaver dissection and the role of memorial ceremonies: a qualitative study. *BMC Med Educ.* 2018;18(1):1–7. doi:10.1186/s12909-018-1358-0.
17. Wisenden PA, Budke KJ, Klemetson CJ, et al. Emotional response of undergraduates to cadaver dissection. *Clin Anat.* 2018;31(2):224–230. doi:10.1002/ca.22992.
18. Abrams MP, Eckert T, Topping D, Daly KD. Reflective writing on the cadaveric dissection experience: an effective tool to assess the impact of dissection on learning of anatomy, humanism, empathy, well-being, and professional identity formation in medical students. *Anat Sci Educ.* 2021;14(5):658–665. doi:10.1002/ase.2025.
19. Guo K, Luo T, Zhou L, et al. Cultivation of humanistic values in medical education through anatomy pedagogy and gratitude ceremony for body donors. *BMC Med Educ.* 2020;20(1):10. doi:10.1186/s12909-020-02292-1.
20. McDonald M. Bodies and cadavers. In Harvey P, Casella EC, Evans G, Knox H, McLean C, Silva EB, et al. eds.

Objects and Materials. Abingdon, Oxon: Routledge; 2014. p. 128–143.

21. Hallam E. Relational anatomy: dissecting and memorialising the dead in medical education. *MAT.* 2017;4(4):99–124. doi:10.17157/mat.4.4.314.

22. Cale AS, Hendrickse A, Lyman M, Royer DF. Integrating a cadaver review session into the existing regional anesthesia training for anesthesiology residents: an initial experience. *Med Sci Educ.* 2020;30(2):695–703. doi:10.1007/s40670-020-00934-z.

23. Rashidian N, Willaert W, Giglio MC, et al. Laparoscopic liver surgery training course on thiel-embalmed human cadavers: program evaluation, trainer's long-term feedback and steps forward. *World J Surg.* 2019;43(11):2902–2908. doi:10.1007/s00268-v019-05103-x.

24. Takayesu JK, Peak D, Stearns D. Cadaver-based training is superior to simulation training for cricothyrotomy and tube thoracostomy. *Intern Emerg Med.* 2017;12(1):99–102. doi:10.1007/s11739-016-1439-1.

25. Lewis CE, Peacock WJ, Tillou A, Hines OJ, Hiatt JR. A novel cadaver-based educational program in general surgery training. *J Surg Educ.* 2012;69(6):693–698. doi:10.1016/j.jsurg.2012.06.013.

26. Kim SC, Fisher JG, Delman KA, Hinman JM, Srinivasan JK. Cadaver-based simulation increases resident confidence, initial exposure to fundamental techniques, and may augment operative autonomy. *J Surg Educ.* 2016;73(6):e33–e41. doi:10.1016/j.jsurg.2016.06.014.

27. Kovacs G, Levitan R, Sandeski R. Clinical cadavers as a simulation resource for procedural learning. *AEM Educ Train.* 2018;2(3):239–247. doi:10.1002/aet2.10103.

28. Yiasemidou M, Gkaragkani E, Glassman D, Biyani CS. Cadaveric simulation: a review of reviews. *Ir J Med Sci.* 2018;187(3):827–833. doi:10.1007/s11845-017-1704-y.

29. Douglas-Jones R. Silent mentors': donation, education, and bodies in Taiwan. *MAT.* 2017;4(4):69–98. doi:10.17157/mat.4.4.454.

30. Balta JY, Cronin M, Cryan JF, O'Mahony SM. Human preservation techniques in anatomy: a 21st century medical education perspective. *Clin Anat.* 2015;28(6):725–734. doi:10.1002/ca.22585.

31. Thiel W. The preservation of the whole corpse with natural color. *Ann Anat.* 1992;174(3):185–195. doi:10.1016/s0940-9602(11)80346-8

32. Hong MK, Chu TY, Ding DC. How the silent mentor program improves our surgical level and safety and nourishes our spiritual life. *Gynecol Minim Invasive Ther.* 2017;6(3):99–102. doi:10.1016/j.gmit.2016.12.003.

33. Levitan RM, Bortle CD, Snyder TA, Nitsch DA, Pisaturo JT, Butler KH. Use of a battery-operated needle driver for intraosseous access by novice users: skill acquisition with cadavers. *Ann Emerg Med.* 2009;54(5):692–694. doi:10.1016/j.annemergmed.2009.06.012.

34. Dyer GSM, Thorndike MEL. Quidne mortui vivos docent? The evolving purpose of human dissection in medical education. *Acad Med.* 2000;75(10):969–979. doi:10.1097/00001888-200010000-00008.

35. Deleuze G, Guattari F. *What is Philosophy?* New York, NY: Columbia University Press; 1991.

36. Nicolini D. *Practice Theory, Work, and Organization: An Introduction.* Oxford, UK: Oxford University Press; 2012.

37. Nicolini D. Practice theory as a package of theory, method and vocabulary: affordances and limitations. In Jonas M, Littig B, Wroblewski A, eds. *Methodological Reflection on Practice-Oriented Theories.* Cham, Switzerland: Springer International Publishing; 2017. p. 19–34.

38. Pink S. *Doing Sensory Ethnography.* 2nd ed. London, UK: Sage; 2015.

39. MacLeod A, Luong V, Cameron P, et al. When I say… human. *Med Educ.* 2021;55(9):993–994. doi:10.1111/medu.14537.

40. Latour B. *Reassembling the Social.* Oxford, UK: Oxford University Press; 2005.

41. Olejaz M. When the dead teach: exploring the postvital life of cadavers in Danish dissection labs. *MAT.* 2017;4(4):125–149. doi:10.17157/mat.4.4.310.

42. Spradley JP. *Participant Observation.* Belmont, CA: Wadsworth Publishing Company; 1980.

43. Paradis E, Sutkin G. Beyond a good story: from Hawthorne Effect to reactivity in health professions education research. *Med Educ.* 2017;51(1):31–39. doi:10.1111/medu.13122.

44. MacLeod A. Six ways problem-based learning cases can sabotage patient-centered medical education. *Acad Med.* 2011;86(7):818–825. doi:10.1097/ACM.0b013e31821db670.

45. Wolcott H. *Transforming Qualitative Data: Description, Analysis and Interpretation.* London, UK: Sage; 1994.

46. Emerson RM, Fretz RI, Shaw LL. *Writing Ethnographic Fieldnotes.* Chicago, IL: University of Chicago press; 2011.

47. May T. When is a Deleuzian becoming? *Cont Philos Rev.* 2003;36(2):139–153. doi:10.1023/A:1026036516963.

48. Carey JM, Rossler K. The how when why of high fidelity simulation. *StatPearls.* May 9 2021. https://www.ncbi.nlm.nih.gov/books/NBK559313/. Accessed October 25, 2021.

49. Hamstra SJ, Brydges R, Hatala R, Zendejas B, Cook DA. Reconsidering fidelity in simulation-based training. *Acad Med.* 2014;89(3):387–392. doi:10.1097/ACM.0000000000000130.

50. Taranikanti V. Is COVID era the beginning of a paradigm shift in anatomy education? *MH.* 2020;15(2):1–2. doi:10.17576/MH.2020.1502.01.

Appendix A

Field notes & memo template

Basics – Please fill out with care

Your Name	
Date of your observation	
Start Time	
End Time	
You are physically present @?	
Which room (number)?	
What program?	
What type of CBS session?	
Is this a stand-alone memo?	
Other notables?	

Research questions

1) How do bodies, learners, tools and spaces come together in everyday practices of CBS?
2) How are these practices situated within wider processes and discourses of simulation learning in the health professions?
3) What is the potential role of CBS in a competency-based postgraduate program?
4) How do social and material dimensions of CBS shape teaching and learning in this context?

Observation Starting Points

9 Dimensions - James Spradley (1980):
1. Space: the physical place or places
2. Actor: the people involved
3. Activity: a set of related acts people do
4. Object: the physical things that are present
5. Act: single actions that people do
6. Event: a set of related activities that people carry out
7. Time: the sequencing that takes place over time
8. Goal: the things people are trying to accomplish
9. Feeling: the emotions felt and expressed

Description:

(Add lines as needed)

Interpretation:

(Add lines as needed)

Thank you for your participation. Please save and rename this document (Field notes_session name_Date_Your initials) and submit to Caine Meyers at caine.meyers@dal.ca.

Appendix B

Interview protocol (human body donation program staff, clinical cadaver program staff)

Note: These are semi-structured, in-depth, open-ended interviews; therefore, the format/conversation will be fluid; however, the interview will follow this general format.

Introduction: The research team is interested in hearing about your experiences working within the Dalhousie [Human Body Donation Program/Clinical Cadaver Program]. I'm going to be asking you a bit about yourself. Then, we'll be talking more about your work experiences.

As a reminder, you are not required to participate in this interview. Also, if you'd like to withdraw at any time, you're free to do so, without prejudice. You do not need to answer any question that makes you feel uncomfortable. Do you have any questions before we begin?

Learning about the participant

Please tell me a bit about yourself.
    When did you first start working within the Program?
    When was your first experience working with/in relation to cadavers?

Please describe your experience with [human body donation/clinical cadaver preparation and teaching] at Dalhousie and elsewhere.

Human body donation/clinical cadaver preparation

How has your experience of facilitating [human body donation/clinical cadaver preparation and teaching] been so far?
    Have you had any emotional reactions to [human body donation/clinical cadaver preparation and teaching]? Please describe.
    Do you feel there are any ethical complexities teaching/working with cadavers? Please explain.
    Complexities of working with human body donation/cadavers
    What are the benefits of [human body donation/clinical cadaver preparation and teaching]?
    What are the challenges of this work?
    Can you describe the physical experience of working with cadavers in this context?
    Imagine you must give instruction to a double who will have to replace you in your professional role. Please walk them through the process of [human body donation/clinical cadaver preparation and teaching] so that the double can fulfill your responsibilities.

Conclusion

Is there anything you'd like to discuss which we did not cover during this interview?
    Thank you for participating. Please feel free to be in contact if you have further questions and/or comments. I'll be sending you, via e-mail, a copy of the transcript of your interview within three weeks. I'll ask you to review your transcript, note any changes/additions/deletions and return it to me within two weeks. If I have not heard from you following the two-week period, I'll assume you have no changes.

Appendix C

Textual/analysis guide & form

Textual/Video Analysis Pointers
Key points to keep in mind as you're reviewing the text:

- Think about what the purpose of this Text/Video might be. What does it accomplish?
- Who (individually or collectively) is involved in producing this Text/Video?
- The Text/Video generates effects. Think about what the effects might be.
- Think about the less obvious (i.e. hidden) meanings communicated through this Text or Video.
- Who and what do these Texts/Videos render visible and/or invisible? How?
- What is explicit? What is implicit?
- What is your 'gut' reaction to the Text/Video?

*Remember: There are no right or wrong ways to review a Text/Video. We're interested in your impressions.

Text/video analysis form (please complete)

Name of Text/Video Reviewed:
Date of Text/Video Review:
Your name:

General

What type of Text/Video are you reviewing (policy, governing document, information document, website, lecture slide, etc.)?

First impression/appearance

Comment on the appearance of the Text/Video (Is it professionally designed? Is it an internal document? Dalhousie brand? What is this text telling you about the institution it is associated with? Etc).

Analytical questions

What do you think the Text/Video is meant to do (purpose)?

- What do you think the Text/Video is actually doing (effects)?
- What was your reaction to the text and why?
- What stands out about the Text/Video and why?

How does your position in the world (personal i.e., mother, son, hiker and professional, i.e., student, academic, photographer, physician) influence how you read this text?

Other comments?

....

Thank you for your participation. Please save and rename this document (something descriptive related to the document reviewed) and email to: caine.meyers@dal.ca

Technical Difficulties: Teaching Critical Philosophical Orientations toward Technology

Benjamin Chin-Yee (iD), Laura Nimmon (iD) and Mario Veen (iD)

ABSTRACT

Issue: Technological innovation is accelerating, creating less time to reflect on the impact new technologies will have on the medical profession. Modern technologies are becoming increasingly embedded in routine medical practice with far-reaching impacts on the patient-physician relationship and the very essence of the health professions. These impacts are often difficult to predict and can create unintended consequences for medical education. This article is driven by a main question: How do we prepare trainees to critically assess technologies that we cannot foresee and effectively use technology to support equitable and compassionate care? ***Evidence:*** We translate insights from the philosophy of technology into a proposal for integrating critical technical consciousness in medical curricula. We identify three areas required to develop critical consciousness with regard to emerging technologies. The first area is technical literacy, which involves not just *knowing* how to use technology, but also understanding its limitations and appropriate contexts for use. The second area is the ability to assess the social impact of technology. This practice requires understanding that while technification creates new possibilities it can also have adverse, unintended consequences. The third area is critical reflection on the relationship between 'the human' and 'the technical' as it relates to the values of the medical profession and professional identity formation. Human and technology are two sides of the same coin; therefore, thinking critically about technology also forces us to think about what we consider 'the human side of medicine'. ***Implications:*** Critical technical consciousness can be fostered through an educational program underpinned by the recognition that, although technological innovation can create new possibilities for healing, technology is never neutral. Rather, it is imperative to emphasize that technology is interwoven with the social fabric that is essential to healing. Like medication, technology can be both potion and poison.

Introduction

When we think of technology, we often think of 'cutting-edge' innovations and 'state-of-the-art' machines. However, it is sobering to realize that, today, most of the objects and practices that make up our day-to-day environment were at one point in human history innovative technologies. For example handwashing was at one time a remarkable technological innovation in global healthcare. Imagine if now, in the context of a global pandemic, this technology—which includes soap, a dispenser, running water, and the associated skills and habits of 'hand

hygiene'—were not available or acceptable to us. Across Europe in the 1840s, "professors, assistants and students often went directly from dissecting corpses to examining patients in the first clinic."[1(p164)] Even in the United States, it was not until the 1980s for the first national handwashing guidelines to emerge.

The development of the Electronic Health Record (EHR) in the 1970s and 1980s that is now ubiquitous in developed countries is a more modern example of a transformative healthcare technology that is often taken for granted. The EHR provides practitioners with external memory about the patient, enabling access to a wealth of information from medical and social history to clinical and laboratory data, before encountering the patient. Just as the EHR reshaped the clinical encounter in many countries, the rapid expansion of eHealth and telemedicine engendered by the COVID-19 pandemic are redefining the nature of the patient-physician relationship in Canada and the Netherlands where the authors are situated.[2]

One challenge is that what counts as 'good' technology depends on issues such as accessibility, resources and infrastructure of a particular location. As authors from Canada and The Netherlands we acknowledge our own positionality, and how our perspectives as researchers and clinicians from the Global North may cause us to focus on healthcare technology as it exists in many countries in this particular context. We are aware that this limited perspective does not address distinctive technological challenges faced elsewhere in the world.

In our modern age, we tend to associate technology with machines; however, human beings have been technical beings since the invention of fire-making, flint tools, and cave art.[3] With rudimentary mortars for smashing medicinal herbs, clay casts for mending broken bones, and evidence for trephination dating back to prehistoric times, the practice of medicine (the art of supporting and healing human beings) has always existed within and been enabled by an evolving *technical* environment. Medication (from penicillin to mRNA vaccines), medical tools (from the surgeon's scalpel to robot-assisted surgery), diagnostic instruments (from the reflex hammer to magnetic resonance imaging) and communication tools (from the rotary phone to videoconferencing) are examples of technologies that have evolved to improve modern medicine.

Philosophy of technology and the pharmakon

In this series on philosophy in medical education, it may seem unclear how technology constitutes a *philosophical* issue rather than just matter for engineering and ethics. However, technology has been a contested issue since Plato and Aristotle, with Plato lambasting the (then modern) technology of writing as a *"pharmakon"*.[4] Consider how while writing a speech guides its near perfect execution, it also erodes the latent ability to remember. The philosophical concept of the *pharmakon* denotes how technology, like a medicine, can be both a potion and poison.[4,5] It can have curative potential but (like the surgeon's scalpel) requires care to avoid causing harm. Several philosophers have since expanded on this nature of technology to exteriorize human abilities such as memory and manual skills.[3,6]

Videoconferencing is a recent example of a *pharmakon*. During the pandemic, particularly in resource-rich countries, videoconferencing has enabled healthcare providers to use visual diagnosis. Whereas, in these contexts, if the pandemic had happened a decade earlier, physicians would have had to rely on just the data and cues from the patient's voice. Modern technology provided a possibility for patient care that would not otherwise have existed. Given the efficiency of remote consultations many initial consultations are now video-mediated.[2] Perhaps one day these consultations will be automated or outsourced to artificial intelligence (AI).[7] However, this raises questions about what unforeseen side-effects this would this have on those qualities that we associate with the face-to-face doctor-patient relationship. Many studies have demonstrated that communication,[8] empathy,[9] connection, and intuition[10,11] have a positive impact on diagnosis and patient adherence.[12]

Applied philosophy of technology

In the twentieth century, philosophy of technology has been applied in Technology Assessment, Science and Technology Studies, and theoretical orientations such as sociomateriality.[13] These orientations concern themselves with, for instance, the question of how to assess the societal benefits and drawbacks of emergent (medical) technologies.[14] In the past few decades, philosophy of technology has expanded as a field by virtue of the acceleration of technological innovation and how technology is impacting our lives.

Innovation is of all ages, but today health care faces unprecedented challenges with accelerating technological innovation. In the time of Hippocrates, there might have been a groundbreaking innovation every century and in the time of Alexander Fleming, every decade. Since the rise of digital technologies it seems that innovations multiply on a daily basis. For example, in the 1980s, there was plenty of time between the introduction of the Personal Computer and its appearance in many doctors' consultation rooms. And with this acceleration, there is also insufficient time to become literate in using a technology and to critically evaluate its impact on patient care, including the relationship between technology and the 'human side' of medicine.

The acceleration of innovation and the reduction of time to master and reflect on emerging technologies is made even more urgent by the degree to which technology intervenes in patient-physician relationships. This acceleration isn't slowing down, which means that it is almost impossible to predict which technologies will have a major impact on medicine in the future. We can educate trainees on the technologies that we see and foresee today, from virtual care platforms to Big Data and AI. However, we cannot educate them on future technologies beyond our horizon of anticipation which is shrinking every year.

At present time, most medical education research tends to focus on existing technologies implemented in education and practice.[15–17] There are, however, inherent challenges assessing the impact of something that is both pervasive and future-based. Here we believe that insights from applied philosophy of technology, specifically from Technology Assessment and sociomateriality, can be especially valuable.

Technical artifacts, techniques, and technics

The first area in which these orientations can contribute is in clarifying the language surrounding technology. Like 'learning' in educational science,[18] the word 'technology' is imprecise. We have already used it to refer to machines, to writing, and to skills such as history-taking. In this paper, we distinguish between three 'levels' of technology. The first is the level of technical artifacts: pencils, smartphones, chairs, and so on. Technical artifacts are always assemblages: 'the EHR' is an assemblage of software code, computer chips, screens. Just as the EHR consists of many different technologies, so it can only function if embedded in a whole network of other technologies (just imagine how useless an EHR would be in an 19th century hospital, or even a 21st century hospital in a location with frequent or unpredictable power outages).

The second level of technology might be better termed *technique*. Technical artifacts are manifestations of techniques. For instance, Artificial Intelligence is a technique, as are software programming and electrical engineering. However, technique also includes human skills. The EHR not only relies on digital techniques to function in the context of clinical practice, but also on abilities to read, reason, and manually operate the device.

In observing how technical devices and techniques blur the traditional distinction between 'the human' and 'the technological', philosophers have enquired into the third level of technology, which we call *technics*.[3] Technics is what allows there to be technology in the first place. It has been called the technosphere (in relation to the geosphere and the biosphere) or "the technical condition", the entanglement of technology, culture and society.[19] Technology is not just an object in our environment, but it has to do with fundamental ways of *being* in the world:[20] from the

technology of writing to technical rationality – a way of relating to the world that aims to minimize input and maximize output. Some even going so far as to assert that there is an originating technicity to being human.[3,6]

In this paper, we draw on applied philosophy of technology to both broaden the concept of technology for medical education and suggest areas where a critical technical consciousness might be integrated into medical curricula. This perspective on technology, we believe, is indispensable for physicians of the future. Just as we strive to not only teach trainees the current state of evidence but also to be critical thinkers, ready to act as "evidence-based practitioners" not simply "evidence users",[21] they should be able to critically assess technology rather than just be technology users. This, we contend, requires not only technical training but also a philosophical orientation.

Positivist and philosophical orientations to technology

The question of technology is intimately related to the question of care that was discussed in an earlier installment in this series.[22,23] In another installment, Fawns and Schaepkens discuss how technology can infringe on basic values in medical education such as trust.[24] In this article, we elaborate the provocative conversations in this series by highlighting how technology concerns not only machines and their instrumental uses, but more fundamentally encompasses how we relate to each other as humans. For example, in medicine touch is not only technical as a diagnostic tool, but also relational in that it can foster empathy and form connection.[25] To emphasize this multiplicity of uses, we contrast a critical view of technology to an implicitly positivist view of technology that is prominent in modern medical education.

According to a positivist view, technology is simply an extension of science: it is rational application of scientific knowledge that allows humans to effectively control and manipulate their environment. From this perspective, technical artifacts are merely tools: a means to an end. While ethical concerns may be acknowledged, the implicit assumption is that technological innovation mirrors scientific progress.[19,26] In medical education, for instance, bedside ultrasound has been promoted despite findings that this technology "was not demonstrated to improve students' understanding of anatomy."[27(p366)] A positivist view does not recognize the entanglement of technology with social and cultural aspects of society and thus can succumb to technological solutionism. But most importantly for teaching in medical education, the positivist sees technology as a steady evolution that is inevitable and extraneous to the core human aspects of medicine, rather than an acceleration of a fundamental component of being human.[26] We suggest an alternative framing that encapsulates how as technology evolves, so does our relationship to patients, the nature of knowledge in the profession, and what it means to be healthy or sick. This is why a basic understanding of philosophy of technology needs to be integrated in medical curricula.

We propose three central ideas to guide teaching on technology in medical curricula that serve as conceptual foundations for fostering critical technical consciousness: how to expand the question of use (technical skill) to technical literacy; how to take into account social impact of emerging technologies; and how to recognize the complex entanglement of the relational (e.g. touch as a technique to form a relationship) and technical (e.g. touch as a technique to gather diagnostic data) aspects of the profession in order to more holistically understand what it is to be a medical expert who provides compassionate and equitable care. This critical philosophical orientation toward technology is not meant to be prescriptive or directive, but rather act as conceptual guide for teaching technology in medical curricula. Thus we will offer broad conceptual ideas that can raise consciousness and have the potential to be integrated creatively into educational initiatives in ways that are sensitive to local context and time.

Fostering critical technical consciousness

Technical literacy

The first and most obvious way to promote a healthy relationship with technology in medical education is to be able to understand how to effectively use technology in service of equitable patient care. Medical curricula might incorporate introductions to emerging technologies, such as Big Data and AI and their various uses in healthcare. However, what health professional learners require is training on how to best apply these technologies in the context of patient care. To this end, we propose an expanded concept of technical literacy.

While a positivist view of technology only focuses on how to use a technology competently, literacy is accompanied by recognizing the appropriate context for its use. This also means recognizing when a particular technology cannot or should not be used. The question is not simply what technical skills are required of physicians but rather what knowledge, skills, and

attitudes are needed for trainees to flexibly apply technology and adapt to local circumstances. Moreover, medical education requires assessing what specific competencies are required in relation to each technology, for instance, knowledge and critical thinking about the risk of bias in use of AI algorithms.[28-30]

Technical literacy includes knowing how a specific technology functions in the assemblage of other technologies to navigate its use in a given practice environment. For instance, an image-based AI algorithm may have demonstrated diagnostic accuracy. However, if additional technical conditions are not present within the target healthcare setting—such as appropriate methods and lighting for image acquisition or the necessary infrastructure to upload and store images—then it may not be the best technology for use in that context.

Flexibility and adaptation to context is especially important in dealing with technical failures. We all have examples of technology *not* working as it should. This is also a common occurrence in healthcare settings. Some hospitals use the term "Code Grey" to designate a new form of medical emergency where critical infrastructure failure, such as disruptions to the EHR, makes it difficult to practice. Technical literacy should involve robustness in the face of such perturbations, guarding against overreliance on use of a particular technology to provide patient care. Arguably, being able to improvise and correct mistakes under pressure is a more valuable competency than in-depth knowledge of a specific technology.[31]

In our times, technical literacy also includes knowledge of the hidden costs. Recently, over 200 health journals called on governments to take emergency action on climate change.[32] Medical technology – from pharmacology to surgery– has a large share in the global carbon footprint, often not advertised by producers.[33,34] Since the industrial revolution, the ecological impact of technology, is now seen as the "greatest threat to global public health."[35(p2)] This shows what happens on a macro-level when we only concentrate on how to produce and use technology, focusing only on the immediate benefits, without considering its implications for our well-being in sociocultural context. Such an example could be used in medical education to support a more encompassing technical literacy that moves beyond the myopic micro-level to recognize the broader context and consequences of technology.

Trainees also require competency to *become literate* in technologies that are still beyond that horizon, yet likely to become the 'cutting-edge' by the time they enter practice. One way to help meet this challenge is to develop curricula not solely focused on the existing technologies that are ready for use, but that also highlight broader trends in technological development and how they interact with the social role and ethical commitments of the healing professions. With the acceleration of technological innovation, it is better to have a head-start in anticipating the human and social impacts of technology in healthcare rather than playing catch-up.

The social construction of technology

Anthropogenic climate change is an extreme example of technology as a *pharmakon*: it has created hitherto unimaginable possibilities for human health but at the same time may also pose its greatest threat.[5] This double-edged nature of technology is not only material but also social. Sometimes these social consequences are obvious but often they can be subtle. Technology Assessment and philosophy of technology helps us to appreciate these subtleties, allowing us to see how technologies are not mere instruments, but rather intimately connected to human activities and the fabric of human relationships.

Technological solutionism is the positivist idea that, since technology has successfully addressed so many problems in human history, any problem has a (purely) technological fix.[36] The trend toward technological solutionism predates COVID-19 but has only been amplified by the pandemic.[37] As mentioned above, although innovations in virtual care have been essential for healthcare delivery during the pandemic, adoption of new technologies is not always done with consideration of the social, political, and ethical side effects.[2,38] Often these side effects are only recognized in retrospect, at a point when technologies have already become embedded within professional norms and practices, making change or resistance difficult. In Technology Assessment,[39] this is referred to as the Collingride Dilemma.[40] This refers to the fact that the social impact of new technologies often only becomes clear when they are already entrenched, leaving little room for adjustment.

In medical education, we strive to train professionals to rigorously appraise evidence for certain medical technologies.[41] This appraisal is largely in the form of diagnostic tests, medications, or procedures. Indeed, the need for critical appraisal of such interventions was the major motivation behind the Evidence-Based Medicine (EBM) movement, which was initially conceived as an initiative in medical education.[41] As debates over merits and pitfalls of EBM continue in medical education,[42] these conversations have inspired calls for more fundamental reflection on medical epistemology in healthcare curricula.[21] Moreover, within this backdrop there remains a collective blind spot in how to teach trainees to critically reflect not only on the epistemic but also the social and ethical dimensions of technology. Three insights in particular from Technology Assessment and Philosophy of Technology[13,26,39,43] can help support critical reflection on the social impact of medical technologies. These include appreciating how the human and the technological are co-constructed, how societal values shape technology, and how these factors intersect with issues of equity.

The first and most basic insight is recognizing the co-construction of the human and the technical: technologies are human creations but also shape our cognition, our interactions, and even our understanding of what it means to be human. Some philosophers have pointed out how this is a basic feature of the human condition,[3] long before smartphones and their digital affordances served as "extended selves". Technology can be seen as an external organ, like the surgeon's knife as an extension of their hand or like the EHR as the extension of their memory. Technology, therefore, cannot be understood as mere extrinsic instruments or artifacts, engineered to rationally and efficiently accomplish distinctively human goals. Rather, technology shapes who and what we are as humans.

Trainees can be made aware of this co-construction to appreciate it in contemporary healthcare. As discussed above, being a physician today increasingly requires leveraging a complex assemblage of technologies, even to perform the most basic "human" aspects of our profession. Consider the example of the EHR, discussed above. In many settings the EHR not only serves as a portal to all medical records, but also as the mode of access to all investigations as well as the means of ordering tests and prescribing therapies. How the EHR has shaped norms of practice, and our growing reliance on this technology, becomes especially apparent when it fails, as in the "Code Grey" scenario. Following a phase of acute disorientation ("You mean I don't know this patient's complete blood count before assessing them?"), the physician, once again, learns to take a history by talking to the patient, rather than sifting through notes from previous encounters. They realize it is in fact possible to measure the vital signs, rather than extracting them from the nursing record and to recall the dose of a commonly ordered drug, rather than ticking off a pre-defined order set. Of course, this is not without its challenges and potential drawbacks in efficiency, accuracy, and safety. All of these factors are what make the EHR a powerful technology, and explain why it has successfully embedded itself into the "core" of our profession. While there is a tendency to pit "human versus machine",[44] a recurrent trope from antiquity to the age of the EHR,[45] trainees must be taught to recognize the co-construction of the human and the technological to better understand the social benefits and drawbacks of technology in clinical practice.

Appreciating this co-construction serves as an entry point into understanding not only how technology shapes human activities, but also how societal values shape technology. A key concept here is the idea of technological underdetermination: technology is not determined solely by considerations of function and efficiency, but also additional social choices.[46] These social choices become subtly incorporated into technologies as "technical code", which introduce biases either from underlying societal prejudices or from the very notion of what makes a rational, well-functioning system.[46,47] Returning to the example of the EHR, while abovementioned considerations such as patient safety may factor into their design, additional considerations such as efficiency in billing or collection of administrative data may also shape their "technical code", serving the interests of certain users over others, which may in turn diverge from the interests of patients.[2] Concerns over bias and discrimination in medical technologies are longstanding,[48] but have been amplified by the rise of machine learning and AI in healthcare, whose allure and power can serve to obscure societal prejudices behind a "veneer of technical neutrality."[49(p422)] Trainees must be taught to scrutinize the social choices that go into technological design and application, and in scrutinizing these choices should learn to ask: Who was included? Who was excluded? What are the unintended consequences? Whose interests do they serve? These questions highlight the need to appraise new technologies with a specific focus on their impact on health equity. Discussion of technological equity is often framed as a problem of access, and indeed access to medical technologies remains a major challenge around the world and barrier to global health.[50]

We acknowledge that our discussion of technical competencies and the examples provided reflect our own privilege as educators and clinicians practicing in high resource settings where problems of access are less common (but certainly still present). Despite this, analysis of technological equity should not stop at issues of access. Rather it should cut across the entire trajectory of technology's social genesis, starting from the power hierarchies that delineate privileged sites of technological design and innovation,[51] which in turn can engender exclusionary definitions of "standard users" and "appropriate" contexts for use.[52] For example, while remote monitoring devices, such as smartwatches, may promise to improve access to healthcare in underserved communities, their current forms are more likely to benefit the already privileged and potentially deepen health disparities.[53] Some might consider this type of appraisal to be beyond the scope of healthcare professions education, dismissed as being more the within purview of the sociologist than the doctor. However, the latter can indeed learn from the former given the tangible links between technology and health equity encountered in day-to-day practice.

The relationship between the "human" and the "technical"

The positivist view presents human and the technical as binary oppositions. But from philosophy of technology orientation we know that they are in fact two sides of the same coin.[3] We are so deeply entangled with technology that it "makes little sense to think of ourselves, our culture, our society as distinctly separate from technology."[19(p7)] A surgeon's scalpel, for instance, requires a whole range of skills, expertise, and interpersonal relationships, such as the relationship between a trainee and supervisor, to function.[54] This assemblage centered around a surgical technology, in this example, creates a new horizon of possibility for human beings, in this case, a longer life-expectancy and better health-related quality of life for patients with hitherto untreatable ailments. So far in this article we have been discussing a critical technological literacy. In the following, we broaden this conversation to discuss the ways medical expertise might be framed as a delicate balance of both technical and relational skills.

In medical education, Nimmon distinguishes *technification* as: "the repurposing of a human social activity to function as a procedural or diagnostic skill designed to gather data about the patient and determine what aspect of the patient requires curing."[25(p380)] This notion critiques the technification of medical expertise, as it is sometimes at the expense of cultivating humanism in practitioners. Technification and humanism are equally responsible for the success of healthcare in our society. Ideally, they can mutually support each other and be employed responsively to context.[55] However, it is myopic to adopt an assumption that everything in healthcare can be technified in the name of data gathering, diagnosis, and efficiency – there is a relational cost. Technology is not just about machines or diagnostic tools, but also language (e.g. touch or non-verbal communication) are a technology that can form or erode human connection. This is exemplified in a paper by de la Croix[56] who reveals how a neurologist gathers and prioritizes technical data about an interaction she has with her disabled son to use as a teaching tool for medical students. De la Croix describes feeling dehumanized and sad about the lack of effort the neurologist makes to build rapport and connection with her.

Individual existence is interwoven in relationships and this interdependence is a necessary condition of being human.[57] The COVID-19 pandemic has shed new light on questions about what aspects of the medical profession can and ought to be mediated or replaced by technology. In the past two years, human connection was suddenly severed at a global and societal level. A collective grappling with the erosion of what it means to be human was captured by an emergency room physician at the Royal Melbourne Hospital in a letter to the New York Times in August 2020.[58] He describes how useful a video chat was to connect a dying patient to loved ones, but underscores his letter by describing how harrowing and soulless the experience is:

> If video chats are soulless to us, how must it feel to say goodbye via video link? A young doctor's voice broke as she described her day to me, going from one sick or dying patient's room to another with her iPad, digitally connecting the patients to their relatives at home and witnessing over and over the families fall apart with grief.

We had a chance to witness the critical need of human connection in healthcare as it played out in the most existentially intimate moments, as in times of death and dying. Writer Sergio Del Molino Sergio encapsulates this sentiment perfectly: "We humans need to touch and be touched; we don't know how to love without it. Distance makes us cold; it makes us care less about one another."[59] In the Netherlands during the first wave of COVID-19 when society was locked down and people were experiencing the effects of social distancing, the term "huidhonger" was popularized,[60] which literally translates as both "hunger for skin" and "hunger of the skin" to capture the intense desire for physical contact and the skin's desire to touch other skin after a sustained period of touch deprivation.

A deeper probing into this tension between technical and humanist expertise and capacity to care can be observed in the context of virtual care. Many patients and practitioners report a strong preference for virtual care (which reduces cost, saves time, and avoids nuisance of travel). However, virtual care also presents challenges for those with limited digital literacy, language barriers, broadband access. Although telehealth provides an essential tool for physicians we must consider the humanistic aspects that may be lost in the doctor-patient relationship. A growing body of work is recognizing that the technology of virtual care can never fully replace the richness of face-to-face encounters. Kelly and colleagues have emphasized how touch is used by healthcare providers to show empathy and demonstrate a shared humanity.[12,61–63] The authors have discovered that in the physical examination physicians use their own bodies to express non-verbal communication and experience the story of patients' illnesses. Underscoring the importance of touch, this body of work describes how in-person physical exams wove a sense of professional identity as a family physician and healer; promoting rapport, continuity, and trust.[12,61,62]

We co-exist with technology in an era of an automated depersonalized society where isolation is a growing epidemic that impacts health and wellbeing.[64,65] What does it mean to be a physician who forms connection and can respond intuitively to patients, not just diagnose and estimate prognosis in a detached automated way? What does it look like to interact sensitively with patients even when this interaction is mediated by technology? There may be an unconscious interference with the healing relationship when healthcare professionals interact mechanically: diagnosing, estimating prognosis, prescribing – emotionally veiled and hidden behind technology. We need to ensure prognosis is more than simply mechanical risk prediction but also serves its humanistic function in helping create narrative continuity between past, present, and future.[66] We are at no better time to engage in philosophical discussion that can deepen our understanding of the therapeutic power of human connection and how this can be sustained in the cultural hype of "progress," "efficiency," and "technological innovation."

Discussion: Difficult technicalities

With the climate crisis, the COVID-19 pandemic, and the increasing technification of the healthcare, there is an urgent need to slow down and reflect on the role of technology in healthcare and the relationship between human and technical aspects of the health professions. One way to stimulate this reflection in education is to ask students to look around and realize how every technology – from chairs to pencils to books – were at one point in human history "cutting edge" while every technology that we now consider new will in the near future seem just as mundane as those old pieces of equipment that have long since lost their technological luster.

The health care professions exist by virtue of old and new technology and it is expected that technological innovation will continue to expand human lifespan with higher health-related quality of life. But technology is a *pharmakon* that requires care.[5] Building on Stiegler's work, others have linked the accelerated evolution of modern technology, especially digital technologies, to a depletion of our capacity to care for and empathize with others.[65] Medical education should therefore not only prepare trainees to take care of patients, but also to master the technical environment that enables them to provide this care. In medical education, perhaps more than in any other field, it is precisely care and humanity that should be at the center. In order to fully embrace the unprecedented possibilities for better health, technology itself needs thoughtful care—a "toxicology" to curb and counter its potential harmful effects on the psychological, social, and ecological context in which healing takes place.

We have argued for integrating a more fundamental shift toward a critical technical consciousness in medical curricula. This shift starts with our own values and attitude. Philosophers have long pointed out that in our technological age, our way of thinking and relating to other human beings can take the form of technical or instrumental rationality, which treats everything (including human beings) as a calculable means to an end, with a focus on efficiency.[3,20,67] Although we may not be using actual tools this instrumental attitude leads us to relate to others as mere tools, treating them as numbers in a calculation, their bodies as mere mechanism. In his autobiography *When Breath Becomes Air*, Kalanithi details his conscious effort to shift away from this attitude of instrumental rationality after an incident during his medical training, when he writes "From that point on, I resolved to treat all my paperwork as patients, and not vice versa."[68(p77)] By proposing a broader conception of technological literacy, we envision a place for technology to support human relationships at the core of the healing professions, which guards against a detached, technical rationality. Just as the clinician who masters the art of blind typing can better maintain eye-contact with the patient, the physician adept in use of videoconferencing can have more meaningful virtual encounters, but, crucially, can also recognize when such encounters are not appropriate and when in-person assessment is required. Medical education today must recognize that technology increasingly intercalates the human interactions of patient care. It is critical to prepare trainees for the realities of practice in a technological age, while equipping them with antidotes against an encompassing technical rationality.

We have outlined three principles that could serve as the starting point of teaching, though the way they are translated into educational practice will depend on the context of each institution. These are promoting technical literacy of current and future technology in context, enabling trainees to assess the impact of emergent technology on the social, psychological, and health-related aspects of patient care, and the awareness that technification can extend to human activities in health care. In teaching, one could take a concrete emergent technology and work through the three ideas related to technology, as we have done in this article with the EHR.

We have focused on what could be implemented in medical curricula to equip future physicians to critically and competently work with technological innovation. We concur that the problems we have discussed also demand more systemic changes in how medicine as a whole relates to technology, situated alongside actions directed at broader issues such as climate change and widening health disparities. Our hope is that health professionals equipped with a critical technical consciousness will be more adept and vocal partners in this larger dialogue, helping to create and support a healthier relationship between the human and the technical for the future of medicine and society at large.

Funding

B.C.Y. acknowledges funding from an AMS Healthcare Fellowship in Compassion and Artificial Intelligence.

ORCID

Benjamin Chin-Yee http://orcid.org/0000-0003-0737-3603
Laura Nimmon http://orcid.org/0000-0002-7291-603X
Mario Veen http://orcid.org/0000-0003-2550-7193

Previous philosophy in medical education instalments

Mario Veen & Anna T. Cianciolo (2020) Problems No One Looked For: Philosophical Expeditions into Medical Education, Teaching and Learning in Medicine, 32:3, 337-344, DOI: 10.1080/10401334.2020.1748634
Gert J. J. Biesta & Marije van Braak (2020) Beyond the Medical Model: Thinking Differently about Medical Education and Medical Education Research, Teaching and Learning in Medicine, 32:4, 449–456, DOI: 10.1080/10401334.2020.1798240
Mark R. Tonelli & Robyn Bluhm (2021) Teaching Medical Epistemology within an Evidence-Based Medicine Curriculum, Teaching and Learning in Medicine, 33:1, 98–105, DOI: 10.1080/10401334.2020.1835666
John R. Skelton (2021) Language, Philosophy, and Medical Education, Teaching and Learning in Medicine, 33:2, 210–216, DOI: 10.1080/10401334.2021.1877712
Zareen Zaidi, Ian M. Partman, Cynthia R.Whitehead, Ayelet Kuper & Tasha R. Wyatt (2021) Contending with Our Racial Past in Medical Education: A Foucauldian Perspective, Teaching and Learning in Medicine, DOI: 10.1080/10401334.2021.1945929
Chris Rietmeijer & Mario Veen (2021) Phenomenological Research in Health Professions Education: Tunneling from

Both Ends, Teaching and Learning in Medicine, DOI:10.10 80/10401334.2021.1971989

Madeleine Noelle Olding, Freya Rhodes, John Humm, Phoebe Ross & Catherine McGarry (2022) Black, White and Gray: Student Perspectives on Medical Humanities and Medical Education, Teaching and Learning in Medicine, 34:2, 223–233, DOI: 10.1080/10401334.2021.1982717

Camillo Coccia & Mario Veen (2022) Because We Care: A Philosophical Investigation into the Spirit of Medical Education, Teaching and Learning in Medicine, 10.1080/10401334.2022.2056744

Tim Fawns & Sven Schaepkens (2022) A Matter of Trust: Online Proctored Exams and the Integration of Technologies of Assessment in Medical Education, Teaching and Learning in Medicine, DOI: 10.1080/10401334.2022.2048832

Anna MacLeod, Victoria Luong, Paula Cameron, George Kovacs, Molly Fredeen, Lucy Patrick, Olga Kits & Jonathan Tummons (2022) The Lifecycle of a Clinical Cadaver: A Practice-Based Ethnography, Teaching and Learning in Medicine, DOI: 10.1080/10401334.2022.2092111

John Humm (2022) Being-Opposite-Illness: Phenomenological Ontology in Medical Education and Clinical Practice, Teaching and Learning in Medicine, DOI: 10.1080/10401334.2022.2108814

Associated Podcast

Let Me Ask You Something (iTunes, Spotify, Google Podcasts and https://marioveen.com/letmeasky ousomething/)

References

1. Gillies D. Hempelian and Kuhnian approaches in the philosophy of medicine: the Semmelweis case. *Stud Hist Philos Biol Biomed Sci.* 2005;36(1):159–181. doi:10.1016/j.shpsc.2004.12.003.
2. Zulman DM, Verghese A. Virtual care, telemedicine visits, and real connection in the era of COVID-19: Unforeseen opportunity in the face of adversity. *Jama.* 2021;325(5):437–438. doi:10.1001/jama.2020.27304.
3. Stiegler B. *Technics and Time, 1: The Fault of Epimetheus.* Stanford, CA: Stanford University Press; 1998.
4. Derrida J. Plato's Pharmacy. In *Dissemination.* Chicago, IL: University of Chicago Press; 1981:61–172.
5. Stiegler B, Ross D. *What Makes Life Worth Living: On Pharmacology.* Cambridge, UK: Polity; 2013.
6. Leroi-Gourhan A. *Gesture and Speech.* Cambridge, MA: MIT Press; 1993.
7. Burki T. GP at hand: a digital revolution for health care provision? *The Lancet.* 2019;394(10197):457–460. doi:10.1016/S0140-6736(19)31802-1.
8. Zolnierek KBH, Dimatteo MR. Physician communication and patient adherence to treatment: a meta-analysis. *Med Care.* 2009;47(8):826–834. doi:10.1097/MLR.0b0 13e31819a5acc.
9. Kim SS, Kaplowitz S, Johnston MV. The effects of physician empathy on patient satisfaction and compliance. *Eval Health Prof.* 2004;27(3):237–251. doi:10.1177/0163278704267037.
10. Stolper E, Van de Wiel M, Van Royen P, Van Bokhoven M, Van der Weijden T, Dinant GJ. Gut feelings as a third track in General Practitioners' diagnostic rea-

soning. *J Gen Intern Med.* 2011;26(2):197–203. doi:10.1007/s11606-010-1524-5.
11. Vanstone M, Monteiro S, Colvin E, et al. Experienced physician descriptions of intuition in clinical reasoning: a typology. *Diagnosis (Berl).* 2019;6(3):259–268. doi:10.1515/dx-2018-0069.
12. Kelly M, Nixon L, Rosenal T, et al. Being vulnerable: a qualitative inquiry of physician touch in medical education. *Acad Med.* 2020;95(12):1893–1899. doi:10.1097/ACM.0000000000003488.
13. Lemmens P, Hui Y. Landscapes of technological thoughts: a dialogue between Pieter Lemmens and Yuk Hui. *Philosophy Today.* 2021;65(2):375–389. doi: 10.5840/ philtoday2021412393.
14. O'Donnell JC, Pham SV, Pashos LP, Miller DW, Smith MD. Health technology assessment: lessons learned from around the world—an overview. *Value in Health.* 2009;12:S1–S5. doi:10.1111/j.1524-4733.2009. 00550.x.
15. Hodges BD. Ones and zeros: Medical education and theory in the age of intelligent machines. *Med Educ.* 2020;54(8):691–693. doi:10.1111/medu.14149.
16. Webster CS. Artificial intelligence and the adoption of new technology in medical education. *Med Educ.* 2021;55(1):6–7. doi:10.1111/medu.14409.
17. van der Niet AG, Bleakley A. Where medical education meets artificial intelligence: 'Does technology care?' *Med Educ.* 2021;55(1):30–36. doi:10.1111/medu.14131.
18. Biesta G, van Braak M. Beyond the medical model: thinking differently about medical education and medical education research. *Teach Learn Med.* 2020;32(4):449–456. doi:10.1080/10401334.2020.1798240.
19. Swierstra T, Lemmens P, Sharon T, Vermaas P, eds. *The Technical Condition: The Entanglement of Technology, Culture, and Society.* Amsterdam: Boom; 2022.
20. Heidegger M. *The Question concerning Technology, and Other Essays.* New York: HarperCollins; 1982.
21. Tonelli MR, Bluhm R. Teaching medical epistemology within an evidence-based medicine curriculum. *Teach Learn Med.* 2021;33(1):98–105. doi:10.1080/10401334. 2020.1835666.
22. Stiegler B. *Taking Care of Youth and the Generations.* Stanford, CA: Stanford University Press; 2010.
23. Coccia C, Veen M. Because we care: a philosophical investigation into the spirit of medical education. *Teach Learn Med.* 2022;34(3):341–349. doi:10.1080/10 401334.2022.2056744.
24. Fawns T, Schaepkens S. A matter of trust: online proctored exams and the integration of technologies of assessment in medical education. *Teach Learn Med.* 2022;34(4):444–453. doi:10.1080/10401334.2022.2048832.
25. Nimmon L. Expanding medical expertise: the role of healer. *Med Educ.* 2020;54(5):380–381. doi:10.1111/medu.14134.
26. Chin-Yee B. The philosophy of technology: on medicine's technological enframing. In: Brown M, Veen M, Finn G, eds. *Applied Philosophy for Health Professions Education.* Singapore: Springer; 2022:251–65.
27. Feilchenfeld Z, Dornan T, Whitehead C, Kuper A. Ultrasound in undergraduate medical education: a systematic and critical review. *Med Educ.* 2017;51(4):366–378. doi:10.1111/medu.13211.
28. Lee Y-M, Cao K, Leech M, De Ponti F. Developing medical artificial intelligence leaders: international

29. McCoy LG, Nagaraj S, Morgado F, Harish V, Das S, Celi LA. What do medical students actually need to know about artificial intelligence? *NPJ Digit Med.* 2020;3(1):86. doi:10.1038/s41746-020-0294-7.

30. Mehta N, Harish V, Bilimoria K, et al. Knowledge of and attitudes on artificial intelligence in healthcare: a provincial survey study of medical students [version 1]. *MedEdPublish.* 2021;10:75. doi:10.1101/2021.01.14.212 49830.

31. Crawford MB. *The World beyond Your Head: On Becoming an Individual in an Age of Distraction.* New York, NY: Farrar, Straus and Giroux; 2015.

32. Wise J. Climate crisis: over 200 health journals urge world leaders to tackle "catastrophic harm". *BMJ.* 2021;374:n2177. doi:10.1136/bmj.n2177.

33. Richie C. Environmental sustainability and the carbon emissions of pharmaceuticals. *J Med Ethics.* 2021;48(5):334–337. doi:10.1136/medethics-2020-106842.

34. Rizan C, Steinbach I, Nicholson R, Lillywhite R, Reed M, Bhutta MF. The carbon footprint of surgical operations: a systematic review. *Ann Surg.* 2020;272(6):986–995. doi:10.1097/SLA.0000000000003951.

35. Atwoli L, Baqui AH, Benfield T, et al. Call for emergency action to limit global temperature increases, restore biodiversity, and protect health. *BMJ.* 2021;374:n1734. doi:10.1136/bmj.n1734.

36. Morozov E. *To save Everything Click Here.* New York, NY: Public Affairs; 2013.

37. Ajjawi R, Eva KW. The problem with solutions. *Med Educ.* 2021;55(1):2–3. doi:10.1111/medu.14413.

38. Wamsley D, Chin-Yee B. COVID-19, digital health technology and the politics of the unprecedented. *Big Data Soc.* 2021;8(1):205395172110194. doi:10.1177/2053 9517211019441.

39. Banta D. What is technology assessment? *Int J Technol Assess Health Care.* 2009;25(S1):7–9. doi:10.1017/S0266462309090333.

40. Collingridge D. *The Social Control of Technology.* New York, NY: St. Martin's Press; 1980.

41. Guyatt G, Cairns J, Churchill D, et al. Evidence-based medicine. A new approach to teaching the practice of medicine. *Jama.* 1992;268(17):2420–2425. doi:10.1001/jama.1992.03490170092032.

42. Thomas A, Chin-Yee B, Mercuri M. Thirty years of teaching evidence-based medicine: have we been getting it all wrong? *Adv Health Sci Educ Theory Pract.* 2022;27(1):263–276. doi:10.1007/s10459-021-10077-4.

43. Franssen M, Lokhorst G, Van de Poel I. Philosophy of technology. In: Zalta EN, ed. *The Stanford Encyclopedia of Philosophy* (Fall 2018 Edition). https://plato.stanford.edu/archives/fall2018/entries/technology/.

44. Mukherjee S. AI versus MD: what happens when diagnosis is automated? *The New Yorker;* 2017:3.

45. Pettman D. *Human Error: Species-Being and Media Machines.* Minnesota: University of Minnesota Press; 2011.

46. Feenberg A. *Critical Theory of Technology.* New York, NY: Oxford University Press; 1991.

47. Feenberg A. *Transforming Technology.* Oxford: Oxford University Press on Demand; 2002.

48. Braun L. *Breathing Race into the Machine.* Minnesota: University of Minnesota Press; 2014.

49. Benjamin R. Assessing risk, automating racism. *Science.* 2019;366(6464):421–422. doi:10.1126/science.aaz3873.

50. Howitt P, Darzi A, Yang G-Z, et al. Technologies for global health. *Lancet.* 2012;380(9840):507–535. doi:10.1016/S0140-6736(12)61127-1.

51. Irani L. "Design thinking": defending Silicon Valley at the apex of global labor hierarchies. *Catalyst.* 2018;4(1):1–19. doi:10.28968/cftt.v4i1.29638.

52. Milan S. Techno-solutionism and the standard human in the making of the COVID-19 pandemic. *Big Data Soc.* 2020;7(2):205395172096678. doi:10.1177/2053951 720966781.

53. Isakadze N, Martin SS. How useful is the smartwatch ECG? *Trends Cardiovasc Med.* 2020;30(7):442–448. doi:10.1016/j.tcm.2019.10.010.

54. Nieboer P, Huiskes M, Cnossen F, Stevens M, Bulstra SK, Jaarsma D. Recruiting expertise: how surgical trainees engage supervisors for learning in the operating room. *Med Educ.* 2019;53(6):616–627. doi:10.1111/medu.13822.

55. Chan M, Nimmon L. Spinning the lens on physician power: narratives of humanism and healing. *Perspect Med Educ.* 2019;8(5):305–308. doi:10.1007/s40037-019-00537-4.

56. de la Croix A. The sense and nonsense of communication (skills) teaching - reflections from a parent and educator. *Patient Educ Couns.* 2022;105(7):2619–2620. doi:10.1016/j.pec.2021.12.004.

57. Reindal SM. Independence, dependence, interdependence: some reflections on the subject and personal autonomy. *Disability Soc.* 1999;14(3):353–367. doi:10.1080/09687599926190.

58. Lokuge A. A doctor asks: is Covid scaring us away from our humanity? *New York Times.* August 28, 2020.

59. del Molino S. What makes me a monster. *New York Times.* December 16, 2021.

60. Boevink W. Huidhonger, je zou een wildvreemde willen omhelzen [Skin-hunger, you would like to hug a stranger]. *Trouw.* March 26, 2020.

61. Kelly M, Svrcek C, King N, Scherpbier A, Dornan T. Embodying empathy: a phenomenological study of physician touch. *Med Educ.* 2020;54(5):400–407. doi:10.1111/medu.14040.

62. Kelly MA, Freeman LK, Dornan T. Family physicians' experiences of physical examination. *Ann Fam Med.* 2019;17(4):304–310. doi:10.1370/afm.2420.

63. Kelly MA, Gormley GJ. In, but out of touch: connecting with patients during the virtual visit. *Ann Fam Med.* 2020;18(5):461–462. doi:10.1370/afm.2568.

64. Murthy VH, Murthy VH. *Together.* New York: Harper Collins Publishers; 2020.

65. Pettman D. *Peak Libido: Sex, Ecology, and the Collapse of Desire.* Cambridge: Polity Press; 2021.

66. Thomas JM, Cooney LM, Jr, Fried TR. Prognosis reconsidered in light of ancient insights: from Hippocrates to modern medicine. *JAMA Intern Med.* 2019;179(6):820–823. doi:10.1001/jamainternmed.2019.0302.

67. Adorno TW. *Negative Dialectics.* London: Routledge; 1973.

68. Kalanithi P. *When Breath Becomes Air.* New York, NY: Random House; 2016.

🔓 OPEN ACCESS

Mind the Gap: A Philosophical Analysis of Reflection's Many Benefits

Sven P. C. Schaepkens 🆔 and Thijs Lijster 🆔

ABSTRACT

Issue: Expectations of reflection run high in medical practice and medical education; it is claimed as a means to many ends. In this article, the authors do not reject the value of reflection for medical education and medical practitioners, but they still ask why reflection can (potentially) yield so many different benefits, and what that implies for the status of reflection in medical education practice. *Evidence:* Based on a conceptual analysis of debates about reflection in the philosophical tradition, the authors argue that there are two quintessential gaps that play a role in the proliferation of (potential) benefits. First, reflection deals with bridging the gap between theory and practice; second, it deals with bridging the gap between the individual sense and communal sense. These gaps prevent the systematization of reflection, and they are fundamental to human thinking and experience in any situated environment, which led contemporary research on reflection to list a wide variety of benefits. *Implications:* The authors argue that if reflection resists systematization, it cannot be learned by following rules or protocols, but only practiced. Then, reflection should no longer be taught and researched as an individual skill one learns, nor as a means to some particular, beneficial end. Rather, one should practice reflection, and experience what it means to be part of a community wherein professionals jump the theory–practice gap constantly in a myriad of situations. Based on their analysis, the authors provide three concrete recommendations for reflection in medical education. First, to give precedence to reflective activities that encompass both gaps wherein situated examples can flourish; second, to use reflective guidelines as sources of inspiration; third, to show reserve about assessing reflection.

Introduction

Expectations of reflection run high in medical practice and medical education; it is claimed as a means to many ends. Reflection can reduce burnout,[1,2] increase empathy,[2] decrease stress,[3] develop professionalism,[4] refine clinical skills,[5–7] help practitioners transition from theory to practice,[8–11] and many more. Albeit various researchers show some reserve about the empirical evidence concerning the benefits of reflection,[12–15] reflection seemingly blossoms with potential. Consequently, some researchers attempt to create order in reflection's proliferated ends, for instance by categorizing reflection's purposes in three domains,[13] while others argue that "reflection has become a generic salve to heal all wounds,"[16(p263)] or has become reductively utilized as purely a means to an end.[17] While we do not reject the value of reflection for

medical education and practitioners, we ask why reflection can (potentially) yield so many different benefits, and what that implies for the status of reflection in medical education practice.

We argue that it is important to critically analyze how reflection relates to its many (potential) benefits because teachers and trainees dedicate much time and many educational resources to reflective activities. In medical curricula, there is a wide variety of ways to reflect, teach, and assess reflection. Reflective activities span written portfolios, essays, journals, mentor programs, training programs, or discussing clinical experience with peers in small groups.[14] Reflective activities receive justification based on the premise that they yield certain benefits.

Our analysis will consist of a philosophical investigation of the concept reflection. We will focus on debates from the philosophical tradition, specifically

---

This is an Open Access article distributed under the terms of the Creative Commons Attribution License (http://creativecommons.org/licenses/by/4.0/), which permits unrestricted use, distribution, and reproduction in any medium, provided the original work is properly cited.

how philosophers connected reflection to the gap between theory and practice, and the gap between an individual sense and communal sense. We will then relate our philosophical considerations to the current research on reflection to determine how researchers conceptually used reflection to pinpoint its benefits. Finally, in the light of our analysis we will formulate three concrete recommendations for reflection in medical practice and education.

A philosophical approach to research on reflection

For this article, we conducted a philosophical, conceptual analysis of reflection.[18-20] We questioned the theoretical presuppositions surrounding reflection, and traced background premises and values that affect this educational practice and its (potential) benefits.[21,22] We drew our philosophical considerations from the continental philosophical tradition, particularly the work of Immanuel Kant, Martin Heidegger, Hannah Arendt and Jacques Derrida. We turned to these philosophers because they map the limits of human knowledge, and critically think about aporias, or how "gaps" play a vital role in human experience and reflection. For them, these aporias should not be understood as problems that are to be solved, but rather as limits that require awareness. Therefore, we started our analysis from the perspective of the gaps to help us understand reflection and its relation to the alleged benefits.

Our analysis consisted of two phases. First, we focused on key philosophical debates on reflection, particularly the gap between theory and practice, and the gap between the individual and communal sense. Second, we related our philosophical considerations to current research on reflection, and scrutinized how researchers conceptually used reflection to pinpoint the benefits. Therefore, we drew insights from literature reviews about research on reflection in medical education or medical practice since the 2000s until 2021.

Phase one: philosophical debates on reflection

The theory–practice gap

In the tradition of philosophy, philosophers regularly contrasted reflection with knowledge acquisition, or blindly following rules and calculation. The ancient Greeks already acknowledged that true wisdom required something more than mere "bookish" knowledge.

Aristotle, for instance, described reflection (sometimes also translated as deliberation) as the ability to connect acquired knowledge with professional experience, or theory with practice.[23] It was the key to "practical rationality" ("*phronèsis*"), which he considered as the highest intellectual virtue, and as an absolute necessity of professionalism in fields such as medicine, politics, law, and military strategy.

The fact that theory can be connected with practice (or knowledge with experience) also implies that there must be a gap between them to begin with. It is precisely this gap that has posed a continuous philosophical problem, to which reflection formed a potential solution. To get a sense of that problem, we can refer to Kant, who in many ways is considered the father of modern philosophy. Kant, too, acknowledged that there exists a gap between theory and practice. One may, within a particular professional field (he mentions law and medicine as examples), *know* all the rules and concepts, but may still be unable to properly apply them in practice. He aptly calls this "stupidity."[24]

The ability to properly apply a rule or concept in a given situation is what Kant calls the power of judgment, but with this power of judgment comes a problem. If judgment means *applying a set of rules to practice*, a second set of rules will always be necessary to determine how the first set of rules should be applied. However, that second set of rules would require a third set of rules to determine how they should be applied, and so forth. In this way, we end up in an infinite regression of formulating rules for applying rules, and we would never bridge the gap from theory to practice. To illustrate this point, consider Kant commentator Henry Allison's explanation of playing chess.[25,26] Formally learning the rules of chess is necessary to play, but making a good move requires complex interpretations of the given, concrete situation. The situation cannot be remedied with devising more rules, since there are always exceptions and alternatives in any given situation. One is not relieved of the necessity "of determining for oneself what the particular situation requires."[25(p206)] Therefore, Kant argues that it must be in principle impossible to formulate, teach, or learn the rules for judgment. In *Critique of Pure Reason*, he concludes that judgment is "a particular talent that cannot be taught at all but can only be practiced."[27(p(A133/B72)14)]

Judgment that cannot be taught seems quite unsatisfactory, and so it was too for Kant, which is why he returned to this problem in his later work *Critique of Judgment*. Judgment, he argues, cannot merely consist in the ability to apply a set of rules to practice (a limited understanding which he now calls "determinative judgment"). As Allison writes: "an account of judgment solely in terms of determination is inherently incomplete, requiring as its complement the activity that Kant terms 'reflection.'"[27(p18)] Besides the ability to apply rules, judgment also consists of the ability to acquire, expand, and develop rules and concepts; people *reflect* on them on the basis of, and in dialogue with, practical experience. This he calls "reflective" judgment.

What reflective judgment does is described by Kant in the following way: "To *reflect* (or consider) is to hold given presentations up to, and compare them with, either other presentations or one's cognitive power [itself], in reference to a concept that this [comparison] makes possible."[28(p400,FI,211)] In other words, reflective judgment involves not so much a "ruling over" the matters at hand, categorizing and determining them in abstract fashion (which would be determinative judgment), but rather "harmonizing" one's (conceptual) thought with the object or situation one is dealing with. Reflective judgment, according to Kant, thus forms the very condition of one's experience, since it assumes that the concepts one uses and the rules with which one applies them are principally related to the world.

The gap between an individual and communal sense

In Section 2.1, we explained that reflection for Kant involves bridging the theory–practice gap, and that it is the very condition of experience. In this section, we show that Kant identified another quintessential gap that plays a role in reflection, and it resides between one's individual sense and a communal sense. Arendt argued that the most important aspect that sets Kant's notion of thinking (as "reflective judgment") apart from his predecessors' is not only the practical, but also the social nature of it. Reflective judgment, for Kant, consists in the *public* use of one's reason, and hence the negotiation of one's considerations with others:

> [Kant] believes that the very faculty of thinking depends on its public use; without 'the test of free and open examination,' no thinking and no opinion formation are possible. Reason is not made 'to isolate itself but to get into community with others'. [29(p40)]

The public nature of reflection is clearly distinguished from mere calculation or rule following, for which one would not need the considerations or recognition of others. Kant illustrates this public nature

of judgment by means of *esthetic* judgments, i.e. statements concerning the beauty of certain objects. One's esthetic judgments, Kant argues, are based on what he calls a *sensus communis*, a shared sense. One considers judgments of beauty not as merely subjective feeling, but rather as a sensation that individuals imagine is shared by all. For example, if I enjoy the sight of a beautiful flower or the sound of a Mozart sonata, I cannot help but expect that others will share my feeling, precisely because there is nothing in particular about me that would distinguish my sensation from that of others. Comparing my judgment with those of others, however, does not mean that I *adjust* my taste to that of the majority. I only presume that my sensation of beauty cannot merely be my own; it must be based on some generally shared sense of beauty.

What Kant says about the nature of esthetic judgment is true for judgments in general, according to Arendt. That one takes the perspective of others into account is a fundamental part of what constitutes thought and even what makes us human. It connects the way one experiences the world with a community. Again, this does not mean that I claim that everyone will *actually* agree with my judgments. Rather, in reflection I relate my judgments to a hypothetical community:

> We compare our judgments not so much with actual as rather with the merely possible judgments of others, and [thus] put ourselves in the position of everyone else, merely by abstracting from the limitations that [may] happen to attach to our own judging. [28(p.160)]

To place oneself in the position of everyone else depends on the power of imagination, but that does not mean that the community is entirely fictitious. "By the force of imagination it makes the others present and thus moves in a space that is potentially public, open to all sides."[29(p43)]

Bridging gaps and the madness of reflection

We saw in the previous sections that reflection concerns two quintessential gaps that play a role in human experience: the theory–practice gap, and the gap between the individual and communal sense. This brings the analysis to the point how practitioners can bridge these gaps, and the pressing question becomes whether and how reflection can be taught and learned.

We return once more to Kant's philosophical analysis of reflection, specifically to two ways reflection fundamentally resists systematization. First, as we have seen, Kant argued that the ultimate rule to connect theory with practice cannot be formulated because that would lead to an infinite regression. To recapitulate briefly, there is a difference between formally learning the rules of chess, and making a good move by interpreting the complex situation at hand, which requires reflective judgment. Therefore, Kant suggested to train reflection with examples, not by formally learning rules like a recipe.[26] Reflection cannot be taught but only practiced as that peculiar talent that brings general rules into dialogue with particular circumstances. From this perspective, reflection fundamentally resists systematization.

The second type of resistance to systematization concerns the gap between the individual and communal sense of reflection. As we explained in Section 1.2, individuals relate their personal judgments to those of the (imagined) community. However, this community is not fully stable but contingent; moreover, the individuals who constitute the community are also viable to change. Thus, the community alters with the passing of time and unique constitution of the community. In the case of reflection, the community's relative instability prevents anyone from definitively formulating what the outcome of reflection should be for everyone, at all times, and everywhere.

After Kant, the resistance to systematization has been much debated in philosophy. In some cases, reflection has even been pitted directly against science, understood as calculative rationality. The philosopher Heidegger provocatively stated that "science does not think,"[30(p8)] which was certainly not meant to disqualify science, but rather to emphasize that (philosophical) reflection does not proceed according to a predetermined methodology, logically inferring on the basis of evident premises. The thinker, according to Heidegger, enters a much more uncertain field: "There is no bridge here – only the leap," and that takes us not only to the other side, but to a totally different place.[30(p8)]

Heidegger's criticism of science is exaggerated, and ignores the fact that scientists regularly tread terrain as uncertain as that of the philosopher. Still, Heidegger's point is relevant for our analysis of reflection in the medical field: if one would know beforehand how to proceed, one would not have to "think." There is, in other words, a fundamental difference between reflecting (or thinking) and calculating or rule following. One could therefore say that reflection resists precise formalization, and that reflection even becomes jeopardized when it is translated into uniform learning-outcomes. If reflection becomes a matter of blindly checking the right boxes, such a process

risks replacing *actual* reflection, and with that the professional attitude.

To consider a professional attitude that encompasses reflection, we take into consideration how the philosopher Derrida argues that the practice of law is never a mere application of the law. He therefore makes the distinction between law and justice. For justice to occur, one must always *decide* whether the law is, in this case, applicable. In other words, a process of professional reflection is needed, which involves the interpretation both of the law and of the case at hand. Were that not so, and justice would consist in the mere following of a rule or protocol, it would be a fully calculable process and we could easily outsource it to a computer. There would, in the strict sense, be no moment of decision or judgment at all. This leads to an interesting paradox for medical professionals. Each decision involves a necessary moment of "undecidability," that is an uncertainty whether the decision is right, or just.[31] "The instant of decision is madness," as Derrida quotes from Søren Kierkegaard.[32(p65)] This might seem exaggerated, but Kierkegaard precisely emphasizes the impossibility of reducing reflection to rule-following or certain knowledge.

The philosophical analysis applied to examples

At this stage, it is helpful to illustrate how our philosophical analysis of reflection and the two gaps could relate to two concrete examples from medical practice and medical education.

Our first example comes from 2008, when patient Elaine Bromiley tragically died after competent and expert anesthetists failed to recognize that they could not intubate and ventilate.[33] "[They] persevered with attempts to intubate and ventilate when they should have changed to another strategy."[34(p61)] Evie Fioratou and colleagues assessed this as a fixation error, or an "unhelpful reliance on past experience to the detriment of the current situation."[34(p61)] They argued that there is no easy fix to prevent this error. Generally, developing routine, following protocols and using checklists are important.[7,35] However, Bromiley's case also showed how fixation is a "natural by-product of (...) rules of thumb."[34(p62)]

Bromiley's case illustrates Kant's problem of bridging the theory–practice gap. Just like Kant, medical practitioners and research experts turn to reflective judgment to pinpoint how practitioners must come to grips with applying rules and standards in particular situations. According to experts this encompasses, for instance, training to accept uncertainty and deliberately seeking out alternatives,[36] embedding moments to "stop and think" (and review checklists in light of the case[7]), and exposing practitioners to routine and non-routine cases to increase their awareness about potential fixations.[34,36] Ultimately, however, the gap between theory and practice will remain, and practitioners must learn to deal with jumping over it.

Elaine Bromiley's case also illustrates the value of bridging the gap between an individual and communal sense.[37] Contrary to the anesthetists, the attending nurses did recognize the problem, but were unable to communicate that to the anesthetists, and failed to "override and change the clinicians' mental model."[35(p116)] Understanding the social dimension and allowing feedback from team members is therefore advized.[36,38,39] It checks practitioners' individual sense (and certainty) about their correct application of procedures.

Our second example comes from a study on weekly group reflection sessions in the Dutch GP specialty training.[40,41] Mario Veen and Anne de la Croix studied how participants themselves make experiences "shared" and "reflectable." One case involves registrar Ilone, who told the group how her supervisor criticized "the way she says her name when she answers the phone, which upset her."[40(p329)] Then, Ilone asked her peers: "I wondered if with you they also observe in such detail? (...) Is this part of it or is it something that my GP trainer suddenly focusses on, very fussy details."[40(p328)] What ensued was a discussion of this experience, which involved exploring (loosely) related themes and giving advice.

Like Bromiley's example, Ilone's example also illustrates reflection and both gaps. Compared to the Bromiley example, however, the two gaps materialize differently. First, GP registrars explore (retrospectively) what general principles (*theory*) play a role while being supervised, and second, how those relate to Ilone's experience (*practice*). The case involved how supervisors should supervise; balancing attention to detail with fussing over details; providing feedback; meta-communication and setting boundaries as a registrar.[40] Moreover, Ilone asked peers about their experiences with supervision. This is a form of shared meaning making,[42] and the registrars (re)constructed their individual and communal sense of being supervised.

In sum, with these two examples we illustrate reflection's *flexibility* to yield value for practitioners, if one understands it as a fundamental human capacity to cross the gaps between theory and practice, and the individual and communal sense in a particular situation. Reflection used for clinical reasoning is different from doing weekly (retrospective) group reflection sessions for the sake of professional development. The situatedness of reflection deserves our critical attention; however, each case transcends mere calculation and blind application of rules that would not require input from others. No decisions or judgments need to be made when everything is clear and certain; then, a computer could execute the tasks. Practice is riddled with minor or major moments of uncertainty. Uncertainty occurs when practitioners face the madness when general principles (captured in rules, procedures, models, theory) do not neatly fit the unique reality.

Phase two: how the philosophical considerations relate to research on reflection

In phase two, we related our philosophical considerations to research that discussed reflection's (potential) benefits. We found that literature reviews about research on reflection since the 2000s listed a wide range of benefits. Meanwhile, many reviews also admonished the lack of a unified theoretical understanding and the paucity of empirical evidence.[12-15] We did not assess theoretical consensus nor empirical evidence in these reports, but used our philosophical considerations to scrutinize the conceptual use of reflection and how that allows researchers to pinpoint various benefits.

The theory–practice gap in research on reflection

In the literature reviews, we saw the following conceptual inclination occur. The research field embraced reflection as a fundamental way to bridge the theory–practice gap. This is, however, the very condition for human experience, and the field ended up listing benefits of reflection that are ubiquitous and multi-applicable. This strategy became especially salient when one kept in mind that practitioners must cross the theory–practice gap on a daily basis, on many different occasions, and for many different reasons.

The literature reviews reported that "reflection helps narrow the gap between theory and practice, ultimately enhancing practice."[10(p495)] Additionally, reviews also used different wordings to describe the transition between theory and practice. For instance, reflection helped practitioners relate experiences from practice to theory,[8] linked or integrated theory with practice,[43,44] handled ambiguity,[45] through contextualization,[13] or exposed how theory is embedded in practice.[9] Reviews also demarcated specific domains wherein reflection helped traverse the theory–practice gap, for instance, clinical reasoning.[46] Take note that within the latter domain different conceptions of reflection exist, which led to variation in its beneficial effects.[7]

The focus on the theory–practice gap led reviewers to report that reflection instigated a variety of changes. For example, reflection transformed behavior and adapted knowledge.[46,47] Another review linked reflection to empowerment and implied various transformations, like more consistently

> using research evidence in practice; taking time to link theory with practice; critically evaluating, questioning, dialoguing about, and problem solving clinical situations and practices; enacting changes in their practice and thinking; debating implications of their actions in practice; taking risks to challenge previously held values, beliefs, and assumptions; and integrating new learning with prior knowledge. [44(p643)]

This quote illustrates the conceptual inclination clearly: contemporary research posited reflection as a central means to address a fundamental problem, which in Kantian terms is bridging the theory–practice gap. Consequently, researchers found how reflection became a beneficial driver for many different but fundamental (behavioral, cognitive, identity) changes that help cross that divide, resulting in many (potential) benefits in a wide range of situations.

The gap between the individual and communal sense in research on reflection

In the literature reviews, we encountered the following conceptual inclination that occurred within the domain of the individual and communal sense. Literature reviews connected the benefits of reflection to self-awareness, which led to a wide array of things one can become self-aware of, with diverse beneficial effects for oneself and the community. This strategy co-occurred often with references to professional development or growth.

The reviews generally reported that reflection impacted professional development,[48] by learning more about oneself.[6] Overall, "established models of reflection propose that personal growth occurs over time, as experiences are examined to produce new understanding that informs future practice."[49(p437)] In particular, reflection helped identify personal beliefs,[13,49-53] gain insight into one's professional strengths and weaknesses,[3,6] recognize personal bias,[4,5,54] and attitudes,[5,52] decrease stress and anxiety,[3,6] and prevent burnout.[1,2] Other beneficial effects for practitioners, by doing for instance reflective writing exercises, include:

> an ameliorated attitude towards work; a development path for [their] job potential; an enhancement of

their introspective knowledge; an enrichment of their expressive capability; an improvement of their interpersonal relationships with patients and colleagues and [it] develop[s] their use of critical and reflective thinking. [6(p8)]

Literature reviews not only listed benefits of reflection for the individual practitioner, but also benefits for the community. It "generate[d] a climate of trust which promoted a sense of community,"[9(p1642)] or supported building a community of practice and better interprofessional relations.[55,56] Reflection helped practitioners understand "other perspectives, medical culture, and the importance of diversity."[49(p.432)] Patients were no longer mere objects of care but practitioners also empathized with them,[2,49,52] and understood "the importance of *why* they were caring for patients."[4(p10)] Reflection kindled altruism,[57] while it also helped practitioners "challenge dominant discourses and oppressive power and social structures."[55(p221)]

The conceptual inclination that underlies the various individual and communal benefits pivots around self-awareness. "Self-awareness may lead to [the] perception that environmental manipulation is needed in one situation and knowledge improvement in another."[46(p387)] Or as some researchers concluded: "'Higher quality' papers identify (...) increased self-awareness and engagement in reflection (...) and continuous professional development."[53(p312)] When researchers turned to reflection that instigates self-awareness, it became a linchpin for many benefits.

The issue at hand is that individuals compare their own judgments with those of others, or confronting their individual sense with the communal one. In effect, they (could) gain awareness of their own position on any given subject. As a result, the literature reviews listed a wide variety of things that one could become (self-)aware of, ranging from one's values, biases, to communication and so forth. The list of things that one could become self-aware of seems potentially endless.

Discussion

With our analysis, we aim to show how two gaps play a role in the benefits of reflection, why there might be so many benefits to reflection, and what that implies for medical education. First, reflection helps practitioners cross the theory–practice gap. Second, reflection helps practitioners cross the gap between the individual and communal sense. Yet, crossing these gaps is so fundamental for human understanding that reflection runs the danger of becoming ubiquitous and generic, indiscriminately relied on for many specific benefits in a wide range of situations. Reflection almost starts behaving like a panacea.[16] In our view, the list to precisely define reflection's benefits for crossing these gaps is potentially endless, also when one takes into consideration that reflection resists systematization. Thus, we advise restraint in pursuing and empirically validating potentially endless specific benefits of reflection.[18]

As Stella Ng and colleagues argued, the pursuit to pinpoint all benefits of reflection plays heavily into a reductive understanding of reflection as a means to utilitarian ends.[12,14] Practitioners "may eventually perceive [reflection] as falling short of its goals because it is difficult to 'prove' reflection 'works.'"[17(p468)] We suggest that the moment of undecidability, or even madness, is difficult to swallow in medical education. Those who cannot accept it, attempt to fill the gaps. These critical observations still leave us with the question how reflection can be practiced if we refuse to "fill the gaps." In the next section, we provide three concrete recommendations for reflection in medical education and medical practice.

Three recommendations

Based on our conceptual analysis of reflection in the tradition of philosophy, and how these relate to contemporary research on reflection, we think that reflection occurs in its situated use.[18] We support that there is no "one-size-fits-all" to reflection.[58] Nonetheless, this does not relieve us from critically approaching reflection, and our philosophical considerations led us to certain preferred recommendations for medical education.

First, we recommend giving precedence to communal reflective activities over solitary ones, wherein situated examples can flourish and come to life. We do not deny that written reflections in the form of reflective essays, written assignments, or portfolios have some merit. For instance, they could train introspection, or "getting a second opinion from your own conscious mind."[36(p550)] Nonetheless, based on our philosophical considerations, we prefer reflective activities that include active and immediate representation of the communal sense that contrasts with one's individual sense when practitioners wrestle with the theory–practice gap. Such exchanges curb practitioners from being "stuck"[59] in their individual sense through solitary reflective activities. Group reflection activities provide more interactive means for calibrating the communal sense of the medical profession based on concrete examples.[42,60] Practically, we take (reflective) discussion groups as a positive example, for instance the Exchange of Experience (EoE) rounds in the Dutch GP specialty training.[40–42] Once a week, a small group of GP registrars under supervision of two teachers come together to discuss their clinical experiences in an open, dialogic environment. Group discussions entice immediate exchanges of diverse perspectives between the individual and communal sense (as represented by other individuals) about concrete experiences.[40–42] Such shared meaning making "promotes the formation of professional identities."[42(p876)]

Second, when it comes to using reflection for one's professional identity, we recommend using formal guidelines and models for reflection as sources of *inspiration* to reflect, and not as normative models that dictate how practitioners *should* reflect.[18,61] We ground our recommendation in the Kantian argument that reflection resists systematization and that formally learning rules is something other than reflection.[26,62] Thus, for Kant, reflection is trained by practice and by being confronted with (situated) examples. Concretely, we take the aforementioned Dutch EoE discussion groups as a case in point once more. In EoE, the experiences take center stage. Registrars tell stories about situated examples that allow them to sharpen their judgments during discussions in a safe environment.[60] These discussions are not dictated, but take shape as "structured spontaneity."[40,42] The discussions become messy,[40] but registrars find that having (guided) freedom to discuss experiences is valuable for professional development.[42]

Third, when we take formal guidelines for reflection as inspiration, then we also must reconsider assessing reflection.[63] Assessment of reflection often comes down to checking if certain rules are followed, and although we understand that clear assessment guidelines for reflection intend to counter problems of arbitrariness and bias, such assessment instigates behavior to correctly follow the recipe and pass the assessment.[62,64] Conversely, reflection in the Kantian sense moves beyond following rules, so assessing whether or not reflection sufficiently took place will necessarily involve moments of "madness" (leaping over the theory–practice gap). Guidelines cannot fill the gap and should be used with caution. Moreover, one is not alone in leaping, and therefore must check one's individual sense against the communal sense of fellow professionals. In sum, the theory–practice gap and the individual–communal sense gap remain in place for assessors too, particularly when it comes to reflection.

Conclusion

The benefits of reflection are (potentially) abundant. While literature reviews about research on reflection attempt to list and validate these benefits, we philosophically analyzed why reflection can have so many benefits. Based on the philosophical tradition, we argued that there are two gaps that play an inherent role in reflection. On the one hand, there is the theory–practice gap that practitioners bridge; on the other hand, practitioners bridge an individual sense opposed to a communal sense of their profession in particular situations.

Philosophers like Kant, Arendt, Heidegger, and Derrida show that reflection can help cross these gaps, which one can practice. However, they also warn us that reflection, by its very condition, resists systematization. There is no definitive set of rules or protocols that form the final keystone to bridge both sides of these divides. Then, reflection also ceases to be merely an individual, learnable skill or an empirically validated means to some particular end. Consequently, if reflection cannot be caught in learnable rules, one should show reserve about assessing it. There only remains the jump from one side to the other. Practitioners can practice jumping, particularly when they are within a community of professionals and exchange their experience while they "mind the gap."

Acknowledgements

We wish to thank Mario Veen for the invitation to write this article.

Disclosure statement

The authors declare no competing interests.

Previous philosophy in medical education installments

Mario Veen & Anna T. Cianciolo (2020) Problems No One Looked For: Philosophical Expeditions into Medical Education, Teaching and Learning in Medicine, 32:3, 337–344, DOI: 10.1080/10401334.2020.1748634

Gert J. J. Biesta & Marije van Braak (2020) Beyond the Medical Model: Thinking Differently about Medical Education and Medical Education Research, Teaching and Learning in Medicine, 32:4, 449–456, DOI: 10.1080/10401334.2020.1798240

Mark R. Tonelli & Robyn Bluhm (2021) Teaching Medical Epistemology within an Evidence-Based Medicine Curriculum, Teaching and Learning in Medicine, 33:1, 98–105, DOI: 10.1080/10401334.2020.1835666

John R. Skelton (2021) Language, Philosophy, and Medical Education, Teaching and Learning in Medicine, 33:2, 210–216, DOI: 10.1080/10401334.2021.1877712

Zareen Zaidi, Ian M. Partman, Cynthia R.Whitehead, Ayelet Kuper & Tasha R. Wyatt (2021) Contending with Our Racial Past in Medical Education: A Foucauldian Perspective, Teaching and Learning in Medicine, DOI: 10.1080/10401334.2021.1945929

Chris Rietmeijer & Mario Veen (2021) Phenomenological Research in Health Professions Education: Tunneling from Both Ends, Teaching and Learning in Medicine, DOI: 10.1080/10401334. 2021.1971989

Madeleine Noelle Olding, Freya Rhodes, John Humm, Phoebe Ross & Catherine McGarry (2022) Black, White and Gray: Student Perspectives on Medical Humanities and Medical Education, Teaching and Learning in Medicine, 34:2, 223–233, DOI: 10.1080/10401334.2021.1982717

Camillo Coccia & Mario Veen (2022) Because We Care: A Philosophical Investigation into the Spirit of Medical Education, Teaching and Learning in Medicine, 34:3, 341–349, DOI: 10.1080/10401334.2022.2056744

John Humm (2022) Being-Opposite-Illness: Phenomenological Ontology in Medical Education and Clinical Practice, Teaching and Learning in Medicine, DOI: 10.1080/10401334.2022.2108814

Anna MacLeod, Victoria Luong, Paula Cameron, George Kovacs, Molly Fredeen, Lucy Patrick, Olga Kits & Jonathan Tummons (2022) The Lifecycle of a Clinical Cadaver: A Practice-Based Ethnography, Teaching and Learning in Medicine, DOI: 10.1080/10401334.2022.2092111

Associated podcast

Let Me Ask You Something (iTunes, Spotify, Google Podcasts and https://marioveen.com/letmeaskyou something/)

Funding

The author(s) reported there is no funding associated with the work featured in this article.

ORCID

Sven Peter Charlotte Schaepkens (ID) http://orcid.org/0000-0001-5513-3554

Thijs Lijster (ID) http://orcid.org/0000-0001-7419-4045

References

1. Bernard AW, Gorgas D, Greenberger S, Jacques A, Khandelwal S. The use of reflection in emergency medicine education. *Acad Emerg Med.* 2012;19(8):978–982. doi:10.1111/j.1553-2712.2012.01407.x
2. Chen I, Forbes C. Reflective writing and its impact on empathy in medical education: systematic review. *J Educ Eval Health Prof.* 2014;11:20. doi:10.3352/jeehp.2014.11.20
3. Contreras JA, Edwards-Maddox S, Hall A, Lee MA. Effects of reflective practice on baccalaureate nursing students' stress, anxiety and competency: An integrative review. *Worldviews Evid Based Nurs.* 2020;17(3):239–245. doi:10.1111/wvn.12438
4. Mitchell KM, Roberts T, Blanchard L. Reflective writing pedagogies in action: a qualitative systematic review.

Review. *International Journal of Nursing Education Scholarship.* 2021;18(1):20210057. doi:10.1515/ijnes-2021-0057

5. Miraglia RA, Asselin ME. Reflection as an educational strategy in nursing professional development. *J Nurses Prof Dev.* 2015;31(2):62–72. doi:10.1097/NND.0000000000000151

6. Artioli G, Deiana L, De Vincenzo F, et al. Health professionals and students' experiences of reflective writing in learning: A qualitative meta-synthesis. *BMC Med Educ.* 2021;21(1):1–14. doi:10.1186/s12909-021-02831-4

7. Mamede S, Schmidt HG. Reflection in medical diagnosis: A literature review. *Health Professions Education.* 2017;3(1):15–25. http://repub.eur.nl/pub/115677 doi:10.1016/j.hpe.2017.01.003

8. Barbagallo MS. Completing reflective practice post undergraduate nursing clinical placements: A literature review. *Teaching and Learning in Nursing.* 2019;14(3):160–165. doi:10.1016/j.teln.2019.02.001

9. Choperena A, Oroviogoicoechea C, Zaragoza Salcedo A, Olza Moreno I, Jones D. Nursing narratives and reflective practice: A theoretical review. *J Adv Nurs.* 2019;75(8):1637–1647. doi:10.1111/jan.13955

10. Ruth-Sahd LA. Reflective practice: a critical analysis of data-based studies and implications for nursing education. *J Nurs Educ.* 2003;42(11):488–497. doi:10.3928/0148-4834-20031101-07

11. Steven A, Wilson G, Turunen H, et al. Critical incident techniques and reflection in nursing and health professions education: Systematic narrative review. *Nurse Educ.* 2020;45(6):E57–E61. doi:10.1097/NNE.0000000000000796

12. Roessger KM. The effect of reflective activities on instrumental learning in adult work-related education: A critical review of the empirical research. *Educational Research Review.* 2014;13:17–34. doi:10.1016/j.edurev.2014.06.002

13. Chaffey L, de Leeuw EJ, Finnigan G. Facilitating students' reflective practice in a medical course: Literature review. *Educ Health (Abingdon).* 2012;25(3):198–203. doi:10.4103/1357-6283.109787

14. Uygur J, Stuart E, De Paor M, et al. A best evidence in medical education systematic review to determine the most effective teaching methods that develop reflection in medical students: BEME Guide No. 51. *Med Teach.* 2019;41(1):3–16. doi:10.1080/0142159x.2018.1505037

15. Mann K, Gordon J, MacLeod A. Reflection and reflective practice in health professions education: a systematic review. *Adv Health Sci Educ Theory Pract.* 2009;14(4):595–621. doi:10.1007/s10459-007-9090-2

16. Hodges BD. Sea monsters & whirlpools: Navigating between examination and reflection in medical education. *Med Teach.* 2015;37(3):261–266. doi:10.3109/0142159x.2014.993601

17. Ng SL, Kinsella EA, Friesen F, Hodges B. Reclaiming a theoretical orientation to reflection in medical education research: a critical narrative review. *Med Educ.* 2015;49(5):461–475. doi:10.1111/medu.12680

18. Schaepkens SPC, Veen M, de la Croix A. Is reflection like soap? A critical narrative umbrella review of approaches to reflection in medical education research.

Adv in Health Sci Educ. 2022;27(2):537–551. doi:10.1007/s10459-021-10082-7

19. Ruitenberg C. Introduction: The question of method in philosophy of education. *Journal of Philosophy of Education.* 2009;43(3):315–323. doi:10.1111/j.1467-9752.2009.00712.x

20. Veen M, Cianciolo AT. Problems no one looked for: Philosophical expeditions into medical education. *Teach Learn Med.* 2020;32(3):337–344. doi:10.1080/10401334.2020.1748634

21. Holma K. The strict analysis and the open discussion. *Journal of Philosophy of Education.* 2009;43(3):325–338. doi:10.1111/j.1467-9752.2009.00696.x

22. Davis A. Examples as method? My attempts to understand assessment and fairness (in the Spirit of the Later Wittgenstein). *Journal of Philosophy of Education.* 2009;43(3):371–389. doi:10.1111/j.1467-9752.2009.00699.x

23. Aristotle. *Nichomachean Ethics.* Ross D, Trans. New York, NY: Oxford University Press; 2009.

24. Kant I. *Critique of Pure Reason.* Pluhar W, trans. Indianapolis, IN: Hacket Publishing Company; 1996.

25. Allison HE. *Kant's Transcendental Idealism: an Interpretation and Defense.* New Haven, CT: Yale University Press; 1983.

26. Procee H. Reflection in education: A Kantian epistemology. *Educational Theory.* 2006;56(3):237–253. doi:10.1111/j.1741-5446.2006.00225.x

27. Allison HE. *Kant's Theory of Taste: A Reading of the "Critique of Aesthetic Judgment".* Cambridge, MA: Cambridge University Press; 2001.

28. Kant I. *Critique of Judgment.* Pluhar W, trans. Indianapolis, IN: Hacket Publishing Company; 1987.

29. Arendt H. *Lectures on Kant's Political Philosophy.* Chicago, IL: University of Chicago Press; 1992.

30. Heidegger M. *What is Called Thinking?.* Gray G, trans. New York, NY: Harper and Row Publishers; 1968.

31. Derrida J. Force of law. The mystical foundation of authority. *Cardozo Law Review.* 1990;11:920–1045.

32. Derrida J. *The Gift of Death.* Wills D, trans. Chicago, IL: University of Chicago Press; 1995.

33. Bromiley M. Have you ever made a mistake? *Royal College of Anaesthetists Bulletin.* 2008;48:2442–2445.

34. Fioratou E, Flin R, Glavin R. No simple fix for fixation errors: cognitive processes and their clinical applications. *Anaesthesia.* 2010;65(1):61–69. doi:10.1111/j.1365-2044.2009.05994.x

35. McClelland G, Smith MB. Just a routine operation: a critical discussion. *J Perioper Pract.* 2016;26(5):114–117. doi:10.1177/175045891602600504

36. Graber ML, Kissam S, Payne VL, et al. Cognitive interventions to reduce diagnostic error: a narrative review. *BMJ Qual Saf.* 2012;21(7):535–557. doi:10.1136/bmjqs-2011-000149

37. Jarzabkowski P, Kaplan S, Seidl D, Whittington R. On the risk of studying practices in isolation linking what, who, and how in strategy research. *Strategic Organization.* 2016;14(3):248–259. doi:10.1177/1476127015604125

38. McIntosh E. The implications of diffusion of responsibility on patient safety during anaesthesia, 'So that others may learn and even more may live' – Martin Bromiley. *J Perioper Pract.* 2019;29(10):341–345. doi:10.1177/1750458918816572

39. Fioratou E, Flin R, Glavin R, Patey R. Beyond monitoring: distributed situation awareness in anaesthesia. *Br J Anaesth.* 2010;105(1):83–90. doi:10.1093/bja/aeq137

40. Veen M, de la Croix A. The swamplands of reflection: using conversation analysis to reveal the architecture of group reflection sessions. *Med Educ.* 2017;51(3):324–336. doi:10.1111/medu.13154

41. van Braak M, Veen M, Muris J, van den Berg P, Giroldi E. A professional knowledge base for collaborative reflection education: a qualitative description of teacher goals and strategies. *Perspect Med Educ.* 2022;11(1):53–59. doi:10.1007/s40037-021-00677-6

42. van Braak M, Giroldi E, Huiskes M, Diemers AD, Veen M, van den Berg P. A participant perspective on collaborative reflection: video-stimulated interviews show what residents value and why. *Adv Health Sci Educ Theory Pract.* 2021;26(3):865–879. doi:10.1007/s10459-020-10026-7

43. Buckley S, Coleman J, Davison I, et al. The educational effects of portfolios on undergraduate student learning: a best evidence medical education (BEME) systematic review. BEME Guide No. 11. *Med Teach.* 2009;31(4):282–298. doi:10.1080/01421590902889897

44. Lethbridge K, Andrusyszyn MA, Iwasiw C, Laschinger HK, Fernando R. Structural and psychological empowerment and reflective thinking: is there a link? *J Nurs Educ.* 2011;50(11):636–645. doi:10.3928/01484834-20110817-02

45. Marshall T. The concept of reflection: a systematic review and thematic synthesis across professional contexts. *Reflective Practice.* 2019;20(3):396–415. doi:10.1080/14623943.2019.1622520

46. Kuiper RA, Pesut DJ. Promoting cognitive and metacognitive reflective reasoning skills in nursing practice: self-regulated learning theory. *J Adv Nurs.* 2004;45(4):381–391. doi:10.1046/j.1365-2648.2003.02921.x

47. Kurt M. Quality in reflective thinking: elicitation and classification of reflective acts. *Qual Quant.* 2018;52(S1):247–259. doi:10.1007/s11135-017-0609-1

48. Bjerkvik LK, Hilli Y. Reflective writing in undergraduate clinical nursing education: a literature review. *Nurse Educ Pract.* 2019;35:32–41. doi:10.1016/j.nepr.2018.11.013

49. Winkel AF, Yingling S, Jones A-A, Nicholson J. Reflection as a learning tool in graduate medical education: a systematic review. *J Grad Med Educ.* 2017;9(4):430–439. doi:10.4300/jgme-d-16-00500.1

50. Ziebart C, MacDermid JC. Reflective practice in physical therapy: a scoping review. *Phys Ther.* 2019;99(8):1056–1068. doi:10.1093/ptj/pzz049

51. Williams B. Developing critical reflection for professional practice through problem-based learning. *J Adv Nurs.* 2001;34(1):27–34. doi:10.1046/j.1365-2648.2001.3411737.x

52. Fragkos KC. Reflective practice in healthcare education: an umbrella review. *Education Sciences.* 2016;6(4):27–16. doi:10.1080/10401334.2017.1392864

53. Jayatilleke N, Mackie A. Reflection as part of continuous professional development for public health professionals: a literature review. *J Public Health (Oxf).* 2013;35(2):308–312. doi:10.1093/pubmed/fds083

54. McGillivray J, Gurtman C, Boganin C, Sheen J. Self-practice and self-reflection in training of psychological interventions and therapist skills development: a qualitative meta-synthesis review. *Australian Psychologist.* 2015;50(6):434–444. doi:10.1111/ap.12158

55. Tretheway R, Taylor J, O'Hara L, Percival N. A missing ethical competency? A review of critical reflection in health promotion. *Health Promot J Austr.* 2015;26(3):216–221. doi:10.1071/he15047

56. Richard A, Gagnon M, Careau E. Using reflective practice in interprofessional education and practice: a realist review of its characteristics and effectiveness. *J Interprof Care.* 2019;33(5):424–436. doi:10.1080/13561820.2018.1551867

57. Prasko J, Mozny P, Novotny M, Slepecky M, Vyskocilova J. Self-reflection in cognitive behavioural therapy and supervision. *Biomed Pap Med Fac Univ Palacky Olomouc Czech Repub.* 2012;156(4):377–384. doi:10.5507/bp.2012.027

58. Platt L. The 'wicked problem' of reflective practice: a critical literature review. *Innovations in Practice.* 2014;9(1):44–53. doi:10.24377/LJMU.iip.vol9iss1article108

59. Lengelle R, Luken T, Meijers F. Is self-reflection dangerous? Preventing rumination in career learning. *Australian Journal of Career Development.* 2016;25(3):99–109. doi:10.1177/1038416216670675

60. Runia E. Constructing a congruent curriculum for the vocational training of GPs. In: Scherpbier AJJA, van der Vleuten MCP, Rethans JJ, van der Steeg AFW, eds. *Advances in Medical Education.* Dordrecht, Netherlands: Springer; 1997: 292–294.

61. Schaepkens SPC, Coccia CQH. In pursuit of time: an inquiry into Kairos and reflection in medical practice and health professions education. In: Brown MEL, Veen M, Finn GM, eds. *Applied Philosophy for Health Professions Education: A Journey Towards Mutual Understanding.* Singapore: Springer Nature; 2022: 311–324.

62. de la Croix A, Veen M. The reflective zombie: problematizing the conceptual framework of reflection in medical education. *Perspect Med Educ.* 2018;7(6):394–400. doi:10.1007/s40037-018-0479-9

63. Veen M, Skelton J, de la Croix A. Knowledge, skills and beetles: respecting the privacy of private experiences in medical education. *Perspect Med Educ.* 2020;9(2):111–116. doi:10.1007/s40037-020-00565-5

64. Birden HH, Usherwood T. "They liked it if you said you cried": how medical students perceive the teaching of professionalism. *Med J Aust.* 2013;199(6):406–409. doi:10.5694/mja12.11827

Conclusions: Envisioning a Philosophy of Medical Education

Anna T. Cianciolo and Mario Veen

Introduction: On This Expedition, What Did We See?

Watching butterflies challenges the mind as well as the senses. When a butterfly alights on a flower, she pauses there just long enough, opening and closing her wings, for the eye to catch but a glimpse of her colors – brilliant blues, royal yellows, passionate oranges, and many others – framed in swirling, black lines. Step closer to examine her more closely, and she is off again, dancing in the air, seemingly in every direction at once. The eye strains to follow – always a step behind – because her path is indirect, unpredictable; one cannot know where she will land or even fly next. Natural historians solved this problem with nets and pins, capturing her lifeless body in glass boxes, retaining the butterfly's likeness, but losing her nature in the attempt to advance human knowledge. But to seek the butterfly's essence, to understand her, one must find a meadow or wetland, retreat with a pair of binoculars, and observe her in action.[1] The butterfly's habitat is shrinking, however, making opportunities to observe and understand her challenging and precious.

Recognizing that the habitat for educators' mindful engagement with medical teaching and learning also is shrinking, subject to increasing time pressures and immediate practical concerns, we started this volume to create opportunities to retreat and observe medical education, framing them as a series of philosophical expeditions. Now we have returned home (at least for now), and it is time to document our experiences and insights and determine what comes next. Cataloging the nature of medical education turns out to be as challenging as watching butterflies. By design, each expedition represented a brief pause to explore philosophically the rushing, interconnected flows of medical education (illness-health, learner-practitioner, classroom-clinic, individual-society, time-space) whereby the beauty of more deeply understanding medical education phenomena tantalized us to approach, only to quickly dart away, raising more questions than it answered. Engaging in the "unnatural and vulgar experience"[2] of forcing stillness upon our object would risk losing the essence of medical

teaching and learning, yet, taken together, what can all this color, this motion mean?

Let us first revisit what is at stake here: helping a field see itself and envisioning a philosophy in medical education. As individual articles in *Teaching and Learning in Medicine*'s Philosophy of Medical Education series, some of the chapters in this volume built on earlier chapters. However, on the whole, they comprise a series of different expeditions undertaken by different people – philosophers, medical educators, and combinations of both. By examining each of these individually, can we hope to identify common themes with respect to philosophy and medical education? What kind of relationship does each chapter promote between philosophy and medical education, and what is its value? Finally, does this collection show us the contours of what a philosophy *of* medical education could look like? There exists a philosophy *of* education (Chapter 2), a philosophy *of* science (Chapter 3), and a philosophy *of* language (Chapter 4), for instance. But while we speak about philosophy *and* medical education, *for* medical education, or *in* medical education, there does not yet exist a philosophy *of* medical education – at least, not in the sense that we have approached philosophy in this series.

In this concluding chapter, we first explore the 'philosophy *of*. What does it mean to have a philosophy *of* something? We then reflect on our experiences so far with considering the role of philosophy for medical education and whether there *should* be a philosophy of medical education. Here we explore the promise of introducing philosophy and the other humanities into medical education research journals. We then summarize how each of the chapters constructs the relationship between philosophy and medical education, and the value of the former for the latter. Hopefully, we will then be able to say something about the contours of a philosophy of medical education, as an open invitation for future explorers of medical teaching and learning. We conclude with reflections on reviewing and publishing philosophical journal articles for an audience of medical educators, exploring who can do philosophy of medical education, and we look toward the future of this community endeavor.

Philosophy of Medical Education: Helping a Field See Itself

A 'philosophy *of* a given field involves creating and maintaining a certain type of relationship to that field, one of posing 'big questions' (Chapter 7), which will evolve as society changes and new insights emerge; philosophy of medical education would reflect that relationship, offering a space for exploring fundamental questions about the field. Toward this end, our introductory chapter (Chapter 1) highlighted the value of identifying "problems no one looked for" in medical education as a way of seeing things anew and catalyzing innovative problem-solving approaches. We proposed philosophy as "the fundamental approach to pausing at times of complexity and uncertainty to ask basic questions about seemingly obvious practices so that we can see (and do) things in new ways"(Chapter 1, p. 338). Philosophy examines the basic concepts on which our everyday (and not so everyday) practices are based. For instance, teaching and learning (Chapter 2) or speaking and listening (Chapter 4) on the one hand, and using cadavers for education on the other (Chapter 11). It involves acknowledging and embracing the ambiguity of real life, resisting the urge to reduce it to a theory or idealized model, and instead try to look at an issue with a beginner's mind and leading it "back to its most fundamental description, prompting assumptions to reveal themselves" (Chapter 1, p. 340). This lays the foundation for what we called in Chapter 1 *disrupting frames of reference*. By introducing a new frame of reference or lens through which to view the world, or by expanding that lens to include multiple other lenses, or by explicitly describing the lenses *as* lenses, philosophy can help a field, including medical education, see itself. This unsettling relationship between questioning and understanding differs from that of scientific research or theory.

The difference between philosophy and good scientific practice is that science uses established methods to examine the correspondence or incongruity between theories or hypotheses on the one hand, and reality on the other, whereas philosophy examines the relationship between the three elements of (1) reality (or experience); (2) the interpretative frameworks that we use to make sense of reality; and (3) the way we relate these interpretative frameworks and reality to each other. In addition, good philosophy is self-reflective, realizing that all philosophical efforts are historically, culturally and positionally embedded. An example from this volume is Chapter 4, where language is examined by disrupting the frame of reference of "communication skills" using the more expansive perspective of philosophy of language. Even though we can examine how "*the limits of my language* mean the limits of my world",[3, p. 7] (emphasis in original) we can only do so by using language.

In Chapter 1, we emphasized that the purpose of philosophy in medical education is not to create "a philosophy" in the sense of a vision or theoretical approach, but rather constantly "shifting frames and turning into objects of analysis the lenses through which we see the world" (Chapter 1, p. 341). Importantly, in the context of medical education this involves recognizing when to connect back to practice and what to offer the field with regard to the question. Sometimes, the chapters in this volume offered specific advice for educational practice, for instance, how to integrate a critical evidence-based approach throughout the curriculum (Chapter 3). But just as often, the advice was about asking certain questions, examining an underexposed issue for oneself, or adopting a different attitude to an issue. We see this as a sign of respect for medical educators, as well as for the context-dependency of educational interventions. For example, Chapter 8 calls attention to care as a concept that medical education approaches from scientific or ethical perspectives (e.g., 'What works to provide patient-centered care?' or 'What should patient-centered care look like?') but which calls for philosophical examination as a concept in itself. The foundational structure of care described in this chapter is 'applicable' in the sense that it can be used to start discussions about care in the classroom, or to unify different modes of care (e.g., technology, health protocols and empathy) in research. Most of all, it serves to instigate dialogue on care, where it is less important that one agrees with the vision laid out in the chapter, and more important that the concept is discussed at this foundational level.

With these thoughts in mind, from teams of philosophers and medical education stakeholders (including students), we solicited analyses that interrogate barriers to the field's progress – and the authors delivered. The analyses probe a variety of constructs that serve as the foundation of medical curriculum and assessment – education, knowledge, language, experience, norms, curriculum, assessment technology, caring, illness, cadaver, medical technology, and reflection – demonstrating that philosophy is relevant to medical education in numerous ways: not just philosophy of education, philosophy of medicine or philosophy of technology, but rather all of these and more. So, a philosophy of medical education would be an *interdisciplinary philosophy*, because medical education is an interdisciplinary field. That medical education is an interdisciplinary field suggests another role for philosophy, as a mediator between different frames, lenses, paradigms, and perspectives. The main way in which this is done is through interrogating, developing, and creating the concepts we use in our field. There is an art and science to doing this, which could be (taught as) part of philosophy of medical education.

By the series authors' own description, our expedition has been taken on in the spirit of promoting human agency over historical, economic, social, and other forces that prioritize certain ways of thinking and being. At a time when medical education is just beginning to come to terms with structural barriers to progress, a philosophy of medical education is needed to identify how educators must change to move the field forward and where the limits of their agency lie. Producing these expeditions as a series of journal articles has made us think about how medical education journals themselves must change to support this progress. Currently, medical education journals are distinct from journals of medical humanities, as if the science and art, the purpose and context, and the technicality and morality of developing physicians are separable. For this series to amount to more than "weak inclusion" (Chapter 7, p. 224) of philosophy or the other humanities in medical education scholarship, we realized that *Teaching and Learning in Medicine*'s publication priorities must adapt to incorporate the humanities, alongside science, into the core of what we publish. This adaptation goes beyond medical educators applying concepts from the humanities, which may mask reinforcement of the conventional assumptions that currently impede progress, to featuring the work of humanities itself.

Envisioning a Philosophy of Medical Education: Reports from Each Expedition

What insights about the essence of medical teaching and learning can we bring back from each expedition? In the pauses we offered to observe medical education in action, what problems did the chapter authors bring to our attention, and how do they prompt us to see medical education anew? Biesta and Van Braak (Chapter 2) launched our expeditions by rejecting the very frame through which we view medical education. Specifically, they rejected the "medical model": the idea of "teaching as an intervention to bring about [i.e., cause] learning in students" (Chapter 2, p. 449). This seems indeed a "problem no one looked for" – for what is more central to the enterprise of medical education than the assumption that the educator's task is to make students learn? Indeed, Biesta and Van Braak's critique is not that learning is irrelevant to medical education, but that

> "the language of learning is not sufficiently precise. After all, students can learn many things when they are in educational settings, just as they can learn many things outside of those settings. The whole point of education,

however, is not to ensure that students learn, but that they learn *something*, learn it *for a reason*, and learn it *from someone*." (Chapter 2, p. 450)

Biesta and Van Braak demonstrate how a branch of philosophy – philosophy of education – can expose the way a fundamental concept in medical education is too limited and imprecise, and they propose a new language that empowers educators to describe what exactly it is we ARE doing, if not causing learning. Instead of 'learning', Biesta and Van Braak posit three purposes of medical education, which they termed collectively as "professional formation": qualification, socialization, and subjectification. Subjectification "denotes the existential dimension of education,"[4, p. 40] developing learners' capacity to act as an agent in their professional life by questioning and evolving.

Every chapter in the series aimed to promote subjectification, an aspect of professional formation that arguably is subverted by medical education's own culture and practices, which prioritize standardization and conformity.[5-7] Tonelli and Bluhm (Chapter 3) argue that it is not enough for students to acquire the knowledge of medical research findings (professional qualification), nor to emulate the 'best clinical practices' informed by nuanced understanding of Evidence-Based Medicine (EBM), which incorporates scientific evidence, clinical experience, and patient preferences into care plans (professional socialization). Rather, students must learn to negotiate between variable, incomplete, and often conflicting sources and kinds of knowledge, which may be seen as an aspect of professional subjectification. Specifically, they argue that students must be able to critically relate to EBM's basic assumptions, which

> "makes strong claims about the *kind of evidence* required and the process of clinical decision making. Examining these claims is important for medical educators and medical students, not just to ensure that clinical practice is based on sound knowledge, but to clarify what EBM does well and what challenges it still faces."(Chapter 3, p. 99, emphasis added)

They introduce a distinction that allows us to think more precisely about what professional subjectification could look like in the context of medical decision-making: students must transform from "evidence users" to "evidence-based practitioners". This latter term indicates that the work of the doctor is not just to *apply* scientific evidence to practice, but that they are *subjects* that bear the freedom and responsibility to assess situations in which there is no rule or guideline that tells them what to do. To achieve this transformation, Tonelli and Bluhm introduce two other ways in which philosophy can relate to medical education.

The first comprises concrete curricular guidelines based on a philosophical argument: instead of first teaching students 'the basics' they need to become qualified (i.e., be able to use scientific evidence in treating patients) and socialized (i.e., become accustomed to the practices and knowledge related to evidence-based practice), Tonelli and Bluhm suggest teaching a critical relationship to evidence throughout medical school, for example, by "having trainees reason out loud, performing an epistemic analysis regarding the knowledge they are utilizing in support of their choices, allow[ing] for a discussion about the relative weight given to different kinds of knowledge in specific cases" (Chapter 3, p. 103).

Second, to do this, Tonelli and Bluhm suggest teaching students the basics of epistemology to allow critical assessment of different kinds of evidence in different contexts:

> "To provide this philosophical foundation, medical educators, with the aid of philosophers of medicine, can incorporate the teaching of language, principles and understanding of medical epistemology into parts of the medical curriculum where they fit naturally. In particular, the curriculum focused on evidence-based medicine represents an ideal opportunity to explore the philosophical questions related to medical knowledge, as EBM represents a school of medical epistemology." (Chapter 3, p. 104)

In other words, philosophy is not an *alternative* to theory or practice, but rather philosophy begins by pointing out that theory and practice in medical education are 'schools' of philosophy. This introduces the possibility to explore alternative ways of doing medical epistemology, and allows students to consciously choose their own path – even if this path is not EBM.

After the first two expeditions demonstrated a need for more precise language, Skelton (Chapter 4) explored how insights from philosophy of language can contribute to medical education. Philosophy of language exemplifies one of philosophy's key characteristics: it addresses the unique challenges that come with the aspects of our life that are so familiar to us we hardly see them and are the hardest to look at with a beginner's mind. Language is like water to fish and air to birds in that it permeates all levels of medical education:

> "Language as a means of exploration, of probing and discussing ideas, of looking at things (perhaps a doctor-patient consultation) and talking about them in a

manner which helps them build and reflect on ideas is a key aspect of education." (Chapter 4, p. 214)

From this perspective, it is easy to see how a more sophisticated philosophy of language – a more precise language to speak about language – would contribute to the quality of medical education. In the context of language, professional subjectification includes judicious use of language, recognizing its purpose and activity. Toward this end, Skelton disrupts the frame of "communication skills" as the model of understanding how language works.

The four ideas Skelton introduces are easy to grasp but take practice and persistence to recognize in all aspects of medical education, including medical education research. First, language is performative: it is *doing things with words* rather than just communicating messages from sender to receiver. Second, meaning is defined by the way words are used in context. Third, beyond 'the data' or 'the evidence', "language offers us a way of thinking about and discussing life as we know it, in all its complexity" (Chapter 4, p. 213). Finally, language and power are intrinsically connected. For instance: "Presumptions about hierarchical position might flow from something as simple as a prestigious accent, or the ability to speak an international language in addition to a local language" (Chapter 4, p. 214). In medicine, this connection may be seen in the power of diagnosis to give language to symptoms and in the distinction between practicing shared–decision-making[8] vs. "mov[ing] the clinic along briskly by getting consent without discussion" (Chapter 4, p. 211).

Power is the central focus of Zaidi et al.'s expedition in Chapter 5. So far, we have discussed medical education, knowledge, and communication as philosophical issues, implying that they are equally accessible to all. By adopting a Foucauldian perspective on systemic racism in medical education, Zaidi et al. introduce the philosophical insight that 'neutral' and 'normal' do not exist but are constructs that hide power relations. Indeed, we can blame much of Western philosophy for the false idea that it is possible to think about and discuss ideas from a neutral, purely rational perspective, abstracted from messy, mundane reality. But education is not equally accessible to all; not everyone can make claims to the same knowledge, and the language one speaks, as Skelton pointed out, engenders presumptions about hierarchical position.

Although we pointed out that the "basic concepts we use in medical education can be traced to philosophy" (Chapter 1, p. 338), one of the reasons why a more critical inclusion of philosophy in medical education is urgent is that many of the classic philosophers 'traditionally' referred to in medical education (e.g., Hume,

Kant,[9] Aristotle[10]) precede the critical turn in philosophy of which Foucault is a part. This includes historical orientations of the philosophers themselves: Hegel claimed that the movement of history skipped over the African continent[11]; Heidegger was a member of the Nazi party;[12] and Flexner contributing to closing all but two black medical schools.[13] But a more critical inclusion also encompasses whose voices were – and to a large extent, still are – excluded from the academic tradition of philosophy: women, LGBTQ+ and people of color.[14] Implicit in Zaidi et al.'s chapter is the deeper idea that if our concepts can be traced back to philosophy, this includes problematic concepts such as the term "underrepresented minorities," it matters which philosophers we include in medical education. Besides Aristotle, Kant, and Hume, we need more Adorno, De Beauvoir, and Foucault.[15] Though the philosophical approaches of these latter three differ tremendously, they share the insight that anything we do, including philosophy and medical education, is historically, culturally, and positionally embedded, and that the fabric of everyday life is permeated with power relations that make it easier (more 'normal') for some voices to be heard than others.

What Zaidi et al. contribute to the relationship between philosophy and medical education is the idea that philosophy can be activist. As the execution of Socrates showed, interrogating established norms and practices is a political and risky activity. Zaidi et al. suggest that:

> "...what is needed is for the profession to interrogate the norms used by institutions. [...] It is the norming practice that must be addressed, so that minoritized physicians can be the kind of physician that upholds their own values, beliefs, and racial norms. [The profession] needs to focus on the recruitment of racially diverse faculty [and to] decolonize medical education and focus on practical wisdom (phronesis) which, when embodied in the physician, links the knowledge and skills of the biomedical and clinical sciences with a moral orientation and call." (Chapter 5, pp. 457, 458, 459)

By addressing racism and other social justice issues in medical education, philosophy can help us take responsibility for and 'own' all aspects of our profession, including its problematic ones. As Biesta and Van Braak note (Chapter 2), education is an open system that is entangled with society, and thereby has to contend with the same problems that society does.

The idea that education is a closed system fits the tradition of regarding science as an objective way to view reality, language as simply a tool to describe that reality, and the very idea that there is an objective reality 'out there' and that it dictates what is considered normal, neutral, factual, and so on. These ideas are foundational for much of medical education research, which is largely based on philosophy of science traditions such as positivism and empiricism. As discussed in Lara Varpio and Anna Macleod's *Philosophy of Science* series, all of our research approaches are based on philosophical ideas about what is considered real (ontology), what constitutes knowledge (epistemology) and what is considered desirable or 'good' practice (axiology).[16] In Chapter 6, Rietmeijer and Veen discuss phenomenology as a philosophical approach that can inform not just 'phenomenological research', but all of medical education research.

In a way, phenomenology is a straightforward approach to research: one can only investigate what one has access to; one should bracket all their assumptions about the mechanisms underlying the phenomenon being examined and instead focus on the phenomenon as something that is worthy of description in its own right and on its own terms. But unlike some of the approaches to research discussed in other expeditions (Chapter 2 and Chapter 3), phenomenology acknowledges that for anything to be an object of research in the first place, it has to occur to *someone* and point to *something*. Said another way, anything we could potentially investigate in medical education only occurs to us in the first place because we have judged it meaningful.

Though all research approaches have philosophical roots, phenomenology is perhaps distinct in that it requires the investigator to keep its philosophical principles in sight throughout all stages of the research, rather than studying them once and then focusing instead on carrying out the research methods. Rietmeijer and Veen argue that this is what makes it possible that 'phenomenological' methods (such as Interpretative Phenomenological Analysis) can be carried out from a non-phenomenological approach, just as methods that are not explicitly labeled 'phenomenological' (such as discourse analysis or ethnography) can be carried out 'phenomenologically' (Chapter 6, p. 118). The rigor of phenomenology is not in denying subjectivity (i.e., bias) in favor of an ideal of objectivity, but rather in embracing one's own unique access to the phenomena as the basis on which we can describe phenomena in medical education meaningfully.

Chapter 6 presents phenomenology as an ongoing search, and the 'tunneling from both ends' metaphor it uses pertains to one researcher coming from medicine and the other from the opposite side of the mountain, the humanities. In Chapter 7, Olding et al. take the humanities as a starting point for medical education, as "much of the early part of the [humanities] course requires an un-learning of the notion that clinical medicine is derived from pure science, devoid of the gray areas medical humanities seeks to understand" (Chapter 7, p. 226). This chapter's authors (all medical students) argued that all medical students should study the arts and humanities, including history, literature, philosophy and ethics, and anthropology, to address these gray areas, deepen understanding and improve care. For instance, Foucault's insights about objectification (Chapter 5), can be used to critically question how medical instruments such as the stethoscope engenders a medical gaze that views patients primarily as objects rather than people with a personal story. As illustrated by Tonelli and Bluhm's recommendations for teaching epistemology throughout medical school (Chapter 3), Olding et al. argue against "weak inclusion" of humanities in medical curricula, for example, as one-off seminars or workshops. They also criticize the absence of the student perspective in discussion about whether medical humanities should be optional or reside at the core of medical curricula.

Regarding the role of philosophy and the humanities for medical education, Olding et al. dispel a common misconception about philosophy, namely, that because it addresses abstract topics and asks fundamental questions, it does not have much to do with (or to offer to) the daily practice of medicine and medical education. Instead, they offer concrete reasons for considering the political, historical, economic, and anthropological contexts that affect medicine:

> "Asking some of these big questions may seem like the opposite of keeping medicine "grounded to reality"; [...] however, this approach provides a wide-angle lens with which to view society and allows us to assess the bigger implications of medical decisions. Medicine is affected by economics, politics, culture, media, and public opinion and in turn it has effects on these sects of society. Yet, as medical students, we can become more and more detached from the outside world as we continue our studies." (Chapter 7, p. 229)

In Chapter 8, Coccia and Veen ask such a big question, perhaps the biggest for medical education. It is also a phenomenological question (Chapter 6): *What is care?* Care can be seen from an instrumental point of view: for instance, using a stethoscope to diagnose symptoms. But caring can also mean empathy, or refer to the whole health care infrastructure. Chapter 8 exemplifies how philosophical questions of the form 'what is X?' can transform them from a container concept into a precise description broad enough to encompass all of its related phenomena. It also anchors care as an essential component of what it means to be human, of which medicine

(taking care of others), medical education (teaching to take care of others), and medical education research (determining the most helpful way to teach care) are extensions. To be professional, in other words, means to take something which all humans can do, and focus on it explicitly.

Philosophy may be an uncomfortable and seemingly unnecessary endeavor because it identifies "problems no one looked for" (Chapter 1). Philosophy gets us into trouble; the moment we acknowledge a problem, we become responsible for it. The problem *assigns* us to engage in an extreme form of bracketing (Chapter 6) or slowing down (Chapter 1), as is illustrated in the previous chapters: the assignment to treat students as subjects with agency instead of objects to be acted upon (Chapter 2); to complicate hierarchies of evidence (Chapter 3); to be mindful of the impact of our words (Chapter 4), and our tendency to objectify others (Chapter 5); to recognize the assumptions about and definitions of an object of research that limit what the investigation can yield before it has even begun (Chapter 6). But "through questioning ideas that are held to be true, we engage more deeply with the information presented to us and as such better our understanding" (Chapter 7, p. 223). Chapter 8 poses such an assignment by challenging us to examine how everything we do in medical education are forms of care, and that care is simultaneously the *raison d'être* of medical education.

Chapter 9 by Fawns and Schaepkens applies the insights of phenomenology to one form of care: sustaining knowledge exam integrity by means of technology. If Chapter 8 demonstrated a way of doing philosophy on foundational structures, in this chapter the pendulum swings to the other side as an empirical form of doing philosophy that zooms in on one example of online proctoring. Much of the reason why the problems identified in previous chapters have been ones no one looked for in medical education has to do with an idea of trust that Chapter 9 confronts head-on. Just as in this chapter trust (that students will not cheat on their exams, that we can rely on exam results) is outsourced to technology, earlier chapters provide an alternative to attempts to outsource learning (Chapter 2), evidence-based practice (Chapter 3), and research (Chapter 6) to 'non-human' and 'objective' sources. But, as Fawns and Schaepkens observe on their expedition, outsourcing produces certain kinds of trust relationships between medical educators and students that risk objectification of learners and their arrested character development.[17]

In a fascinating example of professional subjectification (Chapter 2) and embracing the call of philosophy to involve oneself in inquiry, Humm – a medical student – engages with the fundamental question of what it means to become a doctor in Chapter 10. He performs a first-person phenomenological analysis (Chapter 6) of the clinical encounter from the physician's perspective, supplementing this self-analysis with an analysis of selected literature authored by doctors about their experiences. In so doing, Humm constructs another inroad to exploring the concept of care and ontology (Chapter 8), highlighting tensions that have to do with objectification (Chapters 5 and 7). The result is what Humm calls "being-opposite-illness": a way of characterizing the role of the doctor in the clinical encounter – existing in a liminal space between compassion and objectification that, like technology (as we saw in Chapters 9 and 12), makes health care possible, but requires reflective monitoring or even a form of therapy. Humm does this in a way that is mindful of his own background as a white male, and sensitive to the issues of epistemic authority raised in Chapter 5. Humm's expedition demonstrates the validity and necessity of stimulating research conducted by the 'research object' itself, and strengthens the notion that we should include more students and practitioners as medical education researchers.

The expedition presented in Chapter 11 by MacLeod et al. may be seen as pursuing being-opposite-illness to its logical extreme; it analyzes the philosophical moves involved in using clinical cadavers for medical instruction. In-line with Chapters 5, 7, 8, and 10, MacLeod et al. focus on a locus of ontological ambiguity: in this case, the cadaver having been a person, that is now a dead body, which is used as a tool, in order to simulate a live patient. Such ambiguity between life, death, and instrument can quickly become abstract. However, MacLeod et al. show that philosophy and empirical research methods can complement each other to focus productively on areas of ambiguity that are part of everyday medical education practice (see also Chapter 9).

This expedition prompts us to ask: What would we miss out on if this study had been limited to ethnography, that is, to purely social scientific research rather than a philosophical analysis? We can distinguish two contributions: the first is in MacLeod et al.'s characterization of the cadaver's transformations as ontological. This term, introduced in Chapter 6, literally means 'relating to being'. In line with calls for paying attention in medical education not just to the knowledge, skills, and psychological categories of medical learners, but also to their being[18] – and in contrast to use of the word 'ontology' to simply mean 'worldview'[16, 19] – this chapter demonstrates that the subject–object distinction permeating most of medical education and medical education research does not hold. Conducted from the position of subject–object distinction, his study would have focused

on how students 'subjectively' experienced the 'object' of the cadaver, and how their experience changed over time. But here the term relates to something more fundamental than psychological categories or physical entities. The power of its use here is that anyone who has actually gone through cadaver-based education (or has come face to face with death in another way) will attest that it has an effect (of affect) that cannot just be 'compartmentalized' but involves thinking, feeling, and physical experiences. Ontological fidelity means that more than the sum of its parts, what makes simulation-based education effective is that it gives rise to an experience of 'what it is like' to be in the simulated (clinical) situation, without the associated risks in that situation.

The second contribution of philosophy in this chapter is in its methodology. MacLeod et al. draw on Deleuze and Guattari's distinction between philosophy, science and art,[20] using cadaver-based education as a site for arguing that philosophy's job is creating and forming concepts should be put in practice. These concepts are ontological ambiguity as part of simulation-based education, being-opposite-illness as part of analysis of the clinical encounter, and care as part of discussions about medical education can then become our partner in teaching, curriculum design, and research (Chapter 1). For instance, we could use the meaning of care or the experience of being-opposite-illness as a topic of reflective discussions with students, and we could be guided by the concept of ontological fidelity as a way to make choices in designing simulation-based environments. Chapters 10 and 11 are examples of using philosophy for conceptual innovation in medical education.

In Chapter 11, the ontological ambiguity of the clinical cadaver lies partly in its being used as an instrument. In philosophy, *techne* or *technics* has been described as not quite alive and not quite dead: it is inorganic, like inert objects, but it is organized, like biological (organic) beings.[21] Chapter 6 already highlighted the indispensable aspect of care that pertains to technology and instrumental thinking: without buildings, medical instruments, ways of recording and transferring knowledge, and communication devices it is impossible to have any form of functioning health care, let alone health care education. Chapter 12 by Chin-Yee et al. is a proposal for why and how to include teaching about technology on fundamental as well as applied levels into medical education curricula. It is an example, like Chapters 3 (epistemology) and 4 (linguistics), of how a specific branch of philosophy could be used as a basis for teaching, and how, like Chapters 5, 7, and 9, it is necessary to adequately address a major societal challenge. The challenge in this case is one that philosophers have addressed often, and the awareness of which has been entering all levels of medical education: that of the accelerating innovation of technology and its paradoxical effect of making possible some forms of unprecedented levels of health, prosperity, and connectedness, but at the expense of other forms of health (e.g. planetary health), equality, and human connection.

The key term for this expedition is perhaps integration: Chin-Yee et al. propose to combine teaching literacy of concrete technologies with awareness of the impact of technology on social relations (including the relation between doctor and patient, but also as in Chapter 9, the relationship between students and the medical education institute) and how technological innovation transforms fundamental (i.e., ontological) relationships between human beings. Just like being-opposite-illness, the ability to diagnose and perform medical procedures risks engendering instrumental relationships to the patient as an object (or, as in Chapter 2, to the student as an object of learning). The ability to care empathically has to be integrated with the ability to care effectively (Chapter 8) and based on the most advanced knowledge about care (Chapter 3). Chapter 12 explores how this can be implemented in medical education through teaching a care-full relationship to existing and new technologies, ensuring that technologies' ultimate aim is improved patient care – which is more than curing.[22] The chapter is an attempt to address the dilemma of how to teach *now* about technologies that doctors *in the future* will be dealing with, and that we (as educators) cannot yet foresee. Chin-Yee et al. argue that accompanying all this should be an ongoing reflection on the relationship between doctors and patients, with technology as an indispensable 'third partner'.

Reflection is perhaps most associated with philosophy in medical education, and it was the focus of the final expedition presented in this volume. In Chapter 13, Schaepkens and Lijster combine a traditional literature review approach with a philosophical analysis of this omnipresent but also problematic concept in medical education. If part of a philosophy of medical education is an ongoing reflective practice on all levels, it is fitting to end the book with a reflection on reflection.

In a typical philosophical move, Schaepkens and Lijster refer the question (*What is reflection?*) back to us. Reflection is not a procedure or process for bridging gaps (e.g., between theory and practice), but for minding them. It is a human trait to look for answers and solutions in external authorities, whether these are teachers (Chapter 2), scientific literature (Chapter 3), research methods (Chapter 6), or technology (Chapters 9 and 12). But when we have asked philosophers and/or medical educators to reflect on these issues, they have provided thoughtful and detailed recommendations always accompanied by this assignment: to heed the existential freedom

of students as subjects rather than objects (Chapter 2), to engender their responsibility to weigh different sources of evidence (Chapter 3), and to consider the words they speak (Chapter 4) and their impact on inclusion and exclusion of other perspectives and identities (Chapter 5). All of the expeditions in this volume point to a fundamental freedom, a gap that one should not attempt to bridge or simplify, but rather a gap to exist mindfully in.

In other words, Chapter 13 explicitly points to a gap that all the other chapters refer to either implicitly or by various terms: muddy zones of practice (Chapter 1), ambiguity of meaning and context (Chapter 4), or ontological ambiguity (Chapters 10 and 11). In this gap, we are left to ourselves, with the freedom and responsibility to make choices that reflect our values and professional attitude. Philosophy of medical education is a way of acknowledging the fundamental gaps and ambiguity of our field, but as a starting point for careful, thoughtful, rigorous, and precise analysis, rather than as an endpoint. Precision and rigor in this case does not mean to choose one out of many possible definitions and stick with it, but rather to avoid the temptation to reduce the complex phenomena of medical education to technical definitions, while also recognizing the necessity of technical definitions in other situations.

In line with Chapter 13, we could therefore say that philosophy is not a 'solution' or authority to which medical education can look for ready-made answers, just as our field has perhaps too eagerly looked to medical science and cognitive psychology for these answers. Rather, philosophy is a professional conversation partner for medical education, not unlike a therapist for a client, a doctor for a patient, or a lawyer for a citizen. Philosophy of medical education can be seen as creating, maintaining, and monitoring this specific type of relationship between medical education institutes and professionals and the students and the rest of society.

Who Does Philosophy of Medical Education?

A key challenge for us in editing this series was determining how to present philosophical inquiry (its questions, its language) in a way that was inviting to *Teaching and Learning in Medicine*'s medical educator readers yet also rigorous in the judgment of philosophically trained readers. One strategy we used was to ensure that each article's authors included a trained philosopher and a reflective medical educator; sometimes these were the same person. However, we found that every article required revision to speak more to the listening of medical educators. Example revisions included more concrete examples from medicine to illustrate philosophical concepts; elimination of digressions into philosophical debates that did not move the main argument or demonstration forward; and streamlining the presentation to reduce redundancies. Fundamental to this effort were the questions of: How far can we push *Teaching and Learning in Medicine* readers out of their comfort zone to help them see intractable problems in new, more actionable ways? Can we empower medical educators to see themselves as capable of doing philosophy? More fundamentally, can we help those who engage with this series see that medical education does not exist 'outside' of us, that we are all a part of medical education and the freedom and responsibility that comes with that?

We recognize medical education as an invention. We all continuously (re)create and shape it, so it is our responsibility and our risk. For this reason, we believe that doing philosophy in medical education requires all voices, not just those we hear readily or those we are told we should listen to. Voices typically excluded from shared discourse are ripe for doing philosophy, as they belong to those who question fundamental assumptions and persist in asking "Why?" when others seek the convenience and comfort of closure. Doing philosophy in medical education also involves becoming more literate in philosophy beyond its typical use, for example, as a research reporting requirement or as a lens a researcher swaps into their microscope to examine teaching and learning up close. Given our role in creating and shaping the field, we in the publishing world must acknowledge that doing philosophy of medical education requires inviting voices from the humanities into a space – our academic journals – closely guarded by scientific tradition.

Co-editing the Philosophy in Medical Education Series has had an impact far beyond the articles it produced and the citations and social media attention they have earned. In itself, it has been an act of doing philosophy in medical education, leading us to question what constitutes medical education scholarship and the priority we place on various ways of knowing in our academic journals. Although the initial phase of the series has ended, the expedition lives on in the unsolicited philosophy in medical education submissions *Teaching and Learning in Medicine* now receives. We enthusiastically welcome these submissions and will continue as co-editors to seek peer reviewers who can help the authors maximize their impact on medical education's intractable problems. *Teaching and Learning in Medicine* will also soon welcome submissions from other humanities disciplines as well, including history, language, literature, visual art, poetry, and more. We envision a medical education journal that features, side-by-side, articles that represent the full spectrum of knowing we expect our physicians to engage in when caring for patients. As those with the influence to shape the field, we anticipate role modeling, through our editorial decision-making, the judicious selection of diverse forms of evidence to inform practical problem solving.

Philosophy of Medical Education as an Assignment

We started this series in search of problems no one looked for. From our expeditions, we did not return with maps or gold, but instead with new questions. For example, what does my way of communicating with a patient say about how I perform my work through language (Chapter 4), create a particular relationship of power (Chapter 5), or how I distance or connect emotionally with the illness of the patient (Chapter 10)? What does choosing a particular way of structuring knowledge exams imply about the trust between our students and ourselves (Chapter 9)? It seems we are not finished yet. Indeed, the second phase of the Philosophy in Medical Education series continues at *Teaching and Learning in Medicine* and will include expeditions into the concepts of preparedness and practical wisdom among hopefully many others. Our wish is that other journals will follow suit, also providing a space to approach medical education philosophically.

We acknowledge that we are not the first ones, nor the only ones to claim the relevance of philosophy to medical education. For instance, there has been a series on the philosophy of science published in *Academic Medicine*[16] and a recent edited volume of applied philosophy for health professions education.[15] We also will certainly not be the last, as we see a new appetite for philosophy in medical education. However, with this endeavor, we have aimed to claim philosophy *of* medical education as a sub-field in medical education research and practice and exploring what this field could look like. Questions such as those raised in the previous paragraph represent the first, next steps in that direction.

What is philosophy of medical education? First of all, to claim that there is such a thing means taking ourselves seriously as a field, and taking responsibility for our (imperfect) ways of shaping it. It means constituting ourselves in a particular relationship to our field, not afraid to ask fundamental questions and question basic assumptions. Secondly, we have delineated the field by pointing to issues and questions that it needs to address, such as the dilemma of treating trainees as subjects rather than objects, the tension between technical and human ways of approaching care, and the question of what we mean by fundamental concepts, such as care, identity, and teaching. But most of all, philosophy of medical education is an assignment. It is an assignment to philosophize, which means to have the courage to love and pursue wisdom, to slow down and think deeply, even if it raises problems no one looked for.

References

1. Glassberg J. *A swift guide to butterflies of North America.* Princeton: Princeton University Press; 2017.
2. Renault M. A beginner's guide to butterfly watching. www.popsci.com/beginners-guide-butterfly-watching/. Updated July 6, 2019. Accessed November 30, 2022.
3. Wittgenstein L. *Tractatus Logico-Philosophious, with Introduction by B. Russell.* Kegan Paul, Trench, Trubner, London and Harcourt, Brace and Company, New York. 1922.
4. Biesta G. *World-centred education: A view for the present.* Routledge; 2021.
5. Vanstone M., Grierson L. Thinking about social power and hierarchy in medical education. *Med Educ.* 2022;56(1):91–7. doi: 10.1111/medu.14659
6. de la Croix A., Veen M. The reflective zombie: Problematizing the conceptual framework of reflection in medical education. *Perspect Med Educ.* 2018;7(6):394–400. doi: 10.1007/s40037-018-0479-9
7. Grendar J., Beran T., Oddone-Paolucci E. Experiences of pressure to conform in postgraduate medical education. *BMC Med Educ.* 2018;18(1):4. doi: 10.1186/s12909-017-1108-8
8. Thomas A., Kuper A., Chin-Yee B., Park M. What is "shared" in shared decision-making? Philosophical perspectives, epistemic justice, and implications for health professions education. *J Eval Clin Pract.* 2020;26(2):409–18. doi: 10.1111/jep.13370
9. Donaldson C.M. Using Kantian ethics in medical ethics education. *Med Sci Educ.* 2017;27(4):841–5. doi: 10.1007/s40670-017-0487-0
10. Kinghorn W.A. Medical education as moral formation: An Aristotelian account of medical professionalsim. *Perspect Biol Med.* 2010;53(1):87–105. doi: 10.1353/pbm.0.0145
11. Camara B. The falsity of Hegel's theses on Africa. *J Black Stud.* 2005;36(1):82–96. doi: 10.1177/0021934704268296
12. Safranski R. *Martin Heidegger: Between good and evil.* Harvard: Harvard University Press; 1999.
13. Harley E.H. The forgotten history of defunct black medical schools in the 19th and 20th centuries and the impact of the Flexner Report. *J Natl Med Assoc.* 2006;98(9):1425.
14. Buxton R., Whiting L. *The philosopher queens: The lives and legacies of philosophy's unsung women.* London: Unbound Publishing; 2020.
15. Brown M.E., Veen M., Finn G., eds. *Applied philosophy for health professions education: A journey towards mutual understanding:* Singapore: Springer Nature; 2022.
16. Varpio L., MacLeod A. Philosophy of Science Series: Harnessing the multidisciplinary edge effect by exploring paradigms, ontologies, epistemologies, axiologies, and methodologies. *Acad Med.* 2020;95(5):686–9. doi: 10.1097/ACM.0000000000003142
17. Fatima S. Can doctors maintain good character? An examination of physician lives. *J Medl Humanit.* 2016;37(4):419–33. doi: 10.1007/s10912-016-9385-5
18. Wald H.S. Refining a definition of reflection for the being as well as doing the work of a physician. *Med Teach.* 2015;37(7):696-9. doi: 10.3109/0142159X.2015.1029897
19. Wyatt T.R., Ajjawi R., Veen M. "What does it mean to be?": Ontology and responsibility in health professions education. In: Brown M.E.L., Veen M., Finn G.M., eds. *Applied philosophy for health professions education: A journey towards mutual understanding.* Singapore: Springer Nature; 2022:173–85.
20. Deleuze G., Guattari F. *What is philosophy?* London: Verso; 1995.
21. Stiegler B. *Technics and time, 1: The fault of Epimetheus.* Stanford, Calif.: Stanford University Press; 1998.
22. Nimmon L. Expanding medical expertise: The role of healer. *Med Educ.* 2020;54(5):380–1. doi: 10.1111/medu.14134

Index

Note: Tables are indicated by **bold**.

Adorno, T. W. 131
advocacy 38–9, 58, 64
African American communities 36
Ajjawi R. 43
Allegory of the Cave (Plato) 5
Allison, R. 119
Alpha Omega Alpha Honor Medical Society (AOA) 35
American Association of Medical Colleges (AAMC) 36, 38, 52, 53
anatomisation 91
anthropology 33, 52, 54, 57–8, 91, 132
Anthropology in the Clinic (Kleinman and Benson) 58
anti-Black racism 39
anti-racist medical curriculum 37
Arendt, H. 118, 119, 124
arteriovenous malformations 86
artificial intelligence (AI) 108–10
assessment technology 71–3, 128; medical education 76–7
Assimil 27
Australia 53, 72
Awareness of dying (Glaser and Strauss) 28
axiology 131

Bearman, M. 77
beetle 27, 28
Being and Time (Heidegger) 63–4, 66–8
being-opposite-illness 85–8, 133
Biesta, G. J. J. 18, 52, 129
Big Data 108–9
bioethics 57
biomedicine 82
Birden, Hunter 53
The Birth of the Clinic (Foucault) 54
Black physicians 35–6
Bleakley, Alan 52
Bluhm, R. 27, 130, 132
bodily fragility 85
bookish knowledge 118
bracketing 43, 45, 46
Bromiley, Elaine 120, 121
Bynum, W. 43

cadaver-based simulation (CBS) 90–6, 98–102; limitations 101–2; ontological fdelity 101
Canada 53, 108
care: in everyday life 64; health care education 64–5; medical education 67–8; philosophical encounters 66–7; practice 65–6
Carel, Havi 56
Carless, D. 75
Carnegie Foundation 35
Cartesian Dualism 6
Charon, Rita 56
Chin-Yee, B. 133, 134

chronic obstructive pulmonary disease (COPD) 17
chronic pain syndrome 17
Cianciolo, Anna T. 72, 77
Clinical Cadaver Program (CCP) 92, 94
clinical cadavers 91, 92, 100, 101; stages of the lifecycle **95**
clinical epidemiology 21
Cochrane Collaboration 21
Code Grey 110, 111
Collingride Dilemma 111
communal sense 118–24
communicative competence 25, 26
community meaning 25, 30
Competency Based Medical Education (CBME) 37
congestive heart failure (CHF) 17
conscientização, Portuguese 29
CONSORT Group 21
The Context of Self (Zaner) 84
cookbook medicine 18
coronary artery disease (CAD) 17
Coulehan, Jack 57
Covid-19 pandemic 55, 72, 76, 108, 111, 113
critical appraisal 21, 54, 111
critical consciousness 38
Critique of Judgment (Kant) 118
Critique of Pure Reason (Kant) 118
cultural competence 35, 58
cutting edge 113

Dalhousie CCP 92
The Death of Ivan Illych (Tolstoy) 56
de Beauvoir, S. 81, 87, 131
de Botton, Alain 5
de la Croix, A. 113, 121
Deleuze, G. 4, 91, 92, 101, 102
del Molino, Sergio 113
Derrida, J. 118, 120, 124
Descartes, R. 82
determinative judgment 118–19
Dewey, John 2
differential ontologists 92
digital education platforms 71
digital patient records 71
direct observation (DO) 43, 45–7; patients' experiences 49
disciplinary governmentality 72
Discursive Psychology 48
dividing practices 33–4
Do No Harm (Marsh) 57
Douglas-Jones, R. 91
Doyle, Conan 28

Edson, Margaet 56
educational cadaver 91–3, 95, **95**, 96, 98, 100, 102

138 INDEX

educational ethnography 93
education as open system 13, 15
efficiency 72, 108, 111–14
eidetic reduction 48–9
Electronic Health Record (EHR) 107, 109, 111–12, 114
elite's social hegemony 37
empathy 51, 53, 56–8, 65, 68, 84, 88, 91, 108, 113, 117, 128, 132
epistemology 5, 6, 18, 19, 22, 23, 27, 59, 111, 130–3
Equal Protection Clause 36
essences 44, 51, 53, 127, 129
esthetic judgments 119
ethnographic immersion 92, 93
evidence-based medicine (EBM) 17, 18, 111, 129; clinical
    medicine 20–1; definition 22; fundamentals of 18; medical
    curriculum 18; medical education 21–3; pre-clinical
    studies 19–20
Exchange of Experience (EoE) 123

Fairclough, N. 28
Fawns, Tim 109, 132
fidelity 91, 100, 101, 133
Fioratou, Evie 120
Fitzgerald, Scott 28
Fleming, Alexander 108
Flexner, Abraham 35, 131
Foucault, M. 28, 33, 37–9, 47, 72, 131
Freire, P. 29
*The Fundamental Role of the Arts and Humanities in Medical
    Education* (Howley) 52

Garver, E. 28
Geertz, Clifford 28
general practitioner (GP) 42
giant aneurysms 86
Glaser, B.G. 28
The Great Wave off Kanagawa (Hokusai) 59
Guattari, F. 4, 91, 92, 101, 102
Guyatt, G. H. 21

Halifax Preparation 93
Hallam, E. 91
hard-fixed (traditional) cadavers 91
health care education 63, 68
Health Care Professional (HCP) 68
health professions education (HPE) 42, 49; Chris 43–4; Mario 44;
    phenomenology 49
Heidegger, M. 43, 47, 63, 64, 66, 67, 81, 83, 87, 118,
    120, 124, 131
hidden curriculum 36–7, 53
Higgs, J. 43
Hippocratic Oath 64
Hodges, B. D. 71
Hokusai, Katsushika 59
Hong Kong 53
huidhonger 113
human body donation (HBD) 92–101, 105; body to cadaver
    97–8; cadaver to educational cadaver 98; donor to body 97;
    educational cadaver to teacher 98–9; person to donor 96;
    teacher to loved one and legacy 99–100
humanism 112
humanities 6, 19, 44, 51, 52, 54–9, 67, 77, 84–6, 100, 113, 114, 127,
    129, 131, 132, 135
humanness 102
Hume, D. 2, 27
Humm, J. 132–3
Husserl, E. 47
hyperlipidemia 17
hypertension 17
hypochondria of medical student syndrome 87

Ihde, D. A. 73
indoctrination 13, 15
innovation 108
Inspector of Anatomy (IoA) 97
instrumental thinking 4
intercalated BSc (iBSc) 52
interdisciplinary 3, 38, 42, 52, 54, 128
International Medical Graduates (IMGs) 27
Interpretive Phenomenological Analysis (IPA) 47
interview study 43, 45, 46, 48
intracerebral arterial bypasses 86
Ireland 53

JAMA article 20, 21

Kalanithi, P. 57, 82, 85–7, 114
Kant, I. 44, 63, 118, 119–20, 123, 124
Kelly, M. 113
Kolb, D. A. 2
Kovacs, G. 91
Kripke, S. 27
Kumagai, A. K. 51

Lahdenperä, J. 76
language: doing things with words 26; of learning 10, 12, 14, 129;
    meaning in context 26–7; and power 28–30; reductionism and
    ambiguity 27–8
LGBTQ+ 59, 131
Lijster, Tijs 134
Liu, Y. 52
Locke, J. 2, 29
logico scientific knowledge 56

Macleod, Anna 131, 133
Marshall, Robert 52
Marsh, H. 57, 82, 86–7
McDonald, M. 91
McLachlan, E. 43
McWhinney, I. R. 28
medical admission practices 35
medical education 1–3, 5, 10, 127; curriculum design 14;
    education research 10; existing power structures 37–8; Foucault,
    M. 35–6, 38–9; humanities 51; normalization in 34–5;
    online proctoring 72; philosophy of 128–35; practice
    10, 13; professional qualification, socialization and
    subjectification 11–12; qualification 11; research 10, 14;
    socialization 11; subjectification 11; uncertainty 30
medical humanities (MH) 51, 52, 87–8, 129, 132; AAMC 52;
    definition 52; gray areas 54–8; humanities-sceptic medical
    educators 59; intercalated BSc (iBSc) 52; medical education 52;
    medical student perspective 52–3; strong inclusion 52; "tick-box
    exercise" medical education 58; in the UK 53–4, 59; value of
    51–2, 59; weak inclusion 52
medical model 9, 10, 12, 14–15, 129
medical sociology 28, 33
Medical Student Performance Evaluation letters (MSPE) 35
Merleau-Ponty, M. 47, 87
Mill, J. S. 29
mind-body dualism 6
Mishler, Erwin 25
Mishra, Sundeep 56
mobile phones 71
mode of inquiry 33
Möller, H. 84
mortality 6
muddy zones of practice 1

narrative competency 56
necessary detachment 87

INDEX

Netherlands 108, 113
New Zealand 53
Ng, Stella 123
Nicolini, D. 92
Nieminen, J. H. 76
Nietzsche, F. 67

objectification 33, 82
objective knowledge 75
Olding, M. 132
Ong, L. M. L. 25
On Liberty (Mill) 29
online proctoring 72–7, 132; assessment culture 75–6; economic context 75; historical context 75; integrity, professionalism and surveillance 76; medical education 76–7; MRCP membership exam 73; postphenomology 73–4; scripts and norms 74; trust 74
ontological fidelity 100–1, 133
ontological transitions 91–2

patient-centeredness 29
The Pedagogy of Indignation (Freire) 29
performative 6, 26
perpetuate harmful stereotypes 38
pharmakon 108, 111, 113–14
phenomenology 81, 82; body and illness 83; description 47; in HPE research 47–8; immediate access 45–6; natural attitude 46–7
Phenomenology of Illness (Carel) 56
philosophical analysis 67, 119–21, 133, 134
philosophy of medicine 128
philosophy of science 6, 20, 127, 131, 135
Philosophy of Science (Varpio and MacLeod) 131
phronèsis 118
postdigital 72–6
postphenomenology 72–4, 76
Practical Assessment of Clinical Examination Skills (PACES) 73
practical rationality 118
practice theory 92, 93
pre-reflective experience 43
private capital 72
problem-based learning (PBL) 29, 54
ProctorExam service 73–5
professional identity formation (PIF) 34
professionalism 28
professional qualification 11–15
professional socialization 11–15
professional subjectification 11–15, 18

qualification 11, 14

racism 36–8, 59
randomization 19–20
recursive 13
reflection 30, 48, 49, 51, 52, 57–9, 117, 119, 127, 134; bridging gaps and the madness 119–20; individual and communal sense 119, 122; philosophical analysis 120–1; research 118, 121; theory–practice gap 118–19, 121–2
reflective judgment 119
Regents of California vs. Bakke 36
resistance 12, 111, 120
respiratory monitors 71
Rietmeijer, C. 56
Rothman, David 57
Russo, F. 20

Sackett, D. 21, 22
Sartre, J. 83–5, 87
Schaepkens, Sven P. C. 109, 132, 134
self-preservation 87

Selwyn, N. 72
semiotic system 13
sensus communis 119
Shared decision-making 3, 6, 26
The Sign of the Four (Conan Doyle) 28
Simms, J Marion 55
Skelton, John 56
slowing down 1–2, 4, 72, 108, 132, 135
Smith, Jack 26
socialization 11–15, 52, 129
social media 71, 135
sociomateriality 108
soft-preserved (CBS) cadavers 91, 92
South Africa 53
Speech Act Theory 25, 26, 30
Star Trek 26
Stegenga, J. 20
Stein, C. 84
Strangers at the Bedside (Rothman) 57
Strauss, A. L. 28
strong inclusion 52, 54, 55, 58, 59
structural racism 32
student learning 10, 14
stupidity 118
The Subject and Power (Foucault) 37
subjectification 11–14, 34, 52, 129, 130, 132
sugared snicker doodle 99
systematization 119–20
systemic racism 32, 33, 37–9, 130

tabula rasa 29
Taiwanese Tzu Chi Buddhist Silent Mentor program 91
teach back method 2–3, 5
techne 133
technical code 112
technical literacy 110
technics 109, 133
technification 112–14
technological innovation 107–9, 111, 113, 114, 134
technological literacy 112, 114
technosphere 109
theory–practice gap 118–24
This is Water (Wallace and Kenyon) 5
tick-box exercises 53, 58
Tolstoy, L. 56
Tonelli, M. R. 27, 130, 132
tonsillectomy 26
Toombs, S. 83, 84
Toronto Consensus statement 25
toxicology 114
Tuskegee syphilis study 55
Type II diabetes 17

underrepresented minorities (URM) 33–4
United Kingdom Royal College of Physicians (MRCP) 73, 75–7
United States 107
University Of California Regents vs. Bakke 36
untidy epistemic pluralism 22–3
Usherwood, Tim 53

van Braak, M. 18, 52, 129
van Manen, M. 43
Varpio, Lara 131
Veen, M. 56, 72, 77, 121
Verbeek, P-P. 73
Vermeer, J. 28
View of Delft (Vermeer) 28

Wahlberg, Hansson 26
weak inclusion 52, 54, 55
West Indies 53
What is Philosophy? (Deleuze and Guattari) 91, 102
When Breath Becomes Air (Kalanithi) 57, 86, 114
WHO 63
Williamson, J. 20
Williams, Peter 57
Wit (Edson) 56

Wittgenstein, L. 27, 28
Wolcott, H. 94

Young, I. 87

Zaidi, Z. 55, 130, 131
Zaner, R. 84
Zollikon Seminars (Heidegger and Boss) 67